Language, memory, and aging

Edited by

LEAH L. LIGHT *and* DEBORAH M. BURKE
Pitzer College   *Pomona College*

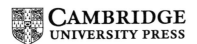 CAMBRIDGE
UNIVERSITY PRESS

CAMBRIDGE UNIVERSITY PRESS
Cambridge, New York, Melbourne, Madrid, Cape Town, Singapore, São Paulo

Cambridge University Press
The Edinburgh Building, Cambridge CB2 8RU, UK

Published in the United States of America by Cambridge University Press, New York

www.cambridge.org
Information on this title: www.cambridge.org/9780521329422

First published 1988
Reprinted 1990
First paperback edition 1993

A catalogue record for this publication is available from the British Library

ISBN 978-0-521-32942-2 hardback
ISBN 978-0-521-44876-5 paperback

Transferred to digital printing 2008

Contents

Contributors

Shirley A. Albertson
Department of Psychology
Claremont Graduate School
Claremont, CA 91711

Deborah M. Burke
Department of Psychology
Pomona College
Claremont, CA 91711

Gillian Cohen
Human Cognition Research Group
The Open University
Milton Keynes, MK7 6AA
England

Olga B. Emery
Departments of Psychology and
    Psychiatry
Case Western Reserve University
Cleveland, OH 44106

Gary Gillund
Department of Psychology
University of Utah
Salt Lake City, UT 84112

Rose Marie Harrold
Department of Psychology
Claremont Graduate School
Claremont, CA 91711

Joellen T. Hartley
Department of Psychology
California State University at Long
    Beach
Long Beach, CA 90840

Lynn Hasher
Department of Psychology
Duke University
Durham, NC 27706

Darlene V. Howard
Department of Psychology
Georgetown University
Washington, DC 20057

F. Jacob Huff
Memory and Cognition Clinic
Alzheimer's Disease Research Center
University of Pittsburgh
Pittsburgh, PA 15213

Susan Kemper
Department of Psychology
University of Kansas
Lawrence, KA 66045

Roberta L. Klatzky
Department of Psychology
University of California
Santa Barbara, CA 93106

Leah L. Light
Department of Psychology
Pitzer College
Claremont, CA 91711

Marion Perlmutter
Institute of Gerontology
University of Michigan
Ann Arbor, MI 48109

Timothy A. Salthouse
School of Psychology
Georgia Institute of Technology
Atlanta, GA 30332

Rose T. Zacks
Department of Psychology
Michigan State University
East Lansing, MI 48824

Elizabeth M. Zelinski
Leonard Davis School of Gerontology
University of Southern California
Los Angeles, CA 90089

Preface

Recent years have seen an upsurge of interest in the psychology of aging, particularly in the area of cognition and aging. Much of the experimental research on cognitive aging has dealt with memory, perhaps because of older adults' proverbial complaints about their memory problems. Relatively little has been published on language in the elderly. However, the overlap in mental operations involved in memory and in language has become clear as cognitive psychologists focus on memory for complex linguistic materials such as texts, and as they develop models of natural language comprehension and production. Within the aging literature, there are findings that implicate age-related changes in language as the source of impairment in other cognitive domains, specifically memory. It has been hypothesized that older adults have decreased ability to understand language and that this deficit in semantic processing is a cause of age-related differences in memory for new information. On the other hand, it has also been hypothesized that memory deficits in old age impair language comprehension and production.

The goals of this book are twofold, to review selected aspects of research on language in old age and to consider the relation between language and memory in old age. Many of us who have contributed to the book come to the study of language after years of research on memory and aging. This fact has influenced our choice of topics. Our emphasis is on those aspects of language that are important for understanding memory in old age and on those aspects of memory that are most heavily involved in language. Thus, we do not offer complete coverage of either memory or language in old age. The reader interested in further discussion of memory and aging should see Craik and Trehub (1982), Kausler (1982), Poon, Fozard, Cermak, Arenberg, and Thompson (1980), and Salthouse (1982). Bergman (1980) offers a thorough treatment of speech perception in old age. Bayles and Kaszniak (1987), Obler and Albert (1980), Beasley and Davis (1981), Hooper and Dunkle (1984), and Ulatowska (1985) discuss a range of topics in normal and pathological language in old age.

The individual chapters in this volume present research involving a range of methodologies, including psychometric and neurolinguistic tests and experimental measures, which isolate specific aspects of language comprehension, production, and memory. The studies compare young and older adults (including both normal and pathological populations), using both between-groups and individual-differences approaches. The theoretical perspectives represented in the volume are drawn from major contemporary models in cognitive psychology, and the issues raised reflect current issues in cognition, such as the role of awareness in memory and language, the relation between semantic and episodic memory, the distinction between automatic and attentional processes, and the usefulness of the levels of processing approach.

The opening chapter, by Klatzky, provides a framework for the issues raised in subsequent chapters by giving an overview of relevant paradigms in contemporary cognitive psychology. The next three chapters deal with individual differences in verbal ability in normal aging. Salthouse reviews literature from psychometric tests and identifies processes and mechanisms underlying age-related changes in verbal ability. Hartley discusses components of verbal ability underlying text memory and presents her research using a factor-analytic approach to determine whether a unique set of verbal skills predicts memory at different ages. Kemper considers the role of memory limitations in syntactic processes involved in language comprehension and production in old age.

The next two chapters deal with automatic and effortful aspects of activation of word meanings. Howard reports studies of semantic and episodic priming that reveal age differences and similarities in the representation of information in memory and that raise the possibility that there are age differences in deliberate recollection but not in memory without awareness. Burke and Harrold evaluate the role of automatic and effortful components of semantic activation in language comprehension and retention and provide evidence for disruption of automatic word retrieval processes in old age.

The next three chapters focus on age-related changes in inferential processes involved in comprehension and memory. Zelinski examines integration processes important for discourse comprehension and reports her research on the role of prior knowledge in discourse level and sentence level comprehension processes. Light and Albertson report research which demonstrates that older adults do not experience problems in drawing inferences except in situations involving heavy demands on working memory and that comprehension problems are themselves due in part to more general memory deficits. Zacks and Hasher present a new version of their processing resource model designed to explain comprehension and memory for discourse and apply it to their research on age declines in drawing inferences from text.

The two chapters that follow present overviews of research on interactions between language and memory and frameworks for understanding age differences. Cohen presents a review of studies, mainly from her own laboratory, which suggests that limitations in processing resources underlie impairments in many linguistic processes. This theme is also taken up by Gillund and Perlmutter, who argue that prior knowledge compensates for reduced processing resources in tasks involving memory.

The penultimate two chapters compare language impairment in normal and pathological aging. Huff reviews evidence from his own and others' research suggesting that impaired naming ability in Alzheimer's disease is largely determined by a semantic deficit. Emery describes her research involving a set of neurolinguistic tests that demonstrates patterns of language impairment in both normal aging and Alzheimer's disease that are unlike those found in aphasia.

In the final chapter, we discuss themes that emerge from a reading of the earlier chapters. In particular, we consider the contributions of different approaches represented in the book to our understanding of patterns of spared and impaired functioning of language and memory in old age.

We are happy to acknowledge the help of several people during the preparation of this book. We thank our families (Don and Kenny MacKay, and Ivan, Matthew, and Nathaniel Light) for their support. We appreciate the help of our graduate students, Shirley Albertson, Debra Valencia-Laver, and Joanna Worthley, with many of the chores that arose during the course of the project. Finally, we are grateful to the National Institute on Aging for its support of our research and to our grant administrator, Leonard Jakubczak, for encouragement and advice over the years.

Deborah Burke
Leah Light
Claremont

References

Bayles, K. A., & Kaszniak, A. W. (1987). *Communication and cognition in normal aging and dementia.* Boston: Little, Brown.

Beasley, D. S., & Davis, G. A. (Eds.). (1981). *Aging: Communication processes and disorders.* New York: Grune & Stratton.

Bergman, M. (1980). *Aging and the perception of speech.* Baltimore, MD: University Park Press.

Craik, F. I. M., & Trehub, S. (Eds.). (1982). *Aging and cognitive processes.* New York: Plenum.

Hooper, C. R., & Dunkle, R. E. (1984). *The older aphasic person.* Rockville, MD: Aspen.

Kausler, D. H. (1982). *Experimental psychology and human aging.* New York: Wiley.

Obler, L. K., & Albert, M. L. (1980). *Language and communication in the elderly.* Lexington, MA: Heath.

Poon, L. W., Fozard, J. L., Cermak, L. S., Arenberg, D., & Thompson, L. W. (Eds.). (1980). *New directions in memory and aging: Proceedings of the George A. Talland Memorial Conference.* Hillsdale, NJ: Erlbaum.

Salthouse, T. A. (1982). *Adult cognition: An experimental psychology of human aging.* New York: Springer-Verlag.

Ulatowska, H. K. (1985). *The aging brain: Communication in the elderly.* San Diego: College-Hill Press.

1   Theories of information processing and theories of aging

Roberta L. Klatzky

The goal of the present chapter is truly introductory. In it, I attempt to provide a theoretical context for the chapters that follow and to raise some general issues. The chapter first outlines a "modal model" of human information processing, particularly that related to memory and language. It then assesses weak and strong contributions that the information-processing approach could make to research on aging.

The modal model

Some 20 years ago, Murdock (1967) used the term "modal model" to describe the then dominant two-store conception of human memory. An important assumption of this model was that there existed two discrete functional units in the memory system, one for active storage and rehearsal of a limited amount of information (short-term memory), the other a more temporally extended, capacious repository of knowledge (long-term memory). This modal model has come under intensive fire, both for its limited perspective on what memory is, and for its rigid partitioning of the memory system. Nonetheless, the fundamental distinction of the model has persisted, in various forms.

In general, human information-processing theory provides two types of description: *Structural* descriptions pertain to the data stored in memory – both the functional components in which they reside, and the nature of the data themselves. *Processing* descriptions pertain to the use of those data – the states they may enter and the transitions between different data representations and stores. Any account of a behavioral phenomenon in information-processing terms must make assumptions about both structures and processes.

In the section that follows, I assume the reader has a general familiarity with cognitive psychology, so that the purpose of this description is primarily to organize theoretical ideas. The discussion considers first the current "modal" model's assumptions about the structural architecture of the system, and then its basic processes.

Structural assumptions

Models of human memory postulate internal structures for representing data – for example, data about the external world, abstractions, or internal states. We can

1

subdivide structural assumptions according to whether they describe the system components in which data resides – the memory stores – or the data themselves. The first type of assumption is exemplified by the early modal model's distinction between short-term and long-term stores. The second type of assumption, about the nature of the data, often takes the form of a binary contrast between data representations. These contrasts include semantic versus episodic, procedural versus declarative, networks versus production systems, propositional versus analogue, lexical versus conceptual, sensorimotor versus cognitive, and more. Only some of these distinctions are relevant to the present chapter, fortunately. The following sections describe assumptions about memory stores and distinctions between types of data representations.

The short-term/long-term assumption, revisited. Early two-store theories of memory were concerned primarily with verbal stimuli. Accordingly, short-term memory was conceived of as a limited set of acoustic/articulatory elements that could be repetitively rehearsed, with each rehearsal incrementing the strength of a corresponding element in long-term memory.

The demise of a strict dichotomy between short- and long-term storage has been virtually complete. At least three major changes can be identified in theories of short-term memory since the late 1960s: (1) Current theory distinguishes among short-term storage systems for different information modalities, especially visual and verbal. (2) Within the verbal domain, there has been a transition from a strict storage-box model of short-term memory to a more complex, modular view that accommodates several different interacting units and a working-memory component. (3) The notion of rehearsal has been reworked, so as to distinguish between its maintenance and learning functions and to relate the learning function to more general theories of encoding.

The first of these changes, modality-specific, short-term memories, was intertwined with theoretical developments in the area of visual imagery. Discussion of these developments would bring in issues that are largely irrelevant to this volume. Kosslyn (1980) has presented a well-developed model of a system for storing and actively processing visual images.

The second type of change, to a multimodule verbal short-term memory with both storage and working functions, is best exemplified by Baddeley's research program. In a fairly recent version (Vallar & Baddeley, 1984), Baddeley describes short-term memory for verbal stimuli as incorporating an auditory/phonological store, an articulatory process, a graphemic (visual) store, and an executive or "working" component. All of these are needed to account for performance on the simple task of repeating back a short list of verbal items.

For example, the importance of the articulatory process is indicated by the finding that performance in a verbatim recall task of this type is inversely related to the pronunciation time for the verbal stimuli. An auditory store is needed to account for interference with the same task by unattended background verbalization. A visual store accounts for above-chance performance when verbal rehearsal is suppressed and for superior performance with visual presentation. The result, in Vallar and Baddeley's term, is a "fractionation" of short-term memory.

The executive component of this system is its controller, with the various stores serving as subsidiaries or "slaves." It is assumed (Baddeley, 1981) that the executive can itself store information as well as control processing. However, "offloading" of storage demands onto the subsidiary systems is needed because the executive has a limited capacity, much of which must be used for controlling the flow of information and performing processes such as reasoning and comprehension. The executive is therefore more like a resource pool than a storage location. Various processes compete for resources, and processing competes with storage, once the limits of the slave systems are exceeded.

Although the fractionated short-term store might be seen as a set of discrete substores, a more general assumption is that performance in a short-term retention task takes advantage of any transient activity in existing verbal representations (e.g., graphemic, lexical, auditory), using this activity to read out and recall. The fractions defined by Baddeley can be taken to reveal the types of representation that can be used in this manner.

Rehearsal has also come under scrutiny since the early duplex model. An important and convincing demonstration has been made by several parties (e.g., Glenberg, Smith, & Green, 1977) to the effect that mere rote repetition of items (essentially, Baddeley's articulatory process) does little to enhance ultimate recall, although it can maintain the items for immediate memory tests. Enhancement of later recall requires elaborative, not just maintenance, rehearsal. In other words, maintenance rehearsal suffices to serve the storage function of short-term memory, whereas elaborative rehearsal exemplifies its function as a "working" memory. Such rehearsal can come in a number of forms: associative chaining, chunking, and imagery, for example. An important distinction among elaborative rehearsal mechanisms has been made within the "levels of processing" theory (Craik & Lockhart, 1972), which stipulates that the more an event is meaningfully and distinctively elaborated, the better it will be remembered.

While short-term memory was undergoing substantial theoretical change, theories of long-term memory were also developing, influenced substantially by computer models of associative memory structures. Among the best known models of long-term memory are those of Collins and Loftus (1975), the UC San Diego group headed by Norman and Rumelhart (1975), and the ACT model of Anderson (1983). All proposed a memory structure in the form of an associative network, in which "nodes" are tied together with linking associations that are differentially weighted to express associative strength.

The associations in network models take specific relational forms. These forms vary from theory to theory, with the San Diegans favoring relations along the lines of case grammar (Fillmore, 1968), and the ACT model adopting a more simplified set. Using these relations in a particular combination allows the network to go beyond the expression of simple connections between knowledge elements. The most critical combination of relations is that which expresses a *proposition* – the internal counterpart of a fact. For example, in ACT, a proposition connects two nodes by a subject–predicate link.

The nodes in a network correspond to mental elements of some fundamental sort. These elements actually exist at several levels. A node might correspond to a single concept like *dog*, but it might also stand for a whole proposition (*My dog has fleas*) or an even larger interrelated structure that expresses a general knowledge framework, variously called a schema, script, or frame.

Before leaving the major structures of human information processing, I should give at least passing reference to a new wave of models that virtually eliminate distinctions of this sort – in fact, that make only minimal assumptions about memory structure (e.g., Grossberg & Stone, 1986; McClelland & Rumelhart, 1985). These "neural net" models adopt a network approach in which the elements and connections are modeled after neurons. Long-term memory, in such a system, is expressed by the weights on interneural links; short-term memory is expressed by a pattern of activation in the links (see below). One striking difference between these models and the networks described previously is that in the neural net, the representation of a given concept is distributed throughout the associative structure. There is no one node or location corresponding to a mental entity; rather, its representation is constituted by the weights within the entire net. As these change with exposure to new patterns, a concept's representation is constantly changing; thus this sort of system is ideally suited to describe such phenomena as categorical abstraction.

We turn now from major architectural structures to the forms of data represented in memory.

Semantic versus episodic data. The distinction between semantic and episodic knowledge was first suggested by Tulving (1972), in response to what he saw as a major shift in the nature of experimental work on memory. This shift was from list-learning procedures that tested autobiographical (episodic) knowledge about the occurrence of events (i.e., list items) in a particular context, to tests of general factual (semantic) knowledge. In fact, Tulving has suggested (1983) that we speak of "semantic memory" and "episodic memory," since the two types of knowledge appear to be formed and used in quite different ways, to have different retention parameters, and to have different degrees of affective association.

Procedural versus declarative knowledge. The distinction between procedural and declarative knowledge has been called one between knowing *how* and knowing *that*. In theory, procedural knowledge underlies people's ability to perform certain acts, or "procedures." The acts might be perceptual (reading a word), motoric (typing), or cognitive (solving equations). Declarative knowledge concerns facts, not acts. The term *declarative* suggests that it can be readily expressed in words. However, there are many procedures (e.g., driving a car) that can also be described verbally at some level, making them declarative, and there are other mental phenomena that are not verbally declarative but also not obviously procedural (e.g., mood states). Despite these blurred aspects of the distinction, it does seem to capture the fact that we can perform many acts – especially skilled ones – but cannot describe how we do so.

Lexical versus conceptual data. With some onomatopoetic exceptions, and Zipf's (1935) law (common concept = short word) notwithstanding, words are generally arbitrary symbols for corresponding concepts. This separation of sign and meaning is acknowledged in network models that place information about the orthographic, phonological, and syntactic properties of words in a "lexicon," distinct from the "concepticon" of semantic memory. This makes clear that there are multiple pathways to conceptual representations. There are distinct lexical pathways through different sensory channels, and there is also direct conceptual access (e.g., through objects) that may bypass the verbal system entirely. Of course, associative connections put the lexical and conceptual systems into direct communication.

Sensorimotor versus cognitive data. This distinction is motivated by the assumption that the processing system represents information at various levels. Information coming from the sense organs is progressively mapped or transformed. Sensory data are those that are achieved early in this sequence of processes. Similarly, motor data are representations that are achieved late in the stream of processing that ends with a motor output. They are commands to the motor system itself, rather than abstract plans or intentions. Cognitive data, in contrast, are not tied to actions or sensory events; they are the representation of more abstract thought. Sensorimotor data are generally placed at the bottom, and cognitive data at the top, in a hierarchical depiction of representations in the processing system, reflecting the assumption that higher-level abstractions subsume a variety of specific instances and their component features.

Process assumptions of the modal model

Any description of human cognitive behavior must adopt assumptions not only about the data structures, but also about the processes that operate on data. Process descriptions can be made at many levels, of course. The appropriate level of analysis depends on the behavior to be explained and the theory to be tested.

At a primitive level, a fundamental process is that of activation. Activation is a state of nodes in the network; it may be modeled as discrete or continuous. A discrete active/inactive distinction (or a cutoff value on continuous activation) is often functionally equated with short-term memory; that is, active elements in the network are equated with elements currently undergoing short-term storage.

When one node is active, its immediate associates are assumed to become active, and their associates in turn. Such a spread of activation between nodes is a theoretical mechanism to describe the retrieval of associated information. Empirical support for such a mechanism is ample. In a classic experiment, Meyer and Schvaneveldt (1976) demonstrated that deciding that a letter string (e.g., butter) is a word is speeded by prior presentation of a related word (e.g., bread). The initial word's activation is assumed to spread to the representations of related words, thus "priming" the second word and speeding its identification. However, estimates of the speed of activation spread indicate that it is virtually instantaneous (e.g., Ratcliff & McKoon, 1981); thus differences between activation spread over weak versus strong links have been attributed to the ultimate level attained rather than to the speed.

Activation not only spreads between concepts like bread and butter; it also travels between different levels of the system. For example, the perception of a printed word has been viewed as a spread of activation from units at the sensory level representing letter features, to letters, and finally to words, with the most active word being the recognized entity. In contrast to this "bottom-up" spread, there is "top-down" spread, which is initiated by activating a concept. For example, in reading *I put the butter on the. . .* , conceptual expectancies about *bread* might lead to the activation of the word, its letters, and their features.

There are a number of important processing distinctions to be made, including automatic versus attentional processing, on-line versus retroactive processing, encoding versus retrieval, retrieval versus decision, and, within language-related processes, decoding versus lexical access versus parsing versus derivation of propositions (involving anaphora and coreference) versus inference. I will deal with these briefly.

Automatic versus attentional processing. The roots of this distinction are in the domain of pattern recognition, where a long-recognized rule is that many incoming channels are ultimately reduced to one recognized channel. We can fully recognize information only from one region in space, one sensory modality, or one information source within a modality. More recent, and controversial, work suggests that many channels are deeply processed, and the limitation is not so much on depth of processing as on conscious access to the results of this processing (Marcel, 1983). In any case, the channel that has privileged access to overt report is called the attended channel.

A more general distinction that goes beyond the perceptual domain can be made between processes that are attention demanding and those that are automatic, or attention free (e.g., Schneider & Shiffrin, 1977). In these terms, conscious pattern recognition demands attention. Earlier stages of perceptual analysis, however, do not. Nor do many nonperceptual processes, apparently, especially those that have been extensively practiced. The criteria for deeming a process "automatic" include evidence that (1) it shows no decrement as it is applied to more and more information (no "workload effect"), (2) it does not interfere with other ongoing processes (no "dual-task interference"), and (3) it is unamenable to conscious intention or control.

The attentional/automatic distinction has been applied to learning as well as performance (Hasher & Zacks, 1979). Specifically, it is assumed that there are certain processes that lay down accessible traces in long-term memory, without demanding attention. Interestingly, rote rehearsal is *not* such a process: Naveh-Benjamin and Jonides (1984) have provided evidence that rote repetition is quickly automated (at which point it does not produce dual-task interference), and that automation coincides with the point at which further repetition produces no changes in memory performance. In contrast, the practices grouped under "elaborative" rehearsal do not become automatic; they consistently demand attention and pay off in retention. As a middle ground between these extremes, there is evidence for automatic processing that does produce accessible traces in memory. Encoding of information about frequency of repetition and modality of input are potential examples (Hasher & Zacks, 1979; Lehman, 1982; Zacks, Hasher, & Sanft, 1982), but there are also contradictory findings (Fisk & Schneider, 1984; Naveh-Benjamin & Jonides, 1986). (One caveat about such automatic learning: It does not mean acquiring information from entirely unattended channels, but rather, "effortless" and incidental learning of information on an attended channel.)

So general is the distinction between automatic and attentional processes that it might best be thought of as orthogonal to the other process distinctions below. That is, any process might, at least theoretically, be attentional or automatic, depending on the data being processed and the experience of the individual.

On-line versus retroactive processes. The term "on-line" derives from computer terminology, referring to events that go on without interruption or intervention from external sources. In reference to humans, on-line generally refers to here-and-now processing, rather than retrieval of the residue or traces of previous events. Actually, the term might better be applied to experimental techniques than to cognitive processing. Measures like eye-fixation time or target detection are on-line; measures of recall are not.

Remembering processes. Remembering is a general term for the retroactive process of uncovering the traces of previous events. A distinction is commonly made between encoding – experiencing the events in the first place, with concomitant rehearsal or automatic learning processes – and retrieval – getting at the residue. Both of these processes, in turn, have various subcomponents. Encoding often involves retrieving concepts and past experiences that are related to the current event. These are used to interpret and expand on the new experience (elaborative rehearsal) and thus influence its representation in memory. Retrieval includes cue encoding (making the context of retrieval into an effective probe of the memory store), search (through the network of associations), decision (editing information found through search), and response generation.

Retrieval may look very different, depending on the nature of the knowledge being retrieved. For example, episodic retrieval requires access to contextual information that specifies the episode of interest. Retrieval of semantic data is more context-free. Retrieval of declarative and procedural data also differ. Declarative data are evidenced in the form of some explicit statement about the contents of memory: I know these particular facts. Procedural data may be retrieved by reenactment, perhaps without conscious awareness of remembering (e.g., Graf, Mandler, & Haden, 1982).

Another variable aspect of retrieval is the extent to which associative search is needed (Mandler, 1980). Some retrieval cues – for example, printed words shown to skilled readers – provide relatively direct access to target nodes in memory. Indirect cues provide general access to memory, but not to specific target locations, necessitating more extensive search. The contrast between these cuing situations is exemplified in the difference between recognition and free recall tests of memory. Recall gives a general cue; recognition, a specific one. The attentional demands of these two retrieval tests are likely to differ considerably (but see Baddeley, Lewis, Eldridge, & Thomson, 1984).

Language comprehension processes. Language is a system for conveying meaning by means of some physically realized signal. Linguistic theory traditionally divides the domain into subareas, concerned with the signal itself (for vocal language: phonology and phonetics), structural units of language embodied by the signal (syntax), and mapping from the signal to "deep structure" or meaning (semantics). More recently, theories of the contextual and functional components of language (pragmatics) have been extensively developed.

Psychology departs from linguistic theory in focusing on the processing of humans as they comprehend and produce language. On a very superficial level (cf. Dell, 1986), these two uses of language, comprehending and producing, can be viewed as similar processes but in reverse order. Comprehension consists of the transition from sensory analysis of the signal to the construction of meaning and ultimate use of language in some communicative context. Production consists of translating meaning and communicative intent into a physical signal. Or, in other words, production is initiated "top-down"; comprehension, "bottom-up."

At a less superficial level, comprehension can be subdivided as follows:

1. *Perceptual decoding and lexical access* include the sensory analysis of the incoming signal, contact with information about words in long-term memory, and ultimate selection of particular meanings as the counterparts of the physical input.

2. *Parsing* is the organization of the incoming language stream into syntactic units of language or surface structure. Particularly important are the units that correspond to propositions. These may be single words, phrases, clauses, or whole sentences. Note, however, that propositional structure is also signaled by nonsyntactic devices, such as stress and semantic features, which may be more important cues than purely syntactic ones (MacWhinney, Bates, & Kliegl, 1984).

3. *Derivation of propositions* from surface units requires assigning fundamental roles, such as action, agent of action, recipient of action, experiencer, and so on, to the concepts expressed in the sentences. Semantic rules express how propositions can be built from these roles. Such subtleties as tense and number must also be extracted from word endings and function words. It is at this stage that *anaphora* – sentence elements that refer back to previous discourse or text (e.g., pronouns) – are critical, because a conceptual entity can be designated by a surface placekeeper that refers back to assignments made previously.

4. *Integration* and *inference* relate the immediately processed proposition to previous content or general knowledge in memory. An important aspect of integration is establishing coreference between concepts that are mentioned in more than one proposition. In an influential model of Kintsch and van Dijk (1978), coreference is used to establish a representation of text as a whole, linking propositions by their shared elements or arguments. Trabasso and van den Broek (1985) have argued that causal relations between elements are critical in constructing an integrated text representation.

Inference extends more broadly beyond the immediate content of a linguistic input, using logical or probable relations between events to construct propositions that were intended (or likely to be so) but not explicitly stated (Harris & Monaco, 1978; Kintsch, 1974).

A distinction related to sentence integration is that between given and new information (Haviland & Clark, 1974). Given information has previously been introduced and incorporated into the ongoing representation of the input, whereas new information pertains to previously unmentioned concepts. Conventional discourse generally presents the given and the new together; the communicative intent is that the existing representation of the given should be linked to a proposition relating it to the new.

On a global level, the content of incoming discourse or text is integrated with existing schematic structures in long-term memory. These structures represent the comprehender's general knowledge about the domain under discussion. The ultimate representation of relevant preexisting knowledge and new content is called a "situation model" by van Dijk and Kintsch (1983).

Memory and language comprehension. The relationship between memory and comprehension is profound and complex. Both short-term memory, in its storage and working guises, and long-term storage are critical, as follows:

1. Short-term memory is assumed to store an input verbatim, during parsing and derivation of an underlying representation. This surface information is critical for anaphoric reference, such as matching antecedents to pronouns and detecting a common argument for two propositions. Daneman and Carpenter (1980, 1983) have linked individual-difference measures of short-term memory capacity to the ability to detect anaphora. In most cases (but not always – e.g., Keenan, MacWhinney, & Mayhew, 1977), surface information is rapidly lost from memory, leaving a representation of content rather than wording (Sachs, 1967).

2. Both short- and long-term memory can store information about the meaning of the current communication or text. This information is used for integrating across propositions and drawing inferences. Which store is operative will depend on the span of the representation, with short-term storage sufficient for shorter, more recent segments, and long-term storage used for the representation of the input as a whole. If the needed information resides in short-term memory and does not have to be retrieved from long-term storage, integration will be speeded (Kintsch & van Dijk, 1978).

3. Long-term memory stores conceptual world knowledge, which is used for inference and construction of a situation model. Of course, long-term memory also stores essential linguistic and logical rules.

4. To the extent that comprehension processes demand attentional capacity (which is likely to be true of later processes like integration and elaboration), they are performed by the "working" component of short-term memory. The connection between comprehension and capacity is made explicit in Baddeley's (1981) model of short-term memory, which assigns to the limited-capacity executive component the burden of interpretive processing. In support of this assumption, Baddeley and Hitch (1974) found that comprehension of an auditory passage was impaired, when listeners simultaneously performed a series of digit-memory tests that imposed substantial short-term storage demands.

Examination of reading times for words in sentences specifically suggests that the integration process is capacity demanding. Reading times generally increase for the final words in sentences and paragraphs and at the end of major clauses. These are points where presentation of propositional components is completed, and hence where integration over propositions is likely to occur (Aaronson & Scarborough, 1976; Haberlandt & Graesser, 1985; Just & Carpenter, 1980).

Other components of comprehension also make attentional demands. Haberlandt, Graesser, Schneider, and Kiely (1986) found that reading time increased as more "new words" – content words introduced for the first time in a text – occurred. In theory, new words require the creation of a corresponding node in the ongoing representation of the text. Apparently, this requires capacity and thus increases comprehension time. Moreover, the new-word effect was particularly pronounced at the end-of-sentence boundary, suggesting that readers reserved processing of at least some new words to this critical point.

5. An end product of comprehension is the representation of some meaningful content in long-term memory. In this sense, comprehension is essentially a form of elaborative rehearsal. In levels of processing terminology, it is a "deep" form of encoding.

Language production. Production is much less studied than comprehension, in part because of the sheer difficulty of obtaining experimental control over the process (but for recent developments, see Dell, 1986). An important source of our understanding of production is the analysis of extended samples of spontaneous speech, including hesitation and pause data and slips of the tongue. Such analyses make it clear that production is not some simple version of comprehension, run backward. However, the gross parallel is not unreasonable. In particular, production appears to include early stages in which intended meanings are organized, intermediate stages in which sentence frames are constructed, and ultimately, lexical selection and output (Clark & Clark, 1975).

By virtue of their similarities, comprehension and production should be sensitive to similar variables measuring the complexity of language. These would include the distance, in surface structure units, between references to a common concept (Daneman & Carpenter, 1980), the number of propositions combined in a single sentence (Kintsch, 1974), the separation of components of a proposition within a sentence (as is evident in *The man that the dog that the grocer owned bit was unharmed* – e.g., Miller & Isard, 1963), and the number of new concepts introduced in discourse (Haberlandt et al., 1986). In both production and comprehension, these variables place loads on memory. For example, if a sentence interrupts some proposition A by interpolating an intervening proposition B, it demands that the first component of A be held temporarily while B is comprehended, and it requires storage of the second component of A while B is produced (assuming that all of A is planned at once).

Language processing issues. A topic of much interest is how independent or interactive language processes are. Fodor (1983) has adopted a theory in which at least some components are quite independent, or "modular." This isolation of processes produces a speed advantage, but its price is stupidity – the failure to take advantage of information from other modules. There is supporting evidence for modularity –

for example, isolation of lexical access from the processing of thematic structure (Kintsch & Mross, 1985). On the other hand, there is evidence that linguistic processes are interactive, at least at relatively late stages (Ferreira & Clifton, 1986). For example, word-level information appears to constrain and guide syntactic parsing (Mitchell & Holmes, 1985).

Another critical issue, discussed to some extent above, is how attention-demanding or automatic these processes are. One manifestation of automaticity is parallel processing. For example, in comprehension, one can ask whether all possible word senses are retrieved simultaneously or whether only the most frequent or contextually expected sense becomes active first. The answer appears to be parallel retrieval followed by selection, in the case of word meanings (e.g., Seidenberg, Tanenhaus, Leiman, & Bienkowski, 1982; Swinney, 1979), but bias toward initial selection of a particular syntactic parse (e.g., Frazier & Rayner, 1982). As a gross generalization, there is greater selectivity in later processing than in early. For example, although multiple word senses may become active in parallel when a word first appears, this process may be followed by selection of a likely sense – which can cause a processing disruption if the selected meaning is ruled out by later context (Rayner & Duffy, 1986).

This concludes the discussion of the "modal model." In the next section, I consider its implications for research on aging.

The modal model and research on aging

Would it be possible to study the effects of aging on cognition, if there were no theory of cognition? The answer would be affirmative, only if we were willing to accept an atheoretical, essentially phenomenological, description of aging. Clearly, some theoretical anchor is needed for aging research, and one is provided by contemporary information-processing theory. The question then becomes, how does the theory contribute to the study of aging?

Research on human information processing can provide a weak or a strong contribution. As its weak contribution, cognitive psychology offers a taxonomy of intellectual phenomena that might show effects of age, tying each phenomenon to some operational definition. This contribution is largely methodological, providing experimental procedures for the study of cognitive components. For example, the verbatim recall of short lists might be proposed as a measure of short-term memory capacity. The natural progression is then to test effects of age on short-term memory by using this task with different age groups.

According to this scenario, cognitive psychology offers no more than a catalog of isolated cognitive phenomena (as operationally defined) that might show effects of age. The catalog would be highly vulnerable to changing methodology and terminology.

To make a stronger contribution, research on information processing must provide a general framework for understanding the effects of aging. Such a framework must serve both an integrating and a predictive function. That is, it must indicate how age-dependent phenomena are related, by coordinating them under a common theoretical construct. And, presented with new research paradigms, it must predict which will show age effects and which will not.

Let me consider some of the forms such a contribution might take. Specifically, I consider several potential loci of aging effects that are consistent with the modal model described above. These loci range from the general – the system as a whole – to very specific cognitive mechanisms. (Note that in the discussion to follow, reference to a chapter of this book indicates that the chapter is relevant, *not* that the authors subscribe to the hypothesis under discussion.)

General systemic effects of aging

According to this hypothesis, aging produces a global change in the information-processing system that affects virtually every structure and process (Emery; Huff, this volume). A particular version of this is a slowing of processing, possibly associated with a slowing in the rate of activation spread in long-term memory (Burke & Harrold; Howard; Light & Albertson; Zacks & Hasher; Zelinski, this volume – but see above for questions about the rate of spread). Other general mechanisms would be a decline in peak activation levels – which would make processing overall less efficient (Salthouse, this volume) – or a decay of stored data.

Effects on a major system component

This hypothesis proposes that a major component of the information-processing system is affected by aging, with other components spared. One important possibility is a decline in short-term memory, particularly working memory capacity, which is for present purposes essentially synonymous with attentional capacity (Cohen; Light & Albertson; Salthouse; Zacks & Hasher; Zelinski, this volume). The outcome would be deficits in attention-demanding tasks, but sparing of highly practiced (or perceptual) tasks, which are likely to be automatic.

One could also consider the possibility of a decline in long-term memory, but this is impossible to distinguish from a decline in the processes that access stored knowledge (see below).

Selective effects on data structures in long-term memory

A set of hypotheses can be considered which propose aging effects on some types of data in long-term memory but not others. For example, one possibility is that general factual knowledge (semantic memory) is unaffected by aging, whereas autobiographical memories (episodic memory) decline (Burke & Harrold; Gillund & Perlmutter; Howard, this volume).

Another notion is that declarative knowledge is affected, whereas procedural knowledge is not. This would lead to greater aging effects on conventional recall and recognition tests than on implicit tests of memory that require "acting out" of knowledge (Howard; Zacks & Hasher, this volume). To the extent that retrieval of procedural knowledge tends to be more automated, this hypothesis is consistent with the idea that aging affects primarily attention-demanding processes, as a result of a loss in capacity. This hypothesis is also consistent with one proposing an age-related loss in conceptual, more than sensorimotor, data. Because retrieval of sensorimotor data occurs through execution of perceptual and movement procedures, it would be unaffected by a decline in declarative knowledge.

Effects on major processing mechanisms

An interesting possibility is that aging has different effects on on-line and retroactive processes, with the former spared and the latter affected (Burke & Harrold; Light & Albertson; Zacks & Hasher; Zelinski, this volume). This means that memory performance would change broadly with age. In contrast, language would be minimally affected, particularly the early stages that do not make heavy demands on retrieval from memory. Later stages of integration and construction of large-scale discourse representations would be likely to show age effects, however, because of the extensive retrieval required. Thus, this hypothesis would be compatible with the notion that aging produces deficits in "deep" levels of processing associated with encoding meaning (Burke & Harrold, this volume).

Selective effects on subprocesses of remembering

A distinction has been made between encoding and retrieval processes in memory. Further distinctions are made among types of encoding processes, particularly elaborative versus attention-free devices, and among subprocesses of retrieval. Aging might affect these subprocesses selectively. Particularly strong candidates are elaborative encoding (or "deep" processing) and the search subprocess of retrieval, which are demanding of system capacity. A selective effect in search would be consistent with a loss in retroactive processing without a deficit in on-line processing.

Selective effects on subprocesses of language

As a major cut point for the effects of aging one might consider aging effects on comprehension alone or production alone. However, the similarity of their subprocesses renders this hypothesis doubtful at the outset (Emery; Kemper; Light & Albertson, this volume).

Any of the subcomponents of language might be affected by aging. Potential deficits include sensory reception (Huff, this volume), motor output, access to the lexicon (Huff, this volume), syntactic parsing during comprehension and surface-structure organization during production (Emery; Huff; Kemper, this volume), and integration within and across propositions (Burke & Harrold; Gillund & Perlmutter; Light & Albertson; Zacks & Hasher; Zelinski, this volume).

Which hypothesis is correct?

The chapters to follow provide a wealth of data that can be used to evaluate the preceding hypotheses. In anticipation of those chapters, I propose the following generalizations:

(1) The cognitive effects of aging are not irrelevant to information-processing theories. The worst that could happen, from the present point of view, is that aging effects would be entirely capricious and unprincipled, and hence unpredictable from any information-processing assumptions. That is not the case. Aging effects are not so omnifarious.

(2) The cognitive effects of aging are selective. The whole-system hypothesis does not seem to apply to normal aging (although more pervasive effects are observed in Alzheimer's patients – Emery; Huff, this volume). Aging effects are not omnipresent.

(3) The cognitive effects of aging are complex. The forthcoming chapters suggest multiple loci for aging effects, rendering suspect any hypothesis that predicts very narrow effects. Aging effects are not simple.

(4) The cognitive effects of aging are related to the concept of capacity. Many of the hypotheses considered above are capacity related, some more directly than others. A generalization that emerges from the present papers is that aging effects become more salient, the greater the demands of the task under study. But note, from (3) above, that no simple capacity hypothesis seems likely to receive full support.

The situation described by (1) to (4) is one in which a general theory of information processing potentially can be of greatest value, to the extent that it can provide an account of the phenomena that do in fact change with age. Were the effects of aging to be unrelated to cognitive theorizing, it would be time to rethink the theory. Were aging effects entirely general, there would be no reason to try to decompose them. The study of aging and of human information processing in general could be merged, because any theoretical organization of human cognition could be imposed on a theory of aging. (This is not to say that general effects would not be of interest; only that the information-processing perspective would be largely irrelevant.) Were aging effects simple, the weak, methodological contribution of cognitive psychology might be sufficient.

The contribution of human information-processing theory to the study of aging, then, is to enable us to organize and predict the complex pattern of functional units affected by age. But at the same time, research on aging provides a test of the theory. If there is no reasonable mapping between cognitive theory and the nature of age-related changes in human performance, the modal model itself is undermined. If there is a reasonable mapping, its value is supported. The chapters to follow demonstrate both sides of this symbiotic relationship. On the one hand, these chapters show how contemporary theory and methodology can be used to generate research. On the other hand, they present results from a broad variety of experimental paradigms. To the extent that these paradigms are thought to assess common components of information processing, the consistency of results reported here provides a test of contemporary models of cognition.

References

Aaronson, D., & Scarborough, H. S. (1976). Performance theories for sentence coding: Some quantitative evidence. *Journal of Experimental Psychology: Human Perception and Performance*, 2, 56–70.

Anderson, J. R. (1983). *The architecture of cognition*. Cambridge, MA: Harvard University Press.

Baddeley, A. (1981). The concept of working memory: A view of its current state and probable future development. *Cognition, 10,* 17–23.

Baddeley, A., & Hitch, G. (1974). Working memory. In G. A. Bower (Ed.), *The Psychology of Learning and Motivation* (Vol. 8, pp. 47–90). New York: Academic Press.

Baddeley, A., Lewis, V., Eldridge, M., & Thomson, N. (1984). Attention and retrieval from long-term memory. *Journal of Experimental Psychology: General, 113,* 518–540.

Clark, H. H., & Clark, E. V. (1975). *Psychology and language.* New York: Harcourt Brace Jovanovich.

Collins, A. M., & Loftus, E. F. (1975). A spreading-activation theory of semantic memory. *Psychological Review, 82,* 407–428.

Craik, F. I. M., & Lockhart, R. S. (1972). Levels of processing: A framework for memory research. *Journal of Verbal Learning and Verbal Behavior, 11,* 671–684.

Daneman, M., & Carpenter, P. A. (1980). Individual differences in working memory and reading. *Journal of Verbal Learning and Verbal Behavior, 19,* 450–466.

Daneman, M., & Carpenter, P. A. (1983). Individual differences in integrating information between and within sentences. *Journal of Experimental Psychology: Learning, Memory, and Cognition, 9,* 561–584.

Dell, G. S. (1986). A spreading-activation theory of retrieval in sentence production. *Psychological Review, 93,* 283–321.

Ferreira, F., & Clifton, C., Jr. (1986). The independence of syntactic processing. *Journal of Memory and Language, 25,* 348–368.

Fillmore, C. J. (1968). The case for case. In E. Bach & R. T. Harms (Eds.), *Universals of linguistic theory* (pp. 1–90). New York: Holt, Rinehart and Winston.

Fisk, A. D., & Schneider, W. (1984). Memory as a function of attention, level of processing, and automatization. *Journal of Experimental Psychology: Learning, Memory, and Cognition, 10,* 181–197.

Fodor, J. A. (1983). *The modularity of mind.* Cambridge, MA: MIT Press.

Frazier, L., & Rayner, K. (1982). Making and correcting errors during sentence comprehension: Eye movements in the analysis of structurally ambiguous sentences. *Cognitive Psychology, 14,* 178–210.

Glenberg, A., Smith, S. M., & Green, C. (1977). Type I rehearsal: Maintenance and more. *Journal of Verbal Learning and Verbal Behavior, 16,* 339–352.

Graf, P., Mandler, G., & Haden, P. E. (1982). Simulating amnesic symptoms in normal subjects. *Science, 218,* 1243–1244.

Grossberg, S., & Stone, G. (1986). Neural dynamics of word recognition and recall: Attentional priming, learning, and resonance. *Psychological Review, 93,* 46–74.

Haberlandt, K. F., & Graesser, A. C. (1985). Component processes in text comprehension and some of their interactions. *Journal of Experimental Psychology: General, 114,* 357–374.

Haberlandt, K. F., Graesser, A. C., Schneider, N. J., & Kiely, J. (1986). Effects of task and new arguments on word reading times. *Journal of Memory and Language, 25,* 314–322.

Harris, R. J., & Monaco, G. E. (1978). Psychology of pragmatic implication: Information processing between the lines. *Journal of Experimental Psychology: General, 107,* 1–22.

Hasher, L., & Zacks, R. T. (1979). Automatic and effortful processes in memory. *Journal of Experimental Psychology: General, 108,* 365–388.

Haviland, S. E., & Clark, H. H. (1974). What's new? Acquiring information as a process in comprehension. *Journal of Verbal Learning and Verbal Behavior, 13,* 512–521.

Just, M. A., & Carpenter, P. A. (1980). A theory of reading: From eye fixations to comprehension. *Psychological Review, 87,* 329–354.

Keenan, J. M., MacWhinney, B., & Mayhew, D. (1977). Pragmatics in memory: A study of natural conversation. *Journal of Verbal Learning and Verbal Behavior, 16,* 549–560.

Kintsch, W. (1974). *The representation of meaning in memory.* Hillsdale, NJ: Erlbaum.

Kintsch, W., & Mross, E. F. (1985). Context effects in word identification. *Journal of Memory and Language, 24,* 336–349.

Kintsch, W., & van Dijk, T. A. (1978). Toward a model of text comprehension and production. *Psychological Review, 85,* 363–394.

Kosslyn, S. (1980). *Image and mind.* Cambridge, MA: Harvard University Press.

Lehman, E. B. (1982). Memory for modality: Evidence for an automatic process. *Memory & Cognition*, *10*, 554–564.

MacWhinney, B., Bates, E., & Kliegl, R. (1984). Cue validity and sentence interpretation in English, German, and Italian. *Journal of Verbal Learning and Verbal Behavior*, *23*, 127–150.

Mandler, G. (1980). Recognizing: The judgment of previous occurrence. *Psychological Review*, *87*, 252–271.

Marcel, A. J. (1983). Conscious and unconscious perception: An approach to the relations between phenomenal experience and perceptual processes. *Cognitive Psychology*, *15*, 238–300.

McClelland, J. L., & Rumelhart, D. E. (1985). Distributed memory and the representation of general and specific information. *Journal of Experimental Psychology: General*, *114*, 159–188.

Meyer, D. E., & Schvaneveldt, R. W. (1976). Meaning, memory structure, and mental processes. *Science*, *192*, 27–33.

Miller, G. A., & Isard, S. (1963). Some perceptual consequences of linguistic rules. *Journal of Verbal Learning and Verbal Behavior*, *2*, 217–228.

Mitchell, D. C., & Holmes, V. M. (1985). The role of specific information about the verb in parsing sentences with local structural ambiguity. *Journal of Memory and Language*, *24*, 542–559.

Murdock, B. B., Jr. (1967). Recent developments in short-term memory. *British Journal of Psychology*, *58*, 421–433.

Naveh-Benjamin, M., & Jonides, J. (1984). Maintenance rehearsal: A two-component analysis. *Journal of Experimental Psychology: Learning, Memory, and Cognition*, *10*, 369–385.

Naveh-Benjamin, M., & Jonides, J. (1986). On the automaticity of frequency coding: Effects of competing task load, encoding strategy, and intention. *Journal of Experimental Psychology: Learning, Memory, and Cognition*, *12*, 378–386.

Norman, D. A., & Rumelhart, D. E. (1975). *Explorations in cognition*. San Francisco: Freeman.

Ratcliff, R., & McKoon, G. (1981). Does activation really spread? *Psychological Review*, *88*, 454–457.

Rayner, K., & Duffy, S. A. (1986). Lexical complexity and fixation times in reading: Effects of word frequency, verb complexity, and lexical ambiguity. *Memory & Cognition*, *14*, 191–201.

Sachs, J. (1967). Recognition memory for syntactic and semantic aspects of connected discourse. *Perception & Psychophysics*, *2*, 437–442.

Schneider, W., & Shiffrin, R. (1977). Controlled and automatic human information processing. I. Detection, search and attention. *Psychological Review*, *84*, 1–66.

Seidenberg, M. S., Tanenhaus, M. K., Leiman, J. M., & Bienkowski, M. (1982). Automatic access of the meaning of ambiguous words in context: Some limitations of knowledge-based processing. *Cognitive Psychology*, *14*, 489–537.

Swinney, D. A. (1979). Lexical access during sentence comprehension: (Re) consideration of context effects. *Journal of Verbal Learning and Verbal Behavior*, *18*, 645–659.

Trabasso, T., & van den Broek, P. (1985). Causal thinking and the representation of narrative events. *Journal of Memory and Language*, *24*, 612–630.

Tulving, E. (1972). Episodic and semantic memory. In E. Tulving & W. Donaldson (Eds.), *Organization and memory*. New York: Academic Press.

Tulving, E. (1983). *Elements of episodic memory*. Oxford: Oxford University Press.

Vallar, G., & Baddeley, A. D. (1984). Fractionation of working memory: Neuropsychological evidence for a phonological short-term store. *Journal of Verbal Learning and Verbal Behavior*, *23*, 151–161.

van Dijk, T. A., & Kintsch, W. (1983). *Strategies of discourse comprehension*. New York: Academic Press.

Zacks, R. T., Hasher, L., & Sanft, H. (1982). Automatic encoding of event frequency: Further findings. *Journal of Experimental Psychology: Learning, Memory, and Cognition*, *8*, 106–116.

Zipf, G. K. (1935). *The psycho-biology of language*. Boston: Houghton-Mifflin.

2 Effects of aging on verbal abilities: Examination of the psychometric literature

Timothy A. Salthouse

From the perspective of laboratory-based cognitive psychologists interested in aging, psychometric tests designed for the comparative evaluation of individuals have both advantages and disadvantages as a means of studying cognition. Most of the advantages are related to the fact that because many such tests are in a paper-and-pencil format and do not require any special apparatus, they are very easy to administer to individuals in large groups. An important consequence of this ease of administration is that data can generally be obtained from very large samples of individuals which allows (1) analyses of the complete age continuum instead of contrasts between only two extreme groups; (2) examination of the influence of variables such as health, socioeconomic status, time of testing, etc.; and (3) determination of how performance on the test relates to performance on other similar and dissimilar tests, that is, identification of how the test fits into a factorial classification of human abilities.

The major criticisms of psychometric tests from the perspective of cognitive psychology are that most tests appear to involve a mixture of theoretically distinct cognitive processes, and frequently provide only coarse assessments of the effectiveness of particular mental abilities. Both of these characteristics are easily understood in light of the nature and purpose of psychometric tests. That is, in most applied settings there is only a limited time in which to obtain as much information as possible, and thus it is generally not practical to devote 30–50 minutes to assess the subtle nuances of one specific ability as is often attempted in psychological laboratories. The available information is necessarily less precise and analytical when the behavior sample is obtained in from $\frac{1}{5}$ to $\frac{1}{10}$ the time of a typical laboratory session.

The grossness with which specific cognitive processes are assessed in psychometric tests is at least partially attributable to the fact that it takes many years to develop a useful psychometric instrument. Applied tests will therefore inevitably lag behind theoretical developments in a given field, and may lead to the impression that the psychometric tests of cognitive abilities are theoretically obsolete. However, in order to establish the viability of a practical test, it is necessary to (1) assemble a collection of items; (2) determine optimal procedures for administration and scoring; (3) refine successive versions to maximize reliability and validity; and finally, (4) obtain normative data. This sequence may easily take several years, and thus even if deliberate attempts were made to incorporate the latest theoretical developments in the psychometric tests they would always be at least several years behind the current research. Furthermore, there is likely to be considerable reluctance among

17

practitioners or test users to abandon a familiar instrument once it is found useful, and thus test developers are probably encouraged to make only minor revisions of earlier tests with updating of norms rather than trying to introduce a completely new test based on the latest developments in cognitive psychology. For all of these reasons it should not be surprising to discover that many of the subtests incorporated in familiar omnibus tests of intellectual ability can be traced back to the early years of mental testing near the beginning of the 20th century.

Despite these perceived weaknesses of most psychometric tests, it is my contention in this chapter that useful information relevant to contemporary theoretical perspectives in the cognitive psychology of aging can be derived from existing psychometric tests by examining the age trends in different tests of a single general ability. In the same manner that an experimental psychologist might contrast two age groups across several different tasks, complete age trends can be contrasted in different psychometric tests in the hopes of identifying conditions that systematically alter the magnitude of the age differences. The degree of control is obviously lessened with psychometric tests, but this shortcoming may in some cases be compensated for by the larger sample sizes typically employed. Comparing age trends in different types of tests is a different form of structural analysis from that used by psychometricians relying on factor-analytic techniques, but a perspective of this type could prove very informative with respect to the nature of age effects in verbal abilities.

The chapter is organized into two distinct sections. The first focuses on an examination and analysis of age trends in psychometric tests of verbal ability with the goal of trying to identify when, and hence by inference, why, age differences occur with such measures. Only cross-sectional data will be considered in this context because there is still relatively little longitudinal or sequential data as compared to that available from cross-sectional studies, and that which does exist represents a very limited sample of verbal ability measures. The second section consists of a proposed integration of the results from an assortment of psychometric verbal ability tests into a conceptual framework that also seems consistent with many of the findings from laboratory investigations of age effects in language and memory. In the third and final section, speculations are offered as to how the conceptual framework might be adapted to a network representation similar to that employed in several recent models of cognition.

Psychometric tests

A variety of psychometric tests involve language and memory functions, but the vast majority designed specifically to evaluate these capabilities fall within the broad category of verbal ability tests. It is rather surprising that although the topic of memory has dominated the interests of laboratory-based cognitive psychologists, very few psychometric tests have been designed to assess aspects of memory. For example, of the three most frequently used psychometric test batteries with adults of varying ages, the Wechsler Adult Intelligence Scales (Wechsler, 1958, 1981), the Primary Mental Abilities Test (Bilash & Zubek, 1960; Schaie, 1983), and the

Army Alpha (Jones & Conrad, 1933; Yerkes, 1921), only one attempts to measure memory. Moreover, this test (in the Wechsler intelligence battery) involves simply determining the sum of forward and backward digit span, a measure that tends to exhibit smaller effects of age than most memory measures of interest to cognitive psychologists. It also seems to be less sensitive to a variety of strategic or organizational factors of great interest in contemporary theoretical perspectives of memory and exhibits relatively low correlations with other measures of memory (e.g., Kelley, 1964; Underwood, Boruch, & Malmi, 1978).

There are some special test batteries designed to assess memory skills, but few have resulted in the availability of extensive data throughout the adult life-span. The Wechsler Memory Scale probably has the greatest amount of data from adults of various ages (e.g., Hulicka, 1966; Kear-Colwell & Heller, 1978; Wechsler, 1945), but it is also not very analytic from the perspective of contemporary cognitive psychology. For example, the measures available from the Wechsler Memory Scale are the digit span, a paired-associates learning measure, a measure of memory for idea units in a paragraph, and a variety of simple measures of general orientation and knowledge. Seven other memory batteries were reviewed by Erikson, Poon, and Walsh-Sweeney (1980), but most were designed for clinical assessment and can be similarly criticized for underrepresenting the variety and intricacies of memory as currently studied by cognitive psychologists.

The situation is considerably better in the area of verbal abilities; nearly every omnibus intelligence test includes one or more measures of verbal ability. The most common test of verbal ability involves some form of vocabulary assessment because determination of word meanings offers an easy and unambiguous means of evaluating the quantity of one's acquired knowledge. Moreover, not only must word meanings be acquired rather than inherited, but also the process of acquisition can be presumed to involve a number of important cognitive operations. That is, in order for a word to be incorporated into one's vocabulary, some type of concept formation must take place to determine the reference of the new word, followed by a form of paired-associate learning of the concept and its associated label. Providing a successful definition of the word at the time of testing also indicates that the concept had been stored and can be retrieved at a later time. Cognitive psychologists might wish that these various processes could be evaluated separately, but the mixture of several presumably important aspects of information processing contributes to the value of vocabulary tests for practical assessments of cognitive functioning.

Most existing vocabulary tests can also be criticized for failing to make potentially important distinctions between active and passive vocabulary, between deliberate and passive acquisition of words, and between high-quality and lower-quality definitions. The active/passive distinction refers to the words actually used in speaking and writing, as opposed to the words for which the meaning is known but which are seldom used in one's own communications. It is possible that increased age has greater effects on the ready accessibility of words than upon the mere existence of the word in one's lexicon, and yet there is no way of making this distinction by means of existing vocabulary tests. (But see Kemper, this volume, for an intriguing analysis of active vocabulary and general language use derived from personal diaries.) Mode of acquisition might also be informative, particularly with words acquired recently, because it would be useful to contrast the efficiency of deliberate learning, as in memorizing entries from the dictionary, with passive abstraction, as when word meanings are inferred from the context in which the word occurs. It is conceivable that aging effects are greater on one of these processes than upon the others, but the lack of an operational means for distinguishing between them on the basis of currently available tests has precluded systematic investigation of this issue.

Several reports (e.g., Botwinick & Storandt, 1974; Botwinick, West, & Storandt, 1975; Looft, 1970) have suggested that older adults provide fewer high-quality definitions (e.g., provision of a synonym, mention of criterial features, indication of the word's classification, etc.; also see the scoring criteria for the Wechsler Vocabulary subtest) than do young adults. One possible explanation for this phenomenon is that the enormous redundancy of the semantic memory system allows a satisfactory definition to be provided even when more optimal definitions are not immediately accessible. In keeping with this interpretation is the finding by Bowles and Poon (1985) that older adults were generally poorer than young adults at identifying a word when given its definition, as though they had greater difficulty in converging on the ideal target item in semantic memory. Unfortunately, because most vocabulary tests do not provide separate measures of quality as opposed to quantity, this promising direction has not been pursued systematically in at least that portion of the psychometric literature concerned with adult age differences.

Many psychometric test batteries also include a test of verbal fluency in which the examinee is requested to generate as many instances of a particular category as possible in a specified period of time. For example, 2 minutes might be allowed to produce as many words as one can generate beginning with the letter *S*. The rationale behind fluency tests is that the ease of accessing and retrieving items from long-term memory is reflected by the number of different items produced in a limited time. Most of the tests rely on the total number of items generated within the allotted time as the fluency score, although other interesting analyses could presumably be conducted. For example, if a record were kept of the number of instances generated in successive temporal intervals, it might be possible to derive separate measures of the access rate and the size of the available item pool from the slope and asymptote, respectively, of the function relating cumulative number of items to time. Inferences about the organization of semantic information might also be possible by examining the sequence in which instances are generated. A pattern such as *sack, sad, safe* would suggest retrieval and/or organization on the basis of alphabetical position, whereas *soup, super, superfluous* would suggest clustering on the basis of acoustic features.

Still another type of verbal ability test often included in psychometric test batteries involves some form of reasoning about previously acquired information. Successful performance on such tests implies that the individual not only has familiarity with the relevant concepts, but also has the ability to carry out the required transformations. On the other hand, poor performance could be due to lack of experience with the concepts, or to an inability to operate on those contents. For the most part, this distinction has been ignored in psychometric tests, and thus precise interpretation of the reasons for a given level of performance on reasoning tests of verbal ability cannot easily be determined.

One of the simplest reasoning tests of verbal ability is the Similarities test in the Wechsler Adult Intelligence Scale, which requires the examinee to specify the manner in which two words are related. Common-word analogy tasks (e.g., thermometer : temperature :: clock : ???) and anagram tasks are also examples of verbal ability tests based on a combination of reasoning and familiarity with verbal material. Tests of proverb interpretation (e.g., Bromley, 1957; also the Comprehension subtest in the Wechsler intelligence battery) might additionally be considered to reflect reasoning from verbal information presumably available to most adults.

Although it is often suggested that verbal abilities do not decline throughout the adult life-span, the data from many tests such as those described above suggest that some decline does occur, particularly in later adulthood. One of the most convincing demonstrations of the cross-sectional decline in vocabulary performance across adulthood was reported by Thorndike and Gallup (1944). These investigators administered a multiple-choice vocabulary test to a nationwide representative sample of 2,906 adults ranging from 21 to over 60 years of age. Median accuracy decreased slightly with each successive decade, with a final level for the adults age 60 and above of 91% of the performance of the adults in their 20s. Although certainly not large in magnitude, and perhaps of little or no practical significance, the age-related reduction in vocabulary score is important because this study probably involved the most representative sample possible in a research study concerned with aging.

However, not all studies report a decline of vocabulary ability, and characteristics of the subject sample seem to influence the nature of the age trend. In particular, people from occupations in which there is continued opportunity for exposure to new words often appear to exhibit significant increases in vocabulary performance with age. For example, studies employing teachers or college professors as subjects typically report that the older adults are superior to the young adults in measures of vocabulary and certain other verbal abilities (e.g., Garfield & Blek, 1952; Lachman, Lachman, & Taylor, 1982; Sorenson, 1933; Sward, 1945). It has also been reported that measures of verbal ability increase with age in groups matched for amount of education (Green, 1969), or in which education is statistically controlled (Birren & Morrison, 1961), suggesting that education is correlated with opportunities for continued exposure to new words. Therefore, because increased age is generally associated with a smaller average amount of education, at least some of the reports of declining vocabulary performance with age (e.g., Thorndike & Gallup, 1944) may be attributable to fewer years of education on the part of the older adults. It would be of considerable interest to determine the relation between age and the cumulative knowledge of an individual when the opportunities for new knowledge acquisition have remained constant, but it seems likely that for most people exposure opportunities decrease as one's cumulative knowledge increases because of the narrowing of interests associated with occupational progress.

Of greater theoretical importance than the increase or decrease with age on certain tests of verbal ability is the fact that the magnitude of the age trend appears to vary systematically with the type of verbal ability test employed. This differential age

TIMOTHY A. SALTHOUSE

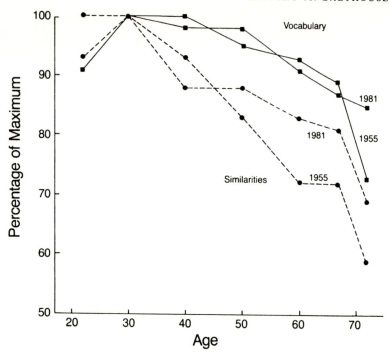

Figure 2.1. Performance at each age range as a function of the maximum performance across all ages in the 1955 and 1981 standardization samples of the WAIS and WAIS-R Vocabulary and Similarities tests.

sensitivity within the domain of verbal ability is illustrated in Figures 2.1 and 2.2. Both figures reflect performance of large numbers of individuals at each age range relative to the best average performance at any age. For example, if the maximum average score of 100 was obtained at age 35 and the average score at age 50 was 80, the 50-year-old range would be represented as 80/100 or 80%.

Figure 2.1 contains raw-score data from the 1955 ($n = 1300$) and 1981 ($n = 1440$) standardization samples of the Wechsler intelligence battery for the Vocabulary and Similarities subtests. The Vocabulary test consists of 40 words which are to be defined by describing the meaning of the word, whereas the Similarities test consists of 13 word pairs for which the examinee is instructed to state the manner in which two words are related. The age trends from these tests are clearly distinct, with a much steeper decline with age on the Similarities test than on the Vocabulary test. Because both sets of results are from the same individuals, it can apparently be inferred that the meanings of words are available to people later in their lives than is the ability to perform relational operations on that information. Jones and Conrad (1933) and Weisenburg, Roe, and McBride (1936) reported a similar divergence between vocabulary and simple reasoning scores in studies involving the administration of a variety of different tests to adults between 20 and 59 years of age. Adults between 55 and 59 years in the Jones and Conrad (1933) study averaged

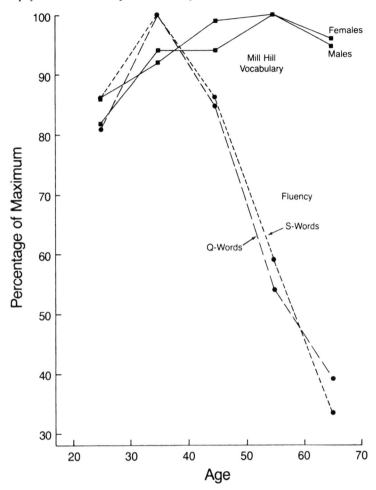

Figure 2.2. Performance at each age range as a function of the maximum performance across all ages for a multiple-choice test of vocabulary (Heron & Chown, 1967), and two measures of verbal fluency (Birren, 1955).

106% of the median performance of 20-year-olds on an antonym test of vocabulary, but only 39% on a test of common-word analogies. The correlations with age in the Weisenburg et al. (1936) study were + .16 and + .33 for two vocabulary tests, but − .37 and − .32 for two common-word analogy tests. Riegel (1959) also found markedly different age trends in vocabulary and verbal analogy tests, with older adults performing at 103% of the average young adult on the vocabulary test, but only at 54.2% on the verbal analogy test.

Another example of different age trends on measures of verbal ability is evident in Figure 2.2. This figure contains data (*n* = 300 males, *n* = 200 females) from Heron and Chown (1967) on the Mill–Hill Vocabulary Test, and fluency data (*n* = 197) from a study by Birren (1955). The Mill–Hill test is commonly used in Great Britain and exists in two versions: a multiple-choice (recognition) synonym test, and a provide-the-definition (recall) test. Primarily for reasons of scoring ease, Heron and Chown used the multiple-choice version in their study. Although not derived from a formal psychometric test, Birren's data are interesting because he examined the speed of generating instances from several different categories, with the displayed data representing the categories having the most entries (words starting with the letter S) and the least (words starting with the letter Q). The parallel functions for the frequent and infrequent categories suggest that the relative ease of accessing different types of categories is maintained throughout adulthood, although there are quite dramatic age-related reductions in the speed of accessing all categories. At least some of the steep age-related decline in the fluency measures reported by Birren are probably attributable to a slower speed of writing with increased age because he also found that there was a substantial reduction with age in the speed of writing digits, and in writing words without any categorical constraints. Furthermore, the age differences, although still quite significant, were less pronounced in a later study by Birren, Riegel, and Robbin (1962) in which oral, rather than written, responses were generated.

Figures 2.1 and 2.2 clearly suggest that the nature and direction of the age trends in measures of verbal ability depend on the particular characteristics of the tests employed. Another illustration of the importance of the specific test characteristics is available by contrasting the trends in Figure 2.2 with the cross-sectional data reported by Schaie (1983) on two tests from the Primary Mental Abilities (PMA) battery. The Verbal Meaning test in this battery assesses vocabulary, whereas the Word Fluency test measures the speed of generating instances from a particular semantic category (words beginning with the letter S). Schaie's data, consisting of cross-sectional samples of adults in 1956, 1963, 1970, and 1977, indicate that the score on the Verbal Meaning test ranged between 78% and 83% of the maximum across all ages at age 67, compared to a range of between 83% and 87% for 67-year-olds on the Word Fluency test. With these particular tests, then, vocabulary appears to exhibit a steeper age-related decline than fluency – exactly the opposite of the pattern in Figure 2.2.

It is likely that this reversal from the pattern represented in Figure 2.2 is attributable to two factors, both undoubtedly related to the fact that the PMA tests used by Schaie (1983) were originally constructed for the assessment of children between 11 and 17 years of age. One factor is that the Verbal Meaning test is a timed multiple-choice test, which probably emphasizes speed more than power. Only 4 minutes are allowed for the examinee to answer 50 items, which is equivalent to a rate of 4.8 seconds per item. This is virtually the same rate reported by Birren (1955) for 25-year-olds generating instances of words starting with the letter S, suggesting that limited time was a major determinant of performance for many individuals. In contrast, the PMA Word Fluency test tends to minimize the role of speed relative to other fluency tests because a relatively long time limit is employed – that is, 5 minutes as opposed to 2 minutes in many other tests. With an increase in the time allowed to retrieve items from the designated category, the critical determinant of performance may be the number of items in the category rather than the speed of locating and retrieving information in long-term memory. Further support for this interpretation of the two PMA tests is that Schaie (1983) reported that a measure of psychomotor speed generally had higher correlations with the Verbal Meaning score than with the Word Fluency score.

The preceding analysis of the effects of age on different tests of verbal ability suggests that the magnitude of the age relationship depends upon the specific demands of the tests, with the greatest age-related reductions on tests requiring operations to be performed on the contents of one's long-term memory. Several different comparisons provide evidence leading to this inference. First are the different age trends in multiple-choice and provide-the-definition vocabulary tests, with the latter (illustrated in Fig. 2.1) apparently declining more rapidly than the former (illustrated in Fig. 2.2). This particular comparison should be made cautiously because the data are from different samples, but there is no a priori reason to suspect that one sample systematically differs from the other. Second is the tendency for the definitions generated by older adults to be of somewhat lower quality than those provided by younger individuals (e.g., Botwinick & Storandt, 1974; Botwinick, West, & Storandt, 1975; Looft, 1970), and for older adults to be poorer at identifying words on the basis of a definition (Bowles & Poon, 1985), as though older adults conducted a less extensive search of semantic memory. The third source of evidence for the inference that age differences are largest when the processing requirements are greatest is that rapid access and retrieval of many different words (as in fluency tests) often results in much more pronounced age trends than when only a single word must be located (as in a vocabulary test). And fourth, the contrast of vocabulary with performance on tests of analogies or reasoning (Fig. 2.1; Jones & Conrad, 1933; Weisenburg et al., 1936) indicates that the magnitude of the age-related differences are greater when the test requires that operations or manipulations be performed on the contents of one's long-term memory.

In the next section an organizational framework is proposed to account for these, and other related, results. The framework is primarily descriptive, but it does seem to provide a reasonably comprehensive basis for integrating existing results.

A proposed integration: The library analogy

Imagine that you have been asked to assess the quality of two libraries, but that all relevant information must be obtained through telephone inquiries rather than from personal visits. Although this would mean that the only available information would concern the accuracy of the answers and the time required to provide those answers, it would still be possible to make very reasonable inferences from astute questioning. For example, a question such as (1), below, could be presumed to require inspection of the relevant book to be answered correctly. Some accurate answers might be supplied from the librarians' personal knowledge, but it is unlikely that many such questions could be answered without direct inspection of the relevant volume. By devising questions from a wide range of topics, therefore, one might be able to obtain an estimate of the number of different books in each library. If the staff of library B is able to answer more of the questions correctly than the staff of library A, it seems plausible to infer that there are more books in library B than in library A. Of course it is possible that factors other than the number of volumes in the library (e.g., organization of the books, workload of the staff, etc.) may result in underestimates of the actual capacities, but influences of this type can presumably be minimized by appropriate incentives and generous time allowances.

(1) Who was James Mortimer in the Sherlock Holmes story "The Hound of the Baskervilles"?

An indication of the efficiency of the staff in each library might be derived by examining the time to provide answers to questions requiring information that could be presumed to be accessible in both libraries. For example, if a variety of questions like (2) were asked of both libraries, and answers were consistently faster from library A than library B, it would seem reasonable to speculate that the staff of library A was somewhat more efficient than that of library B. Many possible factors could be responsible for the differential efficiency – for example, poor organization, incompetence, other higher-priority responsibilities, understaffing, etc. – but a slower average time to respond to a variety of requests would suggest that there is a general difference in the efficiency of the staffs in the two libraries.

(2) How many pages are there in *Gone with the Wind?*

Taken together, accuracy information from questions like (1), and latency information from questions like (2) should allow fairly specific statements about collection size and staff efficiency in different libraries. In particular, on the basis of the information described above, one is probably justified in concluding that library A has a smaller number of volumes, but a more efficient staff, than library B. These two properties are illustrated in Figure 2.3, which also represents the hypothesis that analogous differences characterize the contrast of young and older adults in the domain of verbal abilities. Specifically, it is suggested that because measures of previously acquired knowledge such as vocabulary performance seem to remain stable or increase across adulthood among people with an unrestricted exposure to new words, the size of one's knowledge base tends to increase more or less continuously throughout most of the adult years. However, because fluency measures and performance on tests requiring some form of manipulation or transformation tend to decline with age, it is postulated that the efficiency of carrying out operations on the contents of one's knowledge decreases, beginning in the decade of the 30s. This proposal is very similar to the distinction by Horn and Cattell (e.g., 1967; Horn, 1982) between crystallized and fluid abilities, and the contrasts of past attainments with current potential suggested by many other writers (e.g., Birren, 1955; Bromley, 1974; Foulds & Raven, 1948; Hunt, 1978, Riegel, 1965).

The library analogy has certain advantages over these earlier proposals, however, because it can also be extended to account for a number of other phenomena relating to the effects of age on language and memory. First, like the other proposals, the library analogy leads to the expectation that a variety of age trends would be obtained with tests requiring an uncertain mixture of cumulative knowledge and

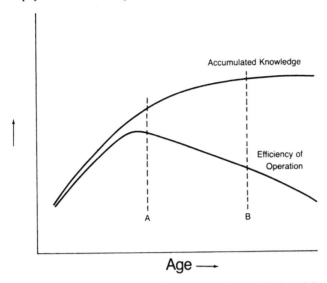

Figure 2.3. Hypothesized relations between age and cumulative knowledge and between age and operation efficiency.

operation efficiency. For example, the pattern of performance with questions like (3) would be difficult to predict; the advantage in accuracy would belong to the library with the most books because more precise estimates could be obtained from larger samples, but the library with the more efficient staff would have the advantage of being better able to carry out the required operations. It is quite conceivable that many psychometric tests (and also laboratory-based experimental tasks) confound the positive effects of cumulative knowledge with the negative effects of impaired basic efficiency in this manner. Virtually any age trend could be produced by devising circumstances that emphasize one or the other of these factors, and hence very confusing patterns would be obtained unless one is careful to distinguish between the contributions of cumulative knowledge, on the one hand, and of the efficiency of operating on that knowledge, on the other hand. Just as one should not expect to obtain a unidimensional index of library quality, so also should one not expect to characterize an individual's level of verbal ability by performance on a single psychometric test.

(3)   What percentage of books published in 1979 had red bindings?

The library analogy also leads to the expectation that certain questions would fail to distinguish between the two libraries because the required information is easily accessible in an automated retrieval system such as a card catalog. Questions such as (4) might therefore be rapidly answered in both libraries because the relevant information is coded in a card catalog that requires minimal expenditure of effort as compared to the process of locating and physically retrieving the book. In this respect, the analogy can incorporate the currently popular distinction in cognitive psychology (e.g., Hasher & Zacks, 1979; Posner & Snyder, 1975; Schneider &

Shiffrin, 1977) between automatic and controlled or effortful processing, and provides an interpretive basis for the distinction – that is, that certain organizational characteristics are intrinsic to particular structural systems such as libraries or cognizing humans.

(4)   When was *Tom Sawyer* published?

Inferences about structural organization can also be derived from the library analogy. In general, questions should be answered rapidly to the extent that they require readily available information. Therefore if a question like (5) is answered faster than one like (6), it would be reasonable to infer that the books are organized on the basis of binding color rather than topic. No definite conclusions would be possible if the speeds do not differ across questions including different types of categories, but a consistent advantage with certain forms of question would suggest a particular type of organization. Moreover, if different libraries exhibited different patterns of superiority for particular forms of questions, they might be considered to employ qualitatively different forms of organization.

(5)   Are there more books with blue covers than books with red ones?
(6)   Are there more psychology books than philosophy books?

Much laboratory research based on reasoning of the type outlined above suggests that young and old adults have similar structural organizations of semantic memory. For example, it has been demonstrated that young and old adults exhibit comparable effects of category typicality (e.g., Byrd, 1984; Eysenck, 1975; Mueller, Kausler, Faherty, & Oliveri, 1980), word frequency (e.g., Bowles & Poon, 1981; Poon & Fozard, 1980; Thomas, Fozard, & Waugh, 1977), and acoustic versus semantic relationship (e.g., Mueller, Kausler, & Faherty, 1980; Petros, Zehr, & Chabot, 1983). Moreover, young and older adults have been reported to generate similar responses in word association tests (e.g., Burke & Peters, 1986; Howard, 1980). Following the earlier argument, these results can be interpreted as indicating that the organization of verbal information appears qualitatively similar across most of the adult years.

It can also be expected from the library analogy that much of the efficiency advantage might be eliminated by asking questions in a specific sequence to capitalize on the common organizational structure. For example, if question (8) followed (7), there might be little difference in response time between libraries A and B because the proximity of the information for question (8) to that for (7) would tend to reduce the effects of any differences in efficiency. There still might be a difference in the time to respond to question (8), but it is likely that in both libraries the response time would be faster than if the preceding question pertained to a different type of information.

(7)   Who was the major protagonist in Arthur Hailey's book *Hotel?*
(8)   Who was the major protagonist in Arthur Hailey's book *Airport?*

The experimental literature on semantic priming effects appears relevant in this connection. It is frequently found that both young and old adults are faster in making a classification decision when the target stimulus is preceded or accompanied by a relevant priming word or context, although the amount of benefit does not appear to be systematically related to age (e.g., Bowles & Poon, 1985; Burke & Harrold, this volume; Burke & Yee, 1984; Cerella & Fozard, 1984; Howard, 1983; Howard, Lasaga, & McAndrews, 1980; Howard, McAndrews, & Lasaga, 1981). This pattern seems reasonable if one assumes that the structural organization remains intact across the life-span, and that although the efficiency of mobilizing one's efforts decreases, variations in efficiency can be minimized by relying on unchanged structural properties of the system.

Another "structural" aspect that might be expected to remain relatively intact is the reliance on familiar and habitual routines of action to aid in complex processing. In the library, this may correspond to the use of automated procedures for checking out books, which would tend to mask any differences in the efficiency of the library staffs. A psychological counterpart of this phenomenon may be the use of scripts or stereotyped event sequences to aid in comprehension and retention, and it is interesting to note that Light and Anderson (1983) found no differences between young and old adults in the effectiveness of using such organizational structures.

The library analogy can also be extended to generate predictions about the advantages of having a more efficient staff, independent of the number of volumes possessed. The efficient librarians should be better able to file and retrieve new materials because they will have more accurate and elaborate cataloging of materials, and perhaps a superior organization of the "information" in their possession. In terms of cognitive psychology, this would probably correspond to "deeper" processing of information with all the advantages that implies for performance on comprehension and memory tasks. More efficient librarians should also be better able to respond to real-time requests, including those that require several activities to be performed concurrently. Superior division of attention in cognitive tasks would thus be expected. Because the efficient staff is not always struggling to avoid falling behind, its members will probably be more receptive to the adoption of new strategies or procedures that facilitate overall productivity. In other words, the ability to consider and adopt new modes of performance may be associated with greater efficiency. And finally, the more efficient staff may even be better at acquiring new volumes because they have more time to engage in fund-raising activities, lobbying efforts, etc., while still handling their normal duties. That is, the rate of increase in new knowledge may be directly dependent upon the current efficiency of one's information processing. Each of these "predictions" seems generally consistent with a broad range of phenomena in the literature concerned with effects of aging on language and memory functions as summarized in Burke and Light (1981), Craik (1977), Craik and Trehub (1982), and Salthouse (1982).

The library analogy does have some limitations, however, and clearly cannot be blindly applied as a blanket characterization of the nature of age differences in verbal (and other cognitive) abilities. For example, the experience assumed to be positively associated with increased age is likely to result not only in a larger accumulation of factual information, but also in the acquisition of more effective strategies for dealing with information within given domains. In other words, both declarative and procedural knowledge can be expected to increase with experience, and yet the library analogy implies that only the declarative knowledge (i.e., the number of books) increases with age.

Another weakness of the library analogy is that it fails to reflect the fact that one's storehouse of knowledge becomes increasingly specialized as one enters and masters a particular occupation. It may therefore be inappropriate to continue to evaluate amount of knowledge and efficiency of operation along general dimensions when it is suspected that interests and expertise become progressively more specialized in a given vocation. Despite these, and probably numerous other, weaknesses of the library analogy, it is useful as a characterization of the effects of age on measures of verbal ability. Age-related increases or age invariances are often found when the variables reflect simple access to cumulative knowledge, whereas slight to severe age-related declines are typically reported when the variables emphasize repetitive operations upon, or transformations of, available information. In this respect, it is reasonable to hypothesize that the experience associated with increased age often results in a greater number of "volumes" in one's library of knowledge, but that the efficiency of carrying out most operations upon that knowledge base gradually declines with age.

From libraries to networks

Although the library analogy provides a useful descriptive basis for understanding the effects of aging on verbal abilities, it does not lead directly to further explanation because of lack of specificity about the representation of knowledge and the nature of variations in efficiency. That is, the library analogy provides no hint as to what the cognitive counterparts are of the size of one's knowledge base and the efficiency of one's operational staff. Some progress in these directions might be possible by considering how the library analogy could be translated into current theoretical concepts in cognitive psychology. Because the most popular form of knowledge representation in contemporary cognitive psychology involves a network of interconnected nodes corresponding to concepts and their postulated interrelationships, this final section explores how the previously discussed age trends in verbal ability might be interpreted in terms of network representations.

If we accept the inferences, derived above, that there is little or no evidence for age-related structural differences in the semantic knowledge system, then it can be postulated that the networks of young and old adults are organized along the same general principles. This assumption greatly simplifies subsequent arguments, but it is important to point out that it can easily be tested. For example, if one were to find a shift with age in the manner in which concepts are related (e.g., from associations based on semantic relationships to associations based on the similarity of the third letter in a concept's name), it would suggest that the structural organization of the network was different across adulthood. However, no convincing evidence of this kind has yet emerged, and thus it seems reasonable to postulate that young and old adults have qualitatively similar types of networks.

The next concern is to determine how variations in the amount of knowledge and degree of efficiency might be represented in a network. No definitive answers to these questions are yet available, but it seems fruitful to speculate about some of the possibilities because discussion of this type may inspire research that will eventually allow the identified alternatives to be distinguished.

Increased experience might be assumed to result in a greater density of nodes and connections such that the network becomes richer and more extensive. Older adults might therefore be expected to have enriched knowledge networks as compared to young adults because of their longer period of knowledge acquisition. However, it is useful to distinguish two different ways in which this greater amount of knowledge might be manifested within the network representations.

One possibility is that the network with the greater knowledge contains more nodes corresponding to different concepts than does the lesser-knowledge network. The availability of a larger number of distinct concepts presumably corresponds to a broader and more extensive knowledge. Perhaps the simplest behavioral assessment of this proposal is a test of vocabulary or some other type of factual knowledge. To the extent that one individual is able to provide more accurate answers to factual questions than another individual can, it seems reasonable to infer that the former has a larger quantity of accessible concepts in the semantic network than the latter.

However, an alternative way of conceptualizing greater knowledge within a network is in terms of more connections among the same number of nodes. For example, the richer network might contain a greater number of connections or linkages from a given concept node to subordinate, coordinate, and superordinate concepts than a more impoverished network. Although this seems to imply that an individual with more connections among nodes should be better able to answer questions about the interrelationships among concepts, there are practical difficulties in investigating this notion. A major problem is that it is often impossible to distinguish between answers based on knowledge already represented in the memory system, and answers based on relationships induced by reasoning at the time of the question.

Despite the practical difficulty of obtaining an assessment of the number of connections among nodes, it is desirable that procedures be devised to allow separate evaluation of the number of nodes (concepts) and of the number of connections (relationships) in an individual's semantic system. This distinction is not only of theoretical interest, because the two forms of knowledge representation are also likely to have different cognitive consequences. That is, the absence of a node is likely to lead to total failure in providing answers to relevant questions, although it might be possible to compensate for fewer connections by circuitous pathways among existing concepts.

Although seldom explicitly discussed, at least three alternative conceptualizations of the limits on efficiency can be identified within network representations. One of these is the number of simultaneously active nodes in the network, which might be considered synonymous with the working-memory capacity of an individual. A major focus of much of cognitive psychology since the mid-1970s has been to establish the importance of working memory for effective cognitive performance, and it is clearly reasonable to speculate that many age-related impairments in cognitive efficiency are attributable to reductions in working-memory capacity.

The limit on efficiency could also be on the total amount of activation throughout the network, which may correspond to what is often referred to as the available attentional capacity. Attentional capacity has never been precisely defined, but a number of theorists (e.g., Craik & Byrd, 1982; Hasher & Zacks, 1979) have hypothesized that a reduction in some type of "mental energy" is responsible for many of the age-related differences observed in cognitive functioning.

And finally, the limit in efficiency of processing within the network might be represented as the time needed to propagate activation from one node to another, a property equivalent to rate of processing information. The effects of processing speed on cognition are still not well understood, but the pervasiveness with which increased age is associated with a slowing of behavior has led to the conjecture that reduced speed may play a causal role in certain cognitive aging phenomena (Salthouse, 1980, 1982, 1985).

It is important that attempts be made to distinguish between these different types of efficiency limitations (or, in current terminology, processing resources). Each is clearly a potentially important source of performance impairment, but we do not yet know the relative importance of each in age-associated impairments, nor whether they have distinguishable consequences in cognitive functioning. Approaches based on formal modeling of the different types of limitations, similar to that begun by Salthouse (1985, pp. 206–214), may be useful with respect to the second issue.

The relative degree of involvement of the different types of efficiency limitations on age differences in cognition could possibly be evaluated by means of partial correlation analyses. That is, if one could obtain an index of each factor proposed as a possible efficiency limitation, then statistical control of that index should eliminate, or at least greatly attenuate, the age differences in a variety of measures of cognitive performance. (See Hartley; Light & Albertson [this volume] and Salthouse [1985, pp. 305–316] for further discussion of this type of reasoning.)

Unfortunately, the correlational approach has not proven very feasible because there are not yet any acceptable operational definitions of the various types of efficiency limitations. For example, although forward digit span, backward digit span, the recency segment of the serial position function in free recall tasks, and numerous other measures have been proposed as indices of working memory, there is still little consensus about how the capacity of working memory is best assessed. There is also a diversity of opinion about how to measure the rate of processing information, with much of the controversy revolving around the issue of simple versus complex tasks. Opponents of simple tasks such as reaction time argue that they may not require sufficient amounts of processing to provide a sensitive assessment of the speed of performing cognitive operations, whereas critics of complex tasks claim that they may introduce qualitative factors into the measurement of what is purported to be a quantitative variable.

Despite its prevalence in the cognitive literature, there are apparently no proposals about how one could directly measure the amount of attentional or mental energy available to an individual. Results from semantic priming studies might eventually prove relevant in this connection if priming is assumed to be mediated by the spreading of activation (or attentional energy) from the representation of the prime item to the representation of the target item. In particular, if in some individuals priming effects are observed for items more remote from the primed item than are observed in other individuals, then it might be inferred that the former had more activation or attentional energy available than did the latter.

However, before data from priming studies can be used to make inferences about the quantity of activation energy available, it must be established or explicitly assumed that the associational structure is identical across the groups being compared (i.e., that the distances traversed are equivalent), and that the groups also do not differ in the rate at which activation is propagated throughout the network. Furthermore, if the dependent variable is latency of a response rather than accuracy of the response, one must either demonstrate or assume that a similar, uniformly monotonic, correspondence between activation amount and latency facilitation exists in each group. It is at least conceivable that a threshold phenomenon exists in which comparable latency facilitation occurs whenever the activation is above a certain amount, and that variations in quantity of activation are detectable only when activation falls below that level. In a situation such as this, it would be impossible to distinguish between different quantities of activation as long as the available activation exceeded the critical amount. Because existing studies have generally failed to satisfy these types of necessary conditions, it appears that they do not directly address the question of the amount of attentional or activation energy available in different age groups.

Distinguishing among the two types of knowledge representation and the three possible determinants of efficiency outlined above may not be feasible on the basis of existing data, but the characterization of age effects on verbal ability developed in this chapter implies that efforts in this direction might be highly productive. To the extent that age trends in measures of verbal ability are produced by a mixture of positive effects of cumulative knowledge and negative effects of declining efficiency, it obviously becomes crucial to understand the exact nature of those knowledge increments and efficiency declines and how they might be remedied or compensated for by further knowledge or adaptive intervention.

References

Bilash, I., & Zubek, J. P. (1960). The effects of age on factorially "pure" mental abilities. *Journal of Gerontology, 15*, 175–182.

Birren, J. E. (1955). Age changes in speed of responses and perception and their significance for complex behavior. In *Old age in the modern world* (pp. 235–247). Edinburgh: Livingstone.

Birren, J. E., & Morrison, D. F. (1961). Analysis of the WAIS subtests in relation to age and education. *Journal of Gerontology, 16*, 363–369.

Birren, J. E., Riegel, K. F., & Robbin, J. S. (1962). Age differences in continuous word associations measured by speed recordings. *Journal of Gerontology, 17*, 95–96.

Botwinick, J., & Storandt, M. (1974). Vocabulary ability in later life. *Journal of Genetic Psychology, 125*, 303–308.

Botwinick, J., West, R., & Storandt, M. (1975). Qualitative vocabulary test responses and age. *Journal of Gerontology, 30*, 574–577.

Bowles, N. L., & Poon, L. W. (1981). The effect of age on speed of lexical access. *Experimental Aging Research, 7*, 417–425.

Bowles, N. L., & Poon, L. W. (1985). Aging and the retrieval of words in semantic memory. *Journal of Gerontology, 40*, 71–77.

Bromley, D. B. (1957). Some effects of age on the quality of intellectual output. *Journal of Gerontology*, *12*, 318–323.

Bromley, D. B. (1974). *The psychology of human ageing*. Harmondsworth: Penguin.

Burke, D. M., & Light, L. L. (1981). Memory and aging: The role of retrieval processes. *Psychological Bulletin*, *90*, 513–546.

Burke, D. M., & Peters, L. J. (1986). Word associations in old age: Evidence for consistency in semantic encoding during adulthood. *Psychology and Aging*, *1*, 283–292.

Burke, D. M., & Yee, P. L. (1984). Semantic priming during sentence processing by young and older adults. *Developmental Psychology*, *20*, 903–910.

Byrd, M. (1984). Age differences in the retrieval of information from semantic memory. *Experimental Aging Research*, *10*, 29–33.

Cerella, J., & Fozard, J. L. (1984). Lexical access and age. *Developmental Psychology*, *20*, 235–243.

Craik, F. I. M. (1977). Age differences in human memory. In J. E. Birren & K. W. Schaie (Eds.), *Handbook of the psychology of aging* (pp. 384–420). New York: Van Nostrand Reinhold.

Craik, F. I. M., & Byrd, M. (1982). Aging and cognitive deficits: The role of attentional resources. In F. I. M. Craik & S. Trehub (Eds.), *Aging and cognitive processes* (pp. 191–211). New York: Plenum.

Craik, F. I. M., & Trehub, S. (Eds.). (1982). *Aging and cognitive processes*. New York: Plenum.

Erikson, R. C., Poon, L. W., & Walsh-Sweeney, L. (1980). Clinical memory testing of the elderly. In L. W. Poon, J. L. Fozard, L. S. Cermak, D. Arenberg, & L. W. Thompson (Eds.), *New directions in memory and aging: Proceedings of the George A. Talland Memorial Conference* (pp. 379–402). Hillsdale, NJ: Erlbaum.

Eysenck, M. W. (1975). Retrieval from semantic memory as a function of age. *Journal of Gerontology*, *30*, 174–180.

Foulds, G. A., & Raven, J. C. (1948). Normal changes in the mental abilities of adults as age advances. *Journal of Mental Science*, *94*, 133–142.

Garfield, S. L., & Blek, L. (1952). Age, vocabulary level, and mental impairment. *Journal of Consulting Psychology*, *16*, 395–398.

Green, R. F. (1969). Age–intelligence relationship between ages sixteen and sixty-four: A rising trend. *Developmental Psychology*, *1*, 618–627.

Hasher, L., & Zacks, R. T. (1979). Automatic and effortful processes in memory. *Journal of Experimental Psychology: General*, *108*, 356–388.

Heron, A., & Chown, S. M. (1967). *Age and function*. Boston: Little, Brown.

Horn, J. L. (1982). The theory of fluid and crystallized intelligence in relation to concepts of cognitive psychology and aging in adulthood. In F. I. M. Craik & S. Trehub (Eds.), *Aging and cognitive processes* (pp. 237–278). New York: Plenum.

Horn, J. L., & Cattell, R. B. (1967). Age differences in fluid and crystallized intelligence. *Acta Psychologica*, *26*, 107–129.

Howard, D. V. (1980). Category norms: A comparison of the Battig and Montague (1969) norms with the responses of adults between the ages of 20 and 80. *Journal of Gerontology*, *35*, 225–231.

Howard, D. V. (1983). The effects of aging and degree of association on the semantic priming of lexical decisions. *Experimental Aging Research*, *9*, 145–151.

Howard, D. V., Lasaga, M. I., & McAndrews, M. P. (1980). Semantic activation during memory encoding across the adult life span. *Journal of Gerontology*, *35*, 884–890.

Howard, D. V., McAndrews, M. P., & Lasaga, M. I. (1981). Semantic priming of lexical decisions in young and old adults. *Journal of Gerontology*, *36*, 707–714.

Hulicka, I. M. (1966). Age differences in Wechsler Memory Scale scores. *Journal of Genetic Psychology*, *109*, 135–146.

Hunt, E. (1978). Mechanics of verbal ability. *Psychological Review*, *85*, 109–130.

Jones, H. E., & Conrad, H. S. (1933). The growth and decline of intelligence: A study of a homogeneous group between the ages of ten and sixty. *Genetic Psychology Monographs*, *13*, 223–298.

Kear-Colwell, J. J., & Heller, M. (1978). A normative study of the Wechsler Memory Scale. *Journal of Clinical Psychology*, *34*, 437–442.

Kelley, H. P. (1964). *Memory abilities: A factor analysis*. Psychometric Society Monographs, No. 11.

Lachman, R., Lachman, J. L., & Taylor, D. W. (1982). Reallocation of mental resources over the productive life-span: Assumptions and task analyses. In F. I. M. Craik & S. Trehub (Eds.), *Aging and cognitive processes* (pp. 279–308). New York: Plenum.

Light, L. L., & Anderson, P. A. (1983). Memory for scripts in young and older adults. *Memory & Cognition, 11*, 435–444.

Looft, W. R. (1970). Note on WAIS vocabulary performance by young and old adults. *Psychological Reports, 26*, 943–946.

Mueller, J. H., Kausler, D. H., & Faherty, A. (1980). Age and access time for different memory codes. *Experimental Aging Research, 6*, 445–450.

Mueller, J. H., Kausler, D. H., Faherty, A., & Oliveri, M. (1980). Reaction time as a function of age, anxiety, and typicality. *Bulletin of the Psychonomic Society, 16*, 473–476.

Petros, T. V., Zehr, H. D., & Chabot, R. J. (1983). Adult age differences in accessing and retrieving information from long-term memory. *Journal of Gerontology, 38*, 589–592.

Poon, L. W., & Fozard, J. L. (1980). Age and word frequency effects in continuous recognition memory. *Journal of Gerontology, 35*, 77–86.

Posner, M. I., & Snyder, C. R. R. (1975). Attention and cognitive control. In R. L. Solso (Ed.), *Information processing and cognition: The Loyola Symposium* (pp. 55–85). Hillsdale, NJ: Erlbaum.

Riegel, K. F. (1959). A study of verbal achievements of older persons. *Journal of Gerontology, 14*, 453–456.

Riegel, K. F. (1965). Speed of verbal performance as a function of age and set: A review of issues and data. In A. T. Welford & J. E. Birren (Eds.), *Behavior, aging, and the nervous system* (pp. 150–189). Springfield, IL: Thomas.

Salthouse, T. A. (1980). Age and memory: Strategies for localizing the loss. In L. W. Poon, J. L. Fozard, L. S. Cermak, D. Arenberg, & L. W. Thompson (Eds.), *New directions in memory and aging* (pp. 47–65). Hillsdale, NJ: Erlbaum.

Salthouse, T. A. (1982). *Adult cognition: An experimental psychology of human aging.* New York: Springer-Verlag.

Salthouse, T. A. (1985). *A theory of cognitive aging.* Amsterdam: Elsevier/North-Holland.

Schaie, K. W. (1983). The Seattle longitudinal study: A 21-year exploration of psychometric intelligence in adulthood. In K. W. Schaie (Ed.), *Longitudinal studies of adult psychological development* (pp. 64–135). New York: Guilford Press.

Schneider, W., & Shiffrin, R. M. (1977). Controlled and automatic human information processing: I. Detection, search, and attention. *Psychological Review, 84*, 1–66.

Sorenson, H. (1933). Mental ability over a wide range of adult ages. *Journal of Applied Psychology, 17*, 729–741.

Sward, K. (1945). Age and mental ability in superior men. *American Journal of Psychology, 58*, 443–479.

Thomas, J. C., Fozard, J. L., & Waugh, N. C. (1977). Age-related differences in naming latency. *American Journal of Psychology, 90*, 499–509.

Thorndike, E. L., & Gallup, G. H. (1944). Verbal intelligence of the American adult. *Journal of Genetic Psychology, 30*, 75–85.

Underwood, B. J., Boruch, R. F., & Malmi, R. A. (1978). Composition of episodic memory. *Journal of Experimental Psychology: General, 107*, 393–419.

Wechsler, D. (1945). A standardized memory scale for clinical use. *Journal of Psychology, 19*, 87–95.

Wechsler, D. (1958). *The measurement and appraisal of adult intelligence.* Baltimore: Williams & Wilkins.

Wechsler, D. (1981). *Manual for the Wechsler Adult Intelligence Scale – Revised.* New York: Psychological Corporation.

Weisenburg, T., Roe, A., & McBride, K. E. (1936). *Adult intelligence.* New York: The Commonwealth Fund.

Yerkes, R. M. (Ed.). (1921). Psychological examining in the United States Army. *Memoirs of the National Academy of Science, 15*, 1–877.

3 Aging and individual differences in memory for written discourse

Joellen T. Hartley

People differ in important and measurable ways along a number of dimensions of human functioning. The study of such *individual differences* has been undertaken traditionally by psychometricians, and their work has shaped current ideas concerning intelligence and personality. Other branches of psychology have been concerned also with the question of individual differences, but from a different point of view: namely, assuring through methods of control that these differences do not obscure or bias the results of experimental studies. Thus, the psychometrician finds *error variance* the focus of interest, whereas the experimental psychologist seeks to minimize it relative to *treatment variance*. The distinction between the two enterprises has been the nature of their respective goals: Psychometrics has concentrated on issues of measurement and structure of proposed dimensions of human difference, whereas experimental psychology has concentrated on general laws of behavior and processes that transcend the boundaries of the individual.

As more traditional views of experimental psychology have been replaced with the newer interests of cognitive psychology, however, there has been an increased interest in the interaction between basic cognitive characteristics of the individual and more complex aspects of cognitive performance. The work of Hunt and his colleagues on components of verbal ability (Hunt, 1978; Hunt, Lunneborg, & Lewis, 1975), for example, has generated a great deal of interest. The appearance of edited volumes devoted to the topic of individual differences in cognitive performance (e.g., Dillon & Schmeck, 1983) further attests to the growing importance of individual-difference concepts in current investigations of human cognition.

This chapter is concerned with the extension of individual-difference concepts to investigations of age differences in memory for written text. Reports of research comparing text memory in older and younger adults began appearing in the mid-1970s (e.g., Gordon & Clark, 1974), and there has since been a steady increase in the number of articles focusing on the topic. With some exceptions (e.g., Harker, Hartley, & Walsh, 1982; Meyer & Rice, 1981; Taub, 1979) the overwhelming ma-

This research was funded by Grant Number AG03362 from the National Institute on Aging. Additional support was provided by the Scholarly and Creative Activities Committee of California State University, Long Beach. Patricia Belluci, James Cassidy, Tomi Graves, Diane Lee, and Thomas Mushaney provided expert assistance in the collection and analysis of the data reported here. Timothy Bigham, Alan Hartley, and Shirley Albertson wrote the computer programs.

36

jority of the research has reported that there are significant age differences in the amount of information that can be recalled from spoken or written texts (e.g., Cohen, 1979; Dixon, Hultsch, Simon, & von Eye, 1984; Dixon, Simon, Nowak, & Hultsch, 1982; Gordon & Clark, 1974; Hartley, 1986; Hultsch & Dixon, 1983; Petros, Tabor, Cooney, & Chabot, 1983; Simon, Dixon, Nowak, & Hultsch, 1982; Spilich, 1983; Zelinski, Gilewski, & Thompson, 1980; Zelinski, Light, & Gilewski, 1984). Older adults recall less information from spoken or written texts than younger adults, and the basic finding remains consistent across a broad range of text types, text lengths, and text processing conditions. Clearly, there is a reliable phenomenon to explain.

There are several reasons for thinking that an individual-differences approach will provide fruitful new information about this age-related phenomenon. First, studies of text memory have found that, although there are marked differences between individuals, a given individual will perform relatively consistently when recall is measured over a number of different texts (e.g., Harker et al., 1982). This pattern of high intraindividual stability, coupled with high interindividual variability, suggests that a significant proportion of text memory performance is related to factors intrinsic to the individual. Second, remembering the contents of a written text is a complex cognitive behavior that must certainly reflect the efficient operation of a set of more basic cognitive skills. Individuals differ in the extent to which they possess those skills (e.g., Frederiksen, 1978; Perfetti, 1983, 1985). Age differences in memory for text may, therefore, be attributed ultimately to a combination of factors, including universal developmental changes in one or more of these basic cognitive abilities, and the interaction of individual and developmental influences on these cognitive abilities. Finally, the results of several existing studies suggest the heuristic value of an individual-differences approach to the investigation of text memory performance in adulthood (Hartley, 1986; Hultsch, Hertzog, & Dixon, 1984; Meyer & Rice, 1983).

The first formal attempt to isolate the effect of individual-difference factors in adult memory for text was reported by Meyer and Rice (1983). Meyer and Rice proposed that verbal ability, indexed by a measure of vocabulary, was an important mediator of text recall and that among adults of high verbal ability there would be few age differences in comprehension and recall of written text. The results from a series of comparisons of old and young groups over a range of vocabulary levels found only equivocal support for this proposition. Other attempts to show a strong effect of relative level of vocabulary on text recall have been equally unsatisfactory (e.g., Dixon et al., 1984; Hartley, 1986).

However, there are both practical and conceptual difficulties in relying on vocabulary score as the single index of verbal ability. At the practical level, there has been no universally used measure of vocabulary in the existing studies of aging and prose memory. In a quick perusal of the relevant literature, I have found reference to five different measures of vocabulary ability. Direct comparison of high verbal ability groups identified in different laboratories may be impossible because different vocabulary measures are used. Certainly, these vocabulary tests differ in difficulty and, consequently, in the success with which they are able to discriminate between ability groups. Perhaps some of the widely used vocabulary measures are not sufficiently demanding to allow for a separation between adults with truly "outstanding" vocabularies and those with only "very good" vocabularies. At the conceptual level, there are several issues concerning the adequacy of the vocabulary score as an index of verbal ability. Salthouse (this volume) discusses conceptual issues related to the different ways that vocabulary is assessed. For example, Salthouse argues that vocabulary tests based on multiple choice among a set of possible synonyms tap an aspect of vocabulary different from that of tests based on production of a satisfactory definition. Further, vocabulary is only one dimension of verbal ability, and it may not be an equally important dimension for indexing verbal skills at different stages in the life-span (Hartley, 1986).

The narrowness of the vocabulary score as an index of verbal ability is apparent when broader definitions of verbal ability are considered. For example, Hunt et al. (1975) considered verbal ability to be a composite of English usage, spelling ability, reading comprehension, and vocabulary (all from the Washington Pre-College Test). In this composite, vocabulary is considered to be no more important than spelling and only slightly more important than reading comprehension. When considered as a part of general intelligence, as measured by the Wechsler Adult Intelligence Scale (WAIS) for example, verbal ability is a composite of six subtests: Information, Comprehension, Arithmetic, Similarities, Digit Span, and Vocabulary. The purpose here is not to choose one of these conceptualizations as the best one, but rather to point out the inadequacy of vocabulary as a single measure of verbal ability. If vocabulary is not an adequate measure of verbal ability, then perhaps we should not expect it to be an infallible predictor of text memory. Clearly, an expanded concept of verbal ability is necessary for more rigorous testing of hypotheses about individual differences in memory for text in adulthood.

In a recent study, Hultsch et al. (1984) stepped beyond a single dimension of individual difference and examined the role of multiple intellectual abilities in text recall. The results of this investigation suggest that text recall in adulthood is determined by more than one ability factor, and that age differences may be traced to declines in more than one specific ability. Although promising from a methodological view, the intellectual abilities measured by Hultsch and his colleagues were not guided by an explicit model of verbal ability or of text processing. Thus, the specific verbal processes that differ with age and that also affect text recall remain unidentified.

In order to look more systematically for developmental differences in specific abilities related to memory for written text, we need a model of text processing and its development. There are several useful models of text comprehension that specify the action of the already developed system (e.g., Just & Carpenter, 1980; Kintsch & van Dijk, 1978), but these models do not include a developmental component. To find a model that includes development, we must look to the literature on the development of reading ability in children. A great deal of research has emerged since the mid-1970s concerning the acquisition of skill in the processing of written text by children. A relatively long period during childhood is devoted to acquiring expertise in reading, and individual differences in level of skill are apparent both early and late in the process.

In a series of experiments, Perfetti and his colleagues have shown that differences in reading skill in children (as measured by tests of reading speed and comprehension) are related to a number of simpler cognitive ability measures (e.g., Perfetti, 1983; Perfetti & Hogaboam, 1975; Perfetti & Lesgold, 1977, 1979). Perfetti (1985) proposed that a set of basic cognitive abilities supports the efficient processing of text, and that the development of reading skill depends in turn upon an increase in the efficiency of these basic verbal processes. When the basic processes in reading become efficient (i.e., require less of the available processing capacity and become "automatic," as defined by Perfetti, 1985), more processing capacity is available for the more difficult components of reading and comprehending text material. The end product of successful development of reading skill is an individual who is considered to have a high level of verbal ability. Children who have a high level of verbal ability tend to have better memory for both written texts (Goldman, Hogaboam, Bell, & Perfetti, 1980) and spoken language (Perfetti & Goldman, 1976). Thus, reading ability – or verbal ability, as defined by Perfetti and his colleagues – is closely correlated with memory measures. Because we are interested in understanding the kinds of individual differences that can help explain age differences in memory for text during adulthood, the theoretical framework that has guided the work described by Perfetti (1983, 1985) might serve as a useful starting point.

In discussing individual differences in the processes that underlie reading ability, Perfetti (1983) proposed that there are three components to verbal ability: (1) simple verbal processes, (2) complex verbal processes, and (3) verbal knowledge. In this conceptualization, a simple verbal process is a cognitive operation on a single linguistic unit such as decoding a word, retrieving the name of a word, or accessing semantic information about a word. Complex verbal processes are those that require access to more than one linguistic unit, or that require the comprehension of a relationship between two or more linguistic units. Verbal knowledge refers to the contents of permanent memory that support simple and complex verbal processes – for example, knowledge about the meaning(s) of a word, grammatical rules, or schemata. The greatest amount of empirical evidence concerns the relationship between simple verbal processes and reading skill. In a series of experiments (described in Perfetti, 1983), Perfetti and his colleagues found that children who were skilled readers were able to decode a word, retrieve its name, and access semantic information about it more rapidly than children who were less skilled readers. These are also the same simple verbal processes that are assumed to become more efficient as reading skill develops (Perfetti, 1985), and the speed with which these processes proceed may remain an important limiting factor for an individual's verbal ability. In his more recent theoretical statements, Perfetti (1985) proposed that inefficiency in simple processes may interfere with text comprehension by (1) competing for processing resources and thus interfering with the assembly of words into propositions in working memory; or (2) producing linguistic information that is of insufficient quality for effective working memory processes.

If the speed of completion of simple verbal processes is a limiting factor in verbal ability, then we might expect that if there were developmental changes in the speed of these processes in late adulthood, these changes would be accompanied by some measurable change in the comprehension and recall of written text. Recent conceptualizations of cognitive aging have proposed that there are such age-related changes in the speed with which basic processing occurs (Birren, Woods, & Williams, 1980; Salthouse, 1980). A study from my own laboratory (Hartley, 1986), has found some evidence that age-related differences in one simple verbal process (word-naming latency) may be correlated with age-related differences in text memory. These data suggest that a systematic exploration of the relationship between measures of simple verbal processes, text memory, and age might provide new information that would bear upon both models of cognitive aging and models of the development of verbal ability.

The remainder of this chapter is devoted to the description of a study concerned with the relationship between a number of individual-difference dimensions and text memory in older and younger adults. In designing the study, I chose to include a number of measures that would tap some of the simple verbal processes described by Perfetti (1983), short-term memory processes (speed and working-memory capacity), and more complex aspects of cognitive functioning (reading comprehension, abstract reasoning, vocabulary). The theoretical underpinnings of the enterprise are admittedly eclectic, but the idea was to cast as broad a net as possible to determine which avenues should be chosen for further studies. First a brief rationale for the various measures is given, followed by the methods and results of the investigation.

Rationale

The model of verbal ability proposed by Perfetti (1983) suggests that lexical access and semantic access are basic skills (simple verbal processes) that become less demanding of cognitive resources as reading skill develops. Measures of the speed of these simple verbal processes were found to be correlated with level of reading skill in young children (Perfetti, 1983). To my knowledge, comparable investigations of the relationship between simple verbal processes and reading/comprehension skill have been conducted only to a limited extent with college-age adults (e.g., Jackson & McClelland, 1979), and not at all with older adults. If simple verbal processes have become rapid and automatic by young adulthood, then they may not be good predictors of text memory in a young adult sample. However, if there is an age-related and progressive slowing of these processes, we might expect that there would be a stronger correlation between text memory and simple processes in an older adult sample that included a wide range of ages. This prediction assumes that slow completion of simple verbal processes would interfere with the success of ongoing, more complex comprehension processes, either by requiring more of the available processing resource or by producing a degraded linguistic code (Perfetti, 1985).

An immediate problem is the measurement of simple verbal processes. It is not clear that these simple processes occur independently, or in such a way that would allow them to be separated cleanly, especially in reasonably skilled adult readers. For example, there is ample evidence that semantic information about a word is activated even in the absence of explicit intent to do so: The phenomenon of semantic priming in lexical decision tasks is well documented (e.g., Meyer & Schvaneveldt, 1976). These issues cannot be ignored, but they are not the primary concern of this paper. In the present study, measures of simple verbal processes similar to those described by Perfetti (1983) were used. Lexical access was indexed with two measures: the speed of word name retrieval and the speed of word identification. Semantic access was indexed by a measure of the speed of identifying a member of a given taxonomic category. The primary reason for choosing these particular indices of simple verbal processes was to maintain some continuity with the existing literature, allowing comparison between the child and adult studies. To some extent, the issue of interdependence among basic processes can be addressed empirically. If these processes are not separable, correlations between their measures should be almost perfect. If they are separable, at least in part, the correlations should be lower.

Two measures of short-term, working memory were included: one a measure of the speed of retrieval from short-term memory, and the other a measure of the capacity of working memory. Models of the comprehension process (e.g., Kintsch & van Dijk, 1978) and also of the reading process (e.g., Perfetti, 1985) almost universally agree that a good reader/comprehender can hold and rapidly access more information in short-term working memory than a poor reader/comprehender. Support for this assumption has been shown by Daneman and Carpenter (1980) in a study that found a strong correlation between a measure of the capacity of working memory and reading comprehension.

It seems intuitively obvious that working-memory capacity should be correlated with the amount of information that can be recalled from a text. However, in an earlier study (Hartley, 1986), a correlation was found between a measure of comprehension and working-memory capacity, but not between discourse recall and working-memory capacity. This result was puzzling and may have reflected the operation of compensating strategies in a self-paced, read-to-remember task. Because the text memory task in the present study was not self-paced, compensating strategies may be less likely to mask the relationship between the text memory measure and the working-memory measure – if it exists.

If current ideas about age-related limitations in working memory are correct (e.g., Light, Zelinski, & Moore, 1982), the capacity of working memory should be smaller in older adults than in younger adults. This expectation was confirmed in a recent study by Light and Anderson (1985) but was not confirmed in my own study (Hartley, 1986). The present investigation provides an opportunity to clarify the discrepant results. Speed of retrieval of information from short-term working memory was also expected to be slower for older adults than for younger adults (e.g., Anders, Fozard, & Lillyquist, 1972).

Three other measures of more complex cognitive behaviors were used in this study. First, a measure of vocabulary was included in order to assess word knowledge. Second, a measure of reading comprehension was included. Because comprehension tests generally ask for recognition only, they provide a measure of understanding of a text that should be independent of retrieval of the information. Third, a measure of abstract reasoning was given. Abstract reasoning tests look at the skill with which a person can manipulate abstract symbols and deduce a relationship. As argued elsewhere (Hartley, 1986), these operations are similar to those that occur when propositions are manipulated in text comprehension tasks. In a previous study (Hartley, 1986), I found that each of these measures was correlated with text memory, and both vocabulary and comprehension were significant unique predictors of text recall in a regression analysis.

Method

Participants

Participants in the study were from three age groups: 24 individuals aged 18–29 years (mean, 22.3 years), 26 individuals aged 44–58 years (mean, 51.5 years), and 44 individuals aged 61–90 years (mean, 73.8 years). There were 12 males and 12 females in the younger group, 7 males and 19 females in the middle-aged group, 22 males and 22 females in the older group. All participants had completed a high school education and most had attended college. The average number of years of education was 13.9, 16.0, and 14.8 for the young, middle, and old groups, respectively. In general, the samples were above average in educational attainment, and were presumed to be above average in intelligence. Young participants were currently in attendance at California State University at Long Beach. Middle-aged participants were a combination of current students and community residents. The old participants were community residents. All participants reported themselves to be in good to excellent health and transported themselves to the university campus for two testing sessions, an indirect measure of their general competence.

General procedure

With the exception of the reading comprehension, vocabulary, and abstract reasoning tests, all tasks were controlled by an Apple II Plus microcomputer equipped with a 40-column, green-screen monitor. Displays were in upper- and lower-case letters. Response latencies were recorded by a John Bell Corporation 6522 peripheral interface card with two on-board timers. The timing routines were machine language programs. During the testing sessions, participants worked with the microcomputer in a small, completely enclosed, quiet cubicle. Experimenters were not present in the cubicle, but progress was monitored frequently through a viewing window. Participants reported that they enjoyed their interactions with the microcomputer, and that they were comfortable with the procedures.

Tasks

Text recall task. Four short descriptive essays (about 175 words) were read and recalled by all participants. Texts were displayed one sentence at a time on the video monitor. Two of the texts were displayed at a relatively fast rate and two at a relatively slow rate that had been determined individually for each participant in an earlier session. Presentation rate did not interact with age; therefore, for purposes of this paper, performance is averaged across presentation rates and this variable will not be considered further. Immediately after each text was read, the participant provided a self-paced, written recall of the content of the text. Verbatim recall was not necessary, and participants were urged to write down as much information from the text as they could remember. Recall protocols were scored according to the system described by Kintsch (1974), using a lenient criterion described by Turner and Greene (1977). Two experienced assistants each scored half of the protocols from each of the age groups. Blind procedures were used to ensure that scoring was uncontaminated by prior expectations. Reliability checks on 10% of the protocols showed that interrater reliability was above .85 for each of the four texts that were scored and intrarater reliability was above .95.

Vocabulary and abstract reasoning tasks. The vocabulary and abstract reasoning subtests of the Shipley–Hartford Scale (Shipley, 1940) were administered in the standard manner, each with a 10-minute time limit. The vocabulary test requires selection of a synonym for a target word from four alternatives. The abstract reasoning test requires the production of an item to complete a sequence of letters, words, or numbers. The maximum score on the vocabulary test is 40, and the maximum score on the abstract reasoning test is 20.

Reading comprehension task. The first half of Form 1B of the Davis Reading Test (Davis, 1944) was administered in half of the time standardly allowed for the whole test. The passages that comprise the test were continuously available for reference, minimizing the contribution of memory. The measure of reading comprehension was the percentage of the number of questions attempted that were correctly answered in the time allowed for the task. This measure expresses comprehension accuracy independently of reading speed.

Memory search task. The rate of search through short-term memory was measured with a version of the task described by Sternberg (1969). A "memory set" consisting of 1, 2, 3, 4, or 5 consonants was inspected for memorization (self-paced). A block of 10 trials followed, during which an individual letter was presented on the video monitor. The subject responded with a button press of "yes" (left hand) or "no" (right hand) to indicate whether the letter was a member of the memory set. Half of the trials in each block presented a memory-set member, and half presented a consonant distractor. Between trials, the memory set was shown for 2 seconds to reduce the possibility that subjects would forget the set. There were two practice blocks followed by two blocks of trials for each of the five memory-set sizes, with each set size tested once before any set size was repeated. Response latency was measured by the microcomputer.

The geometric means of the latencies for correct responses were obtained for each set size. Response latencies were regressed on set size, yielding both a slope and an intercept score for each subject. The slope of the regression line was assumed to represent the rate of search through short-term memory (msec/item), and the intercept was assumed to represent all cognitive and response processes that were independent of set size (Sternberg, 1969).

Word naming task. The speed of word name retrieval was measured with a naming task. This task required that the subject read a printed letter string, retrieve from memory the name associated with the encoded representation, and speak the name of the word out loud. Thus, the task explicitly required the retrieval of the name of the word. On each trial, a question mark was followed in 2 seconds by a word. The words were moderate- to high-frequency nouns, 4–7 letters long, and not more than two syllables. Voice responses were tape-recorded and checked to verify that each latency was associated with a correct response. The latencies for trials in which mispronunciations, extraneous noises, or stuttering occurred were discarded. The final measure was the geometric mean for naming latency computed over all retained trials. A baseline measure of vocal latency that did not require lexical access was also obtained from a series of trials in which the subject verified the presence of a row of four asterisks. In the baseline task, a question mark was followed on half of the trials by asterisks, and on half of the trials by a blank screen. If the asterisks appeared, the subject was instructed to respond "yes." Otherwise, no response was required.

Word search task. The speed of word identification was measured with a version of the word search task described by Perfetti (1983). In this task, a word designated as a target was shown for a time determined by the subject. This study period was followed by eight trials during which a list of words was shown, arranged vertically in the center of the monitor screen. The subject's task was to search the list for the target word and indicate with a button press the presence or absence of the word. Thus, the task required identification of a particular word in a group of words (which were presumed to be identified as well), but retrieval of the name of the word was not an explicit requirement of this task.

The list consisted of 1, 3, 5, or 7 words. For half of the trials the target was present, and for half of the trials the target was absent. Following a practice block, there were eight blocks of eight trials. Each block had a different word designated as the target. To minimize the possibility that a target would become relatively more familiar than the distractor words, each distractor appeared four times in the block of eight trials to which it was assigned. This matched the number of occurrences of the target word. Targets and distractors were all four- and five-letter words. Between trials in a block, the target word was presented for 2 seconds to reduce the possibility that subjects would forget the target.

Data reduction procedures were the same as those described for the short-term memory search task. The slope of the regression line relating set size to response latency represented the rate of word identification in the word search task (msec/item), and the intercept included all other processes that do not vary as a function of set size.

Category search task. The time required to access simple semantic information about a word was measured in a task, described by Perfetti (1983), that was similar to the word search task. Instead of searching for a target word, however, the subject searched a list of words for a member of a designated taxonomic category. The lists were 1, 3, or 5 words long, and a category target was present in half of the lists of each length. Both targets and distractors were moderately frequent members of their respective categories, and the set of words to be used as targets and distractors was drawn from several sources (Battig & Montague, 1969; Hunt & Hodge, 1971; Shapiro & Palermo, 1970). After a practice block of 12 trials, there were seven blocks of 12 trials, with a different category assigned to each block.

The slope of the regression line relating set size to response latency provided a measure of word identification time plus the additional time needed to access specific semantic information about a word (msec/item). The intercept of the regression line was interpreted as described previously.

Reading span. The reading span measure described by Daneman and Carpenter (1980) was used as an estimate of working memory capacity. In this task, a series of sentences at increasing "reading span levels" is read aloud, and the last word of each of the sentences must be reported in correct serial order after the last sentence is read. Thus, the task requires simultaneous processing and storage of information in working memory. A reading span level is defined in terms of the number of sentences that must be processed before memory for the last word of each sentence is tested. The sentences were 12–16 words long, ending with a noun. The levels that were tested were 2 through 6, and each reading span level was tested with three different sets of sentences. Three practice sets were included at level 2. Sentences were presented on the video monitor, but the experimenter controlled the presentation of the sentences. Reading span for the individual was defined as the last level for which the subject recalled, in correct order, all of the items in two of the three sets at that level. If one set was recalled correctly at the next highest level, 0.5 item was added to the estimated span.

Results

For the three tasks that produced both slope and intercept measures (memory search, word search, and category search), the measures obtained on target-present and target-absent trials were averaged to yield a single slope and a single intercept measure for each task. The degree of linearity in the individual regression equations that produced the slope and intercept measures varied from task to task, but age differences in the degree of linearity were absent in five of the six sets of regressions computed. In the word search task, target-absent condition, the regression lines for older adults tended to be less reliably linear than those for the younger adults. Because this one indication of an age difference in degree of linearity of the regression equations was accompanied by age equivalence in all other equations, it was not considered to be a general trend and was not viewed as a problem for analytic procedures. Taken across all participants, the average proportions of variance accounted for by the regression equations were .69, .78, and .97 for the memory search, word search, and category search tasks, respectively. The degree of linearity was judged to be acceptable.

The mean score for each of the age groups on each of the tasks is shown in

Table 3.1. *Mean scores for text memory and
individual-difference tasks*

	Age group			
Task and measure	Young	Middle-aged	Old	Differences
Text recall				
Proportion correct	.38	.32	.27	Y>M>O
Reading comprehension				
Correct (%) of attempted	.65	.68	.55	Y=M>O
Attempted (%)	.79	.66	.52	Y>M>O
Vocabulary	32	36	36	Y<M=O
Abstract reasoning	17	15	13	Y=M>O
Reading span (items)	2.67	3.04	2.67	Y=M=O
Word naming (msec)				
Naming latency	525	526	579	Y=M<O
Baseline voice latency	378	386	417	Y=M=O
Word search (msec)				
Slope of regression line	106	113	126	Y=M=O
Intercept of regression line	424	537	594	Y<M=O
Category search (msec)				
Slope of regression line	214	209	270	Y=M<O
Intercept of regression line	460	586	664	Y<M=O
Memory search (msec)				
Slope of regression line	52	72	80	Y<M=O
Intercept of regression line	457	556	639	Y<M<O

Table 3.1. In addition to the scores for each of the three age groups, the results
of the one-way analysis of variance (ANOVA) for each measure are summarized
in the last column. Notations of group differences or similarities are based on the
outcome of Newman–Keuls analyses that were conducted when the ANOVA showed
a significant group effect ($p < .05$).

The results for the text memory measure were as expected for the old versus
young comparison. Older adults recalled less information from the texts than younger
adults. The middle-aged adults recalled significantly less than the young adults, but
significantly more than the old adults. In general, there was a linear relationship
between age and the amount of information recalled from the texts.

Age differences were found for almost every measure, with three notable exceptions: reading span, baseline voice latency, and the slope of the regression line from
the word search task. The lack of age difference in each of these measures is interesting and warrants comment. First, the results of the reading span measure replicate
the results of an earlier study with a similar sample of subjects (Hartley, 1986):
The capacity of working memory, as measured with the reading span task, did not

differ with age. Second, the equivalence of the baseline voice latency measure suggests that the observed age differences in vocalization latencies for word naming can be attributed to a specific name-retrieval component rather than to a general vocal response-generation component. Third, the equivalence in the slope measure from the word search task suggests that the process of word identification, a very early aspect of reading, may not undergo noticeable age-related slowing in normal, older adults. However, the slope of the regression line for the category search task did show an age difference. Thus, older adults may identify a word as quickly as young adults, but they are slower to access category membership information about the word once it has been identified. Age differences were found for vocabulary, abstract reasoning, and reading comprehension measures as well, confirming the results of a previous study (Hartley, 1986).

Relationship of individual differences to text memory

Although the age differences found in the individual-difference measures were extensive and substantial, the main questions were: (1) Are these measures related to text recall, and if so, (2) can they account for any of the age-related deficit in text memory? The answer to each of these questions appears to be affirmative.

The first step was to examine the correlations between the individual-difference measures and the text memory measure. In order to reduce the number of measures, the following procedures were employed: First, a single measure was constructed to represent the three separate intercept variables. This measure was the average intercept for the memory search, word search, and category search tasks. Because the intercepts derived from each of the tasks were found to be highly correlated for each subject, this procedure seemed justified. Second, the slope of the regression line from the category search task contained two time components, the time to identify a word plus the time to access category information about the word. Because the time to identify a word was assumed to be represented by the slope measure derived from the word search task, the slope of the regression line for the word search task was subtracted from the slope of the regression line for the category search task. The remainder, a variable called "category access rate," represents the component of category search that is presumed to be independent of word identification. Support for the concern about redundancy in the word search and category search rate measures was found in the fact that the correlation between these two measures was .61. The comparable correlation between the word search rate and the derived category access rate was .18. It should be noted, however, that if semantic information about a word is accessed automatically as the word is identified, then the slope of the word search task would retain this automatic component of semantic access speed whereas the category access rate would contain only that component of semantic access that reflects a deliberate assessment of taxonomic category membership. It is this effortful component of the semantic access task that appears to carry the significant age effect. (See Burke and Harrold, this volume, for a more extended discussion of the distinction between the automatic and effortful components of semantic activation and age effects in these components.) The correlations for each of

Table 3.2. *Correlation of text recall with individual-difference measures*

Measure	Whole sample	Age partialed	Young	Middle-aged	Old
Naming latency	−.27*	−.17	−.07	−.15	−.29*
Intercept (combined)	−.37*	−.21*	−.24	−.18	−.33*
Memory search rate	−.24*	−.13	−.06	−.32	−.08
Word search rate	−.23*	−.15	−.04	−.10	−.32*
Category access rate	−.13	−.03	−.01	.06	−.11
Reading span	.33*	.35*	.17	.51*	.44*
Vocabulary	.06	.35*	.50*	.24	.22
Abstract reasoning	.45*	.31*	.19	.37*	.40*
Reading comprehension	.52*	.45*	.65*	.52*	.35*

*$p < .05$.

the individual-difference measures with text recall are shown in Table 3.2 for the whole sample, for the whole sample with age statistically controlled, and for each of the age groups separately.

When the sample was considered as a whole, every measure except for vocabulary and category access rate was correlated reliably with text recall. However, many of these correlations reflect the influence of age. When age was statistically controlled, the pattern of partial correlations was somewhat different. First, the only latency measure that retained a significant correlation with text recall was the intercept measure. Because the intercept measure is a mathematical constant that is derived from the regression of response latency on set size in a task, it is assumed to contain cognitive components that do not vary with the size of the set of stimuli that must be processed, as well as components related to response execution. Thus, the intercept was seen as a measure of more general aspects of processing speed. Each of the nonspeeded measures was correlated with text recall when the influence of age was partialed out, including the vocabulary measure.

An interesting picture emerged from the separate age-group correlations. Consider first the speed measures. In the young and middle-aged subjects, none of the speed measures were related reliably to text recall, although in the middle-aged group the correlations were in the expected direction. In the older group, some of the speed measures were related to text memory and some were not. The naming latency, intercept, and word search rate measures were all correlated reliably with text recall, whereas the memory search and category access rate measures were not.

When the nonspeeded measures were considered, there was some consistency across the age groups, but age-specific relationships were still present. Reading comprehension was correlated with text recall in each of the groups. The relationship between comprehension and text memory has also been found in studies with young children (Goldman et al., 1980) and with older adults (Hartley, 1986). Vocabulary was related to text memory in the young group only. The meaning of this finding is not clear, but it may reflect a ceiling effect in the measure for the two older groups. The final two measures, reading span and abstract reasoning, show interest-

Table 3.3. *Principal component loadings for individual-difference measures*

Measure	Principal component			
	I	II	III	Communality
Word naming	.67	−.03	.34	.56
Intercept	.80	.16	.18	.70
Abstract reasoning	−.75	.37	−.02	.70
Reading span	−.48	.52	.05	.50
Vocabulary	.24	.79	.09	.70
Reading comprehension	−.37	.68	−.17	.63
Memory search	.25	.25	.70	.62
Word search	.37	−.05	.54	.43
Category access	−.07	−.14	.80	.67
Total variance (%)	31.8	18.3	11.1	61.2

ing age-related variations. Both of these measures were correlated with text recall in the middle-aged and older groups only. Reading span was the measure of working-memory capacity, and it did not differ reliably between groups. Nevertheless, the data suggest that in the older adults the capacity of working memory limited the amount of information that could be recalled from a text whereas in the younger adults the capacity of working memory was not limiting. Finally, the relationship between abstract reasoning and text memory suggests that general symbol manipulation and linguistic symbol manipulation are related abilities. Again, a ceiling effect on this measure in the young adults may have masked a consistent, age-invariant correlation with text recall.

When the correlations between the individual-difference measures themselves were examined, it became clear that there were fewer underlying dimensions of difference than were represented with the full set of measures; therefore, a principal components analysis was performed with the set of measures shown in Table 3.2. The principal components analysis was done two ways: (1) with raw scores from the entire sample, and (2) with the correlation coefficients statistically controlled for age. These two separate analyses resulted in similar factor structures; therefore, to simplify the remaining procedures, the result of the analysis with the raw scores from the entire sample was used. The analysis yielded three principal components that accounted for approximately 61% of the variance in the set of measures. These components are shown in Table 3.3. Variables with loadings of .40 or greater on a component were considered to be associated with that component. Using this criterion, with the exception of the reading span measure, each of the variables loaded primarily onto one component. The finding that reading span loaded on two factors replicates a similar result reported by Hartley (1986).

The first principal component (31.8% of the variance) seems to be a general slowness component. Notice that along with slowness in word naming and intercept measures, poor performance on abstract reasoning and a small working-memory capacity were associated with this component. The second component (18.3% of the variance) was a general verbal ability component, with high scores on vocabulary, comprehension, and a large working-memory capacity associated positively with the component. The third and smallest principal component (11.1% of the variance) was one that reflected slowing in the specific processes measured in the study: The rates of word identification, category access, and short-term memory search were most strongly associated with this component.

The pattern of loadings of variables onto the principal components provides a partial answer to the question about the separability of the measures of simple verbal processes. The measure of name retrieval loaded primarily on Component I, but also showed an association with Component III which captured most of the variability in the measures of word identification and category access. The measure of word identification, although showing the strongest association with Component III, also had a reasonable association with Component I. Thus, these two measures seemed to have shared variability along two dimensions. Component I appears to include a motor program aspect: The intercept measure is primarily a motor response measure, and the word naming measure certainly includes a motor response. Perhaps, then, the portion of word identification variability that loads on Component I is a specific, language-based, motor portion associated with a phonological encoding of the words. Component III, on the other hand, has no identifiable motor aspects and seems to reflect central processing speeds. Word identification and word name retrieval clearly include such central, nonmotor processes. However, the measures are not completely redundant because their primary loadings are on different principal components.

The final question concerned the prediction of recall by these structural components. Four separate regression analyses were conducted; one included the whole sample, and the other three corresponded to each of the separate age groups. A two-step hierarchical strategy was used in each of the regressions: The factor scores for the three principal components were entered into the equation as a block in the first step, followed by the age variable in the second step. Table 3.4 shows the results of these analyses. The table is organized to show the total variance accounted for following each step. The significance level of the regression coefficients for each variable at each of the steps in the regression analysis is also shown. It is informative to examine the change in significance level for the variables entered in the regression equation in the first step when age is entered into the equation in the second step. If a variable drops out of the equation (loses its predictive power) when age is added to the equation, it indicates that the variable had been "standing in" or acting as a place-holder for age in the first step. That is, age and the other variable are redundant predictors (Cohen & Cohen, 1975).

In the analysis for the whole sample of 94 individuals, the individual-difference principal components accounted for a modest, but significant, amount of the total variance in the text memory measure. In the first step, each of the components was a unique predictor of text recall, as seen by the presence of significant regression coefficients. When age was entered into the equation in the second step, it accounted for an additional 7% of the variability in text recall; but more importantly,

Table 3.4. *Hierarchical regression of principal component scores and age on text recall*

Predictor	Step I			Step II		
	Beta	F	R^2	Beta	F	R^2
Whole sample (N = 94)						
Principal component I	−.45	27.00**	.32**	−.28	7.14**	.39**
Principal component II	.29	11.34**		.36	17.53**	
Principal component III	−.18	4.46*		−.11	1.51	
Age	—	—		−.34	10.40**	
Young group (N = 24)						
Principal component I	−.07	.15	.28	.05	.09	.42*
Principal component II	.54	7.42*		.78	13.39**	
Principal component III	.10	.26		.06	.10	
Age	—	—		−.47	4.71*	
Middle-aged group (N = 26)						
Principal component I	−.35	3.75	.32*	−.35	3.54	.32
Principal component II	.44	5.99*		.44	5.75*	
Principal component III	−.09	.22		−.08	.15	
Age	—	—		−.03	.03	
Old group (N = 44)						
Principal component I	−.44	9.76**	.33**	−.35	5.67*	.38**
Principal component II	.30	5.06*		.27	4.27*	
Principal component III	−.29	4.47*		−.26	3.76	
Age	—	—		−.24	3.13	

*$p < .05$.
**$p < .01$.

age changed the pattern of prediction associated with the three individual-difference components. First, it appears that the component associated with the speed of specific processes (Component III) was a place-holder for variance associated with age: When age was entered into the equation, the third component dropped out as a significant predictor. An examination of the regression coefficients suggested that some of the variance associated with the general slowness component (Component I) was also standing in for age, but this component remained a significant predictor in the final equation. The variance associated with the verbal ability component (Component II) remained relatively constant in each of the regression steps. The final regression equation in the analysis on the whole sample showed that age and general slowness were significant negative predictors of discourse memory. Verbal ability was a significant positive predictor.

As a whole, the principal components and age accounted for 39% of the observed variability in the text recall measure – approximately 32% on the first step and an additional 7% when age was added to the equation. Did the principal components account for any of the variability that might normally be attributed to age? The question can be answered by reversing the order of entry of the variables into the regression equation, that is, by letting age enter the equation first and the principal components second. When this was done, age accounted for 19% of the variability in text recall and the principal components accounted for the remaining 20%. The difference between the two separate estimates of the effect of age represents the amount of variance in text recall that may be linked to age differences in individual-difference measures. In this study, 12% of the variance in text recall appears to be associated with age-related differences in the individual-difference measures, whereas 7% of the variance is associated with age differences not captured by these measures. In general, this estimate agrees with the results of an earlier study (Hartley, 1986).

The regressions for the separate age groups allowed a closer look at the importance of the individual-difference measures. However, because the groups were relatively small, the results should be seen as suggestive rather than definitive. The final regression equations for the younger and older groups were statistically significant ($p < .05$), but for the middle-aged group the equation was not quite significant ($.05 < p < .10$). The results of these analyses tended to confirm the kinds of relationships that were suggested in the separate correlations shown in Table 3.2. There was one consistent predictor: the verbal ability factor (Component II), which contained variance associated with reading comprehension, vocabulary, and working-memory capacity. In each of the regressions, this factor was a significant, unique, and positive predictor of text memory. In the young and middle-aged groups, neither of the speed components (Components I and III) was a significant predictor, although the negative regression coefficient associated with the general speed factor (Component I) approached significance for the middle-aged group ($.05 < p < .10$). For the older group, the importance of the speed components was clearly seen in the final regression equation: The regression coefficients for the speed components were both negative predictors of text memory, and these relationships were seen even when the age variable was in the equation. However, it should be clear that a sizable proportion of the variance in text recall remained unaccounted for in each of the final equations.

Discussion and synthesis

The results of the study are considered from three overlapping points of view: (1) current theories of cognitive aging, (2) individual differences in cognitive aging and memory for text, and (3) the development of verbal ability.

Two current theories of cognitive aging that have guided this and other research consider either a slowing of central processing speed (Birren et al., 1980; Salthouse, 1980) or a reduction in processing resources (e.g., Craik & Simon, 1980) to be the fundamental failure underlying limitations in cognitive behavior in late adulthood. Although the two positions are not mutually exclusive, they have generally been considered as rival hypotheses. The present results tend to support the hypothesis that there is significant age-related slowing in the speed of mental operations, but do not find direct evidence of a reduction in processing resources.

There was evidence of general slowness in the middle-aged and older groups. This was seen as a significantly longer latency in the intercept measures from the word search, category search, and memory search tasks. Further, there were significant age differences in the speed of specific processes measured by the memory search, category search, and word-name retrieval tasks. Two speed measures did not show a reliable age difference (word search rate and baseline voice latency), although the absolute latencies of these measures were longer in the older group. Taken as a whole, these data provide support for the hypothesis that slowness in central processing is a characteristic of old age.

The single measure of processing resource capacity, reading span, did not vary with age, providing no support for the hypothesis that aging is accompanied by a measurable reduction in capacity components of processing resources. In keeping with the existing literature (Daneman & Carpenter, 1980; Light & Anderson, 1985), the reading span measure was included as an indicator of working memory capacity, a central processing resource that is viewed as critical for complex information processing activities. The present results agree with those from a previous study (Hartley, 1986) but are inconsistent with those reported by Light and Anderson (1985) in which significant age differences in reading span were observed. It is difficult to know for certain the reason for the differing results, but an examination of the span estimates from the discrepant studies suggests that differences in the young subject samples may be a source of the differing conclusions. The estimate of reading span for younger adults was higher in the study reported by Light and Anderson (1985) than it was in either the current study or the study reported by Hartley (1986). Alternatively, there were differences in materials and procedures that may have contributed to the different findings. The sentence lengths used by Light and Anderson (1985) varied from 6 to 12 words whereas the sentence lengths that I have used varied from 12 to 16 words. Whatever the explanation of the discrepancy, the fact remains that in the present study, age differences in working-memory capacity were not observed but age differences in text recall were present.

Significant age differences in basic cognitive abilities are of limited interest, however, unless they are associated with age differences in more complex cognitive abilities. When relationships between the various individual-difference measures were simplified by the principal components analysis, the five different speed measures sorted themselves into two orthogonal components which predicted text recall differentially. The component that contained variance associated with specific processing rates (Component III) was a substitute for more than half of the age-related variance in the whole sample regression equation and was a marginally significant predictor of recall in the old group regression equation. Naming latency and the intercept measures were associated with a component (Component I) that also included variance related to abstract manipulation of symbols and working-memory capacity, suggesting that this component (called a general slowing component) may be tapping processing resources in some general way. This component was a more powerful predictor of text memory overall, and was a significant predictor of text memory in both middle-aged and older groups. However, neither of the principal components that incorporated variance associated with speed of processing (Components I and III) was a significant predictor of text memory in the young group. Although complex, the gist of the pattern of relationships suggests that both general and specific slowing may be a limiting factor in text memory in older adults.

The measure of working-memory capacity was associated with text recall in an interesting pattern which suggests that this cognitive ability has a stable, and less age-dependent role in text memory performance. First, as seen in Table 3.2, the reading span measure of working-memory capacity was correlated with text recall in every case, except for the young sample. (Although not shown, separate correlation analyses found that the reading span measure was strongly correlated with the reading comprehension measure, which was in turn correlated with text memory, in all age groups.) Second, the reading span measure was associated with two of the principal components, suggesting two mechanisms of influence, one of which was independent of age. Estimates of larger working-memory capacity were associated with high scores on both vocabulary and reading comprehension measures (Component II). This component was a significant predictor of text memory in each of the regression analyses, suggesting that its influence was independent of age. Estimates of small working-memory capacity were associated with general slowing and poor scores on the abstract reasoning test (Component I). This component assumed an increasing role in prediction of recall as age increased, suggesting that its influence was dependent on age. Clearly then, the absence of significant age differences in the reading span measure does not tell the entire story about the importance of this ability in the maintenance of text memory performance in older adults. It is possible that as basic activity of the information processing system slows, the capacity of working memory may assume greater importance in determining the outcome of the comprehension process.

In general, the individual-difference measures were better predictors of text memory with increasing age. This pattern is consistent with that reported by Hultsch et al. (1984), although the sets of measures were different. The importance of this converging evidence should not be lost amidst the details of the various relationships. The broader picture suggests a changing pattern across the ages studied. In the young group, the limiting abilities were revealed as more complex, integrated cognitive skills such as reading comprehension and vocabulary skills. In middle age, symbol manipulation and working-memory capacity were added to the list. Finally, in old age, speed measures assumed importance as well.

Can this pattern of changing relationships be explained? Hultsch et al. (1984) have suggested that such a shift in correlational patterns might be observed if some members of the older group of subjects have experienced a decline in processing skills relevant to text memory whereas others have not. Such a differential loss would then increase the likelihood that these variables would predict recall. Young individuals, on the other hand, are presumed to have intact processing skills that do not vary systematically with text recall. One way to view the younger adults is to assume that they have sufficient raw processing power so that the components of the discourse processing system are not overextended by the text memory task. The present data are consistent with this interpretation.

As a final point of discussion, the relationship of the present data to the model of the development of verbal ability proposed by Perfetti (1983, 1985) will be considered briefly. Perfetti (1983) has summarized the results of a number of experiments with high- and low-ability readers at differing stages in the development of reading skills. In general, the speed of word-name retrieval and word identification are two simple verbal processes that consistently correlate with reading ability level in the early stages of skill acquisition. If we assume that text recall is an indicator of reading ability in adulthood, then we can compare the results from the adult samples in the present study with the child samples described by Perfetti (1983). First, there was no evidence that the speed of execution of any of the simple verbal processes was correlated with text recall in the young adult sample. However, in the old adult sample, measures of both word-name retrieval and word identification rate were correlated with text recall, in a manner similar to that observed with young children. Whether similarities in the data obtained for children and older adults can be explained with a single mechanism, or whether different limitations are present at either end of the life-span remains to be determined.

In conclusion, the work reported here suggests that individual differences in the basic processes underlying text comprehension and memory assume greater importance in an older group of adults, when compared to a younger group of adults. The results are consistent with other reports of individual differences in text memory in older adults (Hartley, 1986; Hultsch et al., 1984). The specific abilities that are related to text recall in older adults are nominally the same as those that are related to reading ability in young children (e.g., Perfetti, 1983, 1985). Changes in these abilities in childhood and late adulthood may reflect similar, but oppositely working, developmental events. I believe that the effort to characterize the development of verbal ability across the life-span and to isolate the key individual-difference variables in verbal ability will continue to be of benefit to researchers interested in both cognitive aging and language development.

References

Anders, T. R., Fozard, J. L., & Lillyquist, T. D. (1972). Effects of age upon retrieval from short-term memory. *Developmental Psychology, 6,* 214–217.

Battig, W. F., & Montague, W. E. (1969). Category norms for verbal items in 56 categories: A replication and extension of the Connecticut category norms. *Journal of Experimental Psychology Monograph, 80* (3, Part 2).

Birren, J. E., Woods, A. M., & Williams, M. V. (1980). Behavioral slowing with age: Causes, organization, and consequences. In L. W. Poon (Ed.), *Aging in the 1980s: Psychological issues* (pp. 293–308). Washington, DC: American Psychological Association.

Cohen, G. (1979). Language comprehension in old age. *Cognitive Psychology, 11,* 412–429.

Cohen, J., & Cohen, P. (1975). *Applied multiple regression/correlation analysis for the behavioral sciences.* Hillsdale, NJ: Erlbaum.

Craik, F. I. M., & Simon, E. (1980). Age differences in memory: The roles of attention and depth of processing. In L. W. Poon, J. L. Fozard, L. S. Cermak, D. Arenberg, & L. W. Thompson (Eds.), *New directions in memory and aging: Proceedings of the George A. Talland Memorial Conference* (pp. 95–112). Hillsdale, NJ: Erlbaum.

Daneman, M., & Carpenter, P. A. (1980). Individual differences in working memory and reading. *Journal of Verbal Learning and Verbal Behavior, 19,* 450–466.

Davis, F. B. (1944). Fundamental factors in reading. *Psychometrica, 9,* 185–197.

Dillon, R. F., & Schmeck, R. R. (Eds.). (1983). *Individual differences in cognition* (Vol. 1). New York: Academic Press.

Dixon, R. A., Hultsch, D. F., Simon, E. W., & von Eye, A. (1984). Verbal ability and text structure effects on adult age differences in text recall. *Journal of Verbal Learning and Verbal Behavior, 23,* 569–578.

Dixon, R. A., Simon, E. W., Nowak, C. A., & Hultsch, D. F. (1982). Text recall in adulthood as a function of level of information, input modality, and delay interval. *Journal of Gerontology, 37,* 358–364.

Frederiksen, J. R. (1978). Assessment of perceptual, decoding, and lexical skills and their relation to reading proficiency. In A. M. Lesgold, J. W. Pellegrino, S. D. Fokkema, & R. Glaser (Eds.), *Cognitive psychology and instruction* (pp. 153–169). New York: Plenum.

Goldman, S. R., Hogaboam, T. W., Bell, L. C., & Perfetti, C. A. (1980). Short-term retention of discourse during reading. *Journal of Educational Psychology, 68,* 680–688.

Gordon, S. K., & Clark, W. C. (1974). Application of signal detection theory to prose recall and recognition in elderly and young adults. *Journal of Gerontology, 29,* 64–72.

Harker, J. O., Hartley, J. T., & Walsh, D. A. (1982). Understanding discourse: A lifespan approach. In B. A. Hutson (Ed.), *Advances in reading/language research* (pp. 155–202). Greenwich, CT: Jai Press.

Hartley, J. T. (1986). Reader and text variables as determinants of discourse memory in adulthood. *Psychology and Aging, 1,* 150–158.

Hultsch, D. F., & Dixon, R. A. (1983). The role of pre-experimental knowledge in text processing in adulthood. *Experimental Aging Research, 9,* 17–22.

Hultsch, D. F., Hertzog, C., & Dixon, R. A. (1984). Text processing in adulthood: The role of intellectual abilities. *Developmental Psychology, 20,* 1193–1209.

Hunt, E. (1978). Mechanics of verbal ability. *Psychological Review, 85,* 109–130.

Hunt, E., Lunneborg, C., & Lewis, J. (1975). What does it mean to be high verbal? *Cognitive Psychology, 7,* 194–227.

Hunt, K. P., & Hodge, M. H. (1971). Category-item frequency and category-name meaningfulness (*m'*): Taxonomic norms for 84 categories. *Psychonomic Monograph Supplements, Vol. 4* (6, whole No. 54).

Jackson, M. D., & McClelland, J. L. (1979). Processing determinants of reading speed. *Journal of Experimental Psychology: General, 108,* 151–181.

Just, M. A., & Carpenter, P. A. (1980). A theory of reading: From eye fixations to comprehension. *Psychological Review, 87,* 329–354.

Kintsch, W. (1974). *The representation of meaning in memory.* Hillsdale, NJ: Erlbaum.

Kintsch, W., & van Dijk, T. A. (1978). Toward a model of text comprehension and production. *Psychological Review, 85,* 363–394.

Light, L. L., & Anderson, P. A. (1985). Working memory capacity, age, and memory for discourse. *Journal of Gerontology, 40,* 737–747.

Light, L. L., Zelinski, E. M., & Moore, M. (1982). Adult age differences in reasoning from new information. *Journal of Experimental Psychology: Learning, Memory, and Cognition, 8,* 435–447.

Meyer, B. J. F., & Rice, G. E. (1981). Information recalled from prose by young, middle and old adult readers. *Experimental Aging Research, 7,* 253–268.

Meyer, B. J. F., & Rice, G. E. (1983). Learning and memory from text across the adult life span. In J. Fine & R. O. Freedle (Eds.), *Developmental studies in discourse* (pp. 291–306). Norwood, NJ: Ablex.

Meyer, D. E., & Schvaneveldt, R. W. (1976). Meaning, memory structure, and mental processes. *Science, 192,* 27–33.

Perfetti, C. A. (1983). Individual differences in verbal processes. In R. F. Dillon & R. R. Schmeck (Eds.), *Individual differences in cognition* (Vol. 1, pp. 65–104). New York: Academic Press.

Perfetti, C. A. (1985). *Reading ability.* New York: Oxford University Press.

Perfetti, C. A., & Goldman, S. R. (1976). Discourse memory and reading comprehension skill. *Journal of Verbal Learning and Verbal Behavior, 14,* 33–42.

Perfetti, C. A., & Hogaboam, T. (1975). The relationship between single word decoding and reading comprehension skills. *Journal of Educational Psychology, 67,* 461–469.

Perfetti, C. A., & Lesgold, A. M. (1977). Discourse comprehension and sources of individual differences. In M. A. Just & P. A. Carpenter (Eds.), *Cognitive processes in comprehension* (pp. 141–183). Hillsdale, NJ: Erlbaum.

Perfetti, C. A., & Lesgold, A. M. (1979). Coding and comprehension in skilled reading and implications for reading instruction. In L. B. Resnick & P. W. Weaver (Eds.), *Theory and practice of early reading* (Vol. 1, pp. 57–84). Hillsdale, NJ: Erlbaum.

Petros, T., Tabor, L., Cooney, T., & Chabot, R. J. (1983). Adult age differences in sensitivity to semantic structure of prose. *Developmental Psychology, 19,* 907–914.

Salthouse, T. A. (1980). Age and memory: Strategies for localizing the loss. In L. W. Poon, J. L. Fozard, L. S. Cermak, D. Arenberg, & L. W. Thompson (Eds.), *New directions in memory and aging: Proceedings of the George A. Talland Memorial Conference* (pp. 47–66). Hillsdale, NJ: Erlbaum.

Shapiro, S. I., & Palermo, D. S. (1970). Conceptual organization and class membership: Normative data for representatives of 100 categories. *Psychonomic Monograph Supplements, Vol. 3* (11, whole No. 43).

Shipley, W. C. (1940). A self-administering scale for measuring intellectual impairment and deterioration. *Journal of Psychology, 9,* 371–377.

Simon, E. W., Dixon, R. A., Nowak, C. A., & Hultsch, D. F. (1982). Orienting task effects on text recall in adulthood. *Journal of Gerontology, 31,* 575–580.

Spilich, G. J. (1983). Life-span components of text processing: Structural and procedural changes. *Journal of Verbal Learning and Verbal Behavior, 22,* 231–244.

Sternberg, S. (1969). Memory-scanning: Mental processes revealed by reaction-time experiments. *American Scientist, 57,* 421–457.

Taub, H. A. (1979). Comprehension and memory of prose by young and old adults. *Experimental Aging Research, 5,* 3–13.

Turner, A., & Greene, E. (1977). *The construction and use of a propositional text base.* Technical Report No. 63. Boulder, CO: University of Colorado, Institute for the Study of Intellectual Behavior.

Zelinski, E. M., Gilewski, M. J., & Thompson, L. W. (1980). Do laboratory memory tasks relate to everyday remembering and forgetting? In L. W. Poon, J. L. Fozard, L. S. Cermak, D. Arenberg, & L. W. Thompson (Eds.), *New directions in memory and aging: Proceedings of the George A. Talland Memorial Conference* (pp. 519–544). Hillsdale, NJ: Erlbaum.

Zelinski, E. M., Light, L. L., & Gilewski, M. J. (1984). Adult age differences in memory for prose: The question of sensitivity to passage structure. *Developmental Psychology, 20,* 1181–1192.

4　Geriatric psycholinguistics: Syntactic limitations of oral and written language

Susan Kemper

Geriatric psycholinguistics has largely neglected to examine the basic psycholinguistic abilities of adults. Although rarely made explicit, traditional models of language acquisition assume that linguistic skills, once acquired, do not vary across the lifespan (cf. Clark & Clark, 1977; Menyuk, 1977; Owens, 1984; Slobin, 1981). Obler (1985) has emphasized the expansion of vocabulary and acquisition of pragmatic skills as central characteristics of adult language development. The expanded pragmatic skills of adults include the acquisition of multiple speech registers or stylistic shifts in phonology and syntax reflecting differences in audience, context, or topic. Nevertheless, age-related declines in basic linguistic skills have been found in normative studies of the many standardized tests of adult language (Albert, 1981; Borod, Goodglass, & Kaplan, 1980; Duffy, Keith, Shane, & Podraza, 1976; Emery, this volume; Gleason et al., 1980; Schuell, 1965). These norms indicate that linguistic skills deteriorate in old age in otherwise healthy and active adults.

Obler and her colleagues (1980, 1985; Obler & Albert, 1985; Gleason et al., 1980) reported that young and elderly adults responded differently when asked to tell a story about a picture; she concluded that elderly adults are more loquacious than middle-aged adults and that elderly adults' speech is more "elaborate" in that their speech is characterized by more repetition and redundancy, metalinguistic comments, and personalizations.

Other studies by Walker, Hardiman, Hedrick, and Holbrook (1981) and Emery (1985, 1986, this volume) support the conclusion that elderly adults' language skills are impaired relative to those of young adults. Walker et al. (1981) examined select aspects of natural conversations by young and elderly adults. The elderly adults used fewer words per *T unit* – words per clause – and clauses per T unit than did the younger adults. (A T unit is a main clause and all subordinate or embedded clauses linked to it [Hunt, 1970].) Emery (1985, 1986, this volume) has reported that elderly adults are impaired, relative to younger adults, on a wide range of tests of sentence repetition and comprehension.

This research was supported in part by Biomedical Research Support Grant RR07037 to the University of Kansas. Preparation of this chapter was supported by National Institute on Aging Grant AG06319. I thank Donna Kynette, Marsha Ambler, Jeff Hine, and Hiromi Morikawa for their assistance with these studies, and Walter Crockett, Nancy W. Denney, and John Belmont for their comments on this research.

Recently, I suggested that a syntactic processing deficit may generally limit elderly adults' performance on many different psycholinguistic tasks (Kemper, 1986, 1987; Kynette & Kemper, 1986). My research has demonstrated that some types of syntactic structures are difficult for elderly adults to produce and imitate. The structures that pose special difficulty for elderly adults are ones that involve sentence embeddings that increase processing demands. Similar processing limitations on sentence embeddings are commonly assumed by researchers developing models of automatic syntactic parsing (Berwick & Weinberg, 1984; Church, 1982; Frazier & Fodor, 1978; Kimball, 1973).

Multiclause sentences can involve two general types of embeddings: left-branching structures in which the embedded clause interrupts the main clause, and right-branching structures in which the two clauses are successive. An asymmetry in the processing of left- and right-branching constructions is commonly incorporated in models of sentence production or comprehension although the various models are formally distinguished by the precise mechanisms evoked to account for this asymmetry. For example, left-branching structures are assumed to be more difficult to produce because the main clause constituents must be anticipated while those of the embedded clause are being produced; right-branching structures are easier to produce because the constituents of the main and embedded clauses are produced successively (Bock, 1982).

One explanation for the left-/right-branching asymmetry for sentence comprehension is given by the parsing model of Frazier and Fodor (1978). They assume that syntactic analysis involves two stages. First, small groups of words are analyzed as to part of speech and then packaged together into likely noun phrases (NPs), verb phrases (VPs), or prepositional phrases (PPs). Second, these phrases are assembled into clauses. Frazier and Fodor further assume that the first-stage parser is "shortsighted" in that it can process only short strings of up to six words at one time; the second-stage parser is not so restricted but has access to all the phrase packages produced by the first stage. The left-/right-branching asymmetry is explained as a result of this "shortsightedness" of the first-stage parser.

In the right-branching sentence (1), the first five words would be initially segmented into three phrases: a NP (*the girl*), a verb (*loved*), and a second NP (*the man*). Words six to eleven would be segmented as a NP (the relative pronoun *who*), a verb (*met*), a NP (*the woman*), another NP (the second relative pronoun), and a final verb (*died*). During the second stage, these phrases could be correctly assembled as a main NP–verb–NP clause (*the girl loved the man*), an embedded NP–verb–NP clause (*the man who met the woman*), and a doubly embedded NP–verb clause (*the woman who died*).

(1) The girl loved the man who met the woman who died.

In contrast, in the left-branching sentence (2), the first six words would be segmented into one phrase: a conjoined NP consisting of three iterated NPs (*the woman, the girl,* and *the man*). Words seven through nine would be segmented into one phrase: a conjoined VP consisting of three iterated verbs (*loved, met,* and *died*). The second-stage parser would be required to reanalyze these phrases to establish the correct constituent structure by determining both the subject and object NP for each verb. Note that the conjoined NP and conjoined VP phrases must be broken up in order to assign subjects and objects correctly to each verb.

(2)   The woman the man the girl loved met died.

Alternatively, the first-stage parser might yield six phrases (three NPs and three verbs) and the second-stage parser would have to assign the correct subjects and objects to each verb. This account is not consistent with Blumenthal's (1966) demonstration that young adults tend to impose a conjoined NP interpretation on multiply-embedded left-branching relative clauses. In either case, the "shortsightedness" of the first-stage parser results in more work for the second-stage parser for left-branching constructions than for right-branching ones.

Frazier and Fodor (1978) assume that the "shortsightedness" of the first-stage parser results from working-memory capacity limitations. Working memory is generally assumed to be a limited capacity component of the human information processing system (Baddeley & Hitch, 1974). In working memory, the manipulation, organization, elaboration, and combination of new information with old information is limited by the amount of attention that can be allocated to these tasks. Individual differences in sentence and text comprehension have been linked to working-memory capacity and the ability to manipulate lexical, syntactic, and semantic information mentally (Daneman & Carpenter, 1980; Dempster, 1980; Hunt, 1978, 1985; but see Light & Anderson, 1985). Further, age group differences have been frequently reported for a variety of tasks requiring the storage and manipulation of information in working memory although it is unresolved whether these differences are due to absolute capacity limitations or to strategic differences in the allocation of attentional resources (e.g., Cohen, this volume; Craik & Simon, 1980; Salthouse, 1982; Smith, 1980; Spilich, 1985; Stine, Wingfield, & Poon, in press; Zacks & Hasher, this volume).

In a series of studies, I have investigated how age group differences in working memory may affect adults' production and imitation of complex syntactic constructions. In general, I made within-subject comparisons of adults' use of complex sentences with left- or right-branching embeddings. I have assumed that elderly adults' working-memory capacity is exceeded by complex structures, particularly left-branching structures, such as those in Table 4.1. In contrast, simple structures, including right-branching structures, also illustrated in Table 4.1, do not appear to exceed elderly adults' working-memory capacity. Branching direction, provided only a single level of embedding is used, does not appear to affect the performance of young and middle-aged adults.

Oral production

Kynette and Kemper (1986) undertook a detailed investigation of the spontaneous speech of active, healthy adults between the ages of 50 and 90 years. All adults were asked to relate oral narratives about significant events in their lives. Their topics included getting married, leaving home for the first time, and going off to war. A

Table 4.1. *Examples of left- and right-branching sentences*

Left-branching sentences

Subordinate clause:	Because Bill left the party without his coat, John was upset.
Infinitive:	For Bill to leave the party without his coat was odd.
That-clause:	That Bill left the party without his coat upset John.
Gerund:	Bill's leaving the party without his coat upset John.
Wh-clause:	When Bill left the party without his coat upset John.
Relative clause:	The news that Bill left the party without his coat upset John.

Right-branching sentences

Subordinate:	John was upset because Bill left the party without his coat.
Infinitive:	John told Bill to leave the party without his coat.
That-clause:	John was upset that Bill left the party without his coat.
Gerund:	John was upset by Bill's leaving the party without his coat.
Wh-clause:	John was upset about when Bill left the party without his coat.
Relative clause:	John was upset by the news that Bill left the party without his coat.

20-minute sample of speech was selected from the middle portion of these narratives to avoid effects of initial nervousness or fatigue. The analysis tallied the incidence of different syntactic structures, verb tenses, and form classes (parts of speech) as well as measures of sentence length, lexical diversity, and the incidence of speech disfluencies such as sentence fragments and filled pauses.

Across this age range, there was a reduction in the variability and accuracy of the adults' production of syntactic structures, verb tenses, and form classes. The 50- and 60-year-olds produced some syntactic structures that the 70- and 80-year-olds did not use. These included simple syntactic structures with modal auxiliary verbs, gerunds, participles, subject-relative clauses, coordinate subjects, subordinate clauses, and noun-phrase complements. The 50- and 60-year-olds also produced a greater range of complex structures with multiple embeddings, embeddings plus coordination, and complex combinations of structures. The 50- and 60-year-olds produced more different grammatical forms and used them more correctly than did the 70- and 80-year-olds. The 70- and 80-year-olds made more errors including the omission of obligatory grammatical morphemes, such as articles, possessives, complementizers, and relative pronouns, and the use of incorrect past-tense inflections and mismatched subjects and verbs.

Despite these changes in syntax, mean length of utterance did not change with age nor was there any change in the measures of lexical diversity or speech disfluency. Further, the age groups were matched in terms of educational history and performance on a shortened version of the vocabulary test from the Wechsler Adult Intelligence Scale (Wechsler, 1945). Consequently, it appears that the observed changes reflect age-related changes in the production of complex syntax per se. Many of the constructions that were not used by the 70- and 80-year-olds involved left-branching grammatical structures. The 70- and 80-year-olds did use right-branching structures which enabled them to preserve the length of their utterances. The 70- and 80-year-olds' grammatical errors also seemed to be associated with their attempts to produce complex, left-branching structures.

It is likely that the age-related changes in adults' oral production of syntactic structures reflect changes in working-memory capacity. The nature of these changes was explored more carefully in two further studies investigating the role of working memory in elderly adults' speech production.

Working memory and syntactic complexity

Converging evidence for the hypothesis that working-memory capacity limitations affect elderly adults' ability to produce complex syntactic structures comes from two further studies: I previously studied how accurately adults could imitate sentences varying in complexity (Kemper, 1986); a follow-up study investigated the interrelationship among measures of working-memory capacity, the complexity of spontaneous speech, and sentence imitation.

Imitations

In my study of adult imitation (Kemper, 1986), elderly adults between 70 and 89 years and younger adults between 30 and 49 years were asked to imitate a variety of prompts. The prompts included both a main clause and an embedded clause. The prompts varied in grammatical correctness and in the length and the position of the embedded clause. The task required the adults to hold a prompt in memory long enough to detect and correct a grammatical error, if there was one, and to produce orally a grammatically correct imitation (McNeill, 1966). Working-memory capacity was assumed to limit the adults' ability to retain, monitor, and, if necessary, correct the prompts. Examples of the prompts and adults' responses, taken from Kemper (1986), are given in Tables 4.2 and 4.3.

Four categories were used to score the adults' responses: (1) grammatically correct imitations of both grammatical and ungrammatical prompts, (2) grammatically correct paraphrases that preserved the semantic content but altered the syntactic form of the originals, (3) grammatically correct sentences that abridged the semantic content of the original prompts by omitting one or more phrases, and (4) other types of changes that distorted the syntactic form or semantic content of the originals.

The younger adults had no difficulty imitating the prompt sentences regardless of their grammatical correctness, or the length or position of the embedded clause; 86% of their responses were grammatically correct imitations, and 12% were grammatically correct paraphrases. Compared to the younger adults, the elderly adults had more difficulty responding to the ungrammatical sentences; 32% were abridged or otherwise distorted during imitation. Further, the length and the position of the embedded clause also affected their ability to imitate the sentence prompts. Whereas the elderly adults correctly imitated or paraphrased 97% of the prompts with short embedded clauses, they correctly imitated or paraphrased only 48% of those with long embedded clauses; 52% of the long embedded clauses were abridged or otherwise distorted by the elderly adults. The elderly adults correctly imitated or paraphrased sentence-final embeddings 89% of the time, but they correctly imitated or

Table 4.2. *Examples of imitation prompts*

Left-branching prompts		
Short	Grammatical:	What I did interested my grandchildren.
	Ungrammatical:	What I have did interested my grandchildren.
Long	Grammatical:	What I took out of the oven interested my grandchildren.
	Ungrammatical:	What I have took out of the oven interested my grandchildren.
Right-branching prompts		
Short	Grammatical:	My grandchildren watched what I did.
	Ungrammatical:	My grandchildren watched what I have did.
Long	Grammatical:	My grandchildren watched what I took out of the oven.
	Ungrammatical:	My grandchildren watched what I have took out of the oven.

Source: Adapted from Kemper (1986) by permission of *Applied Psycholinguistics*, published by Cambridge University Press.

Table 4.3. *Examples of imitation responses*

Ungrammatical prompt	*Grammatical prompt*
My grandchildren enjoyed the cookies that I did baked.	That the ginger cookies were golden brown surprised me.
Grammatical imitation	
My grandchildren enjoyed the cookies that I baked.	That the ginger cookies were golden brown surprised me.
Grammatical paraphrases	
I baked the cookies that my grandkids enjoyed.	I was surprised that the ginger cookies were golden brown.
I baked some cookies and my grandchildren enjoyed them.	The ginger cookies were golden brown. This surprised me.
My grandchildren liked the ginger cookies I made.	The cookies, ginger ones, surprised me by being golden brown.
Grammatical abridgment	
My grandchildren enjoyed the cookies.	The cookies were brown.
I baked some cookies.	The cookies surprised me.
I baked cookies for my grandchildren.	I baked ginger cookies.
Other	
My grandchildren baked me some cookies.	I didn't like them.
I have six grandchildren.	The cookies were burnt.

Source: Adapted from Kemper (1986) by permission of *Applied Psycholinguistics*, published by Cambridge University Press.

paraphrased sentence-initial ones 56% of the time and abridged or distorted them 44% of the time.

The results clearly demonstrated that elderly adults have an impairment of their ability to imitate complex syntactic structures. The elderly adults had difficulty imitating sentences with long or sentence-initial embedded clauses, yet they could

Table 4.4. *Examples of prompts used to measure left- and right-branching imitative span*

Left-branching span

Span	Prompt
1	Running impresses me.
2	John's running impresses me.
3	Running long distances impresses me.
4	John's running long distances impresses me.
	.
	.
	.
12	How John's running long distances every week has helped his mental concentration impresses me.
13	How John's running long distances every week has helped his mental concentration improve impresses me.

Right-branching span

Span	Prompt
1	I like running.
2	I like John's running.
3	I like running long distances.
4	I like John's running long distances.
	.
	.
	.
12	I like how John's running long distances every week has helped his mental concentration.
13	I like how John's running long distances every week has helped his mental concentration improve.

---

accurately imitate sentences with short or sentence-final embeddings. These interactions suggest that with old age there are processing capacity limitations that limit elderly adults' ability to retain long or sentence-initial embeddings and to monitor and correct grammatical violations. Such capacity limitations may also constrain other discourse processes including those of semantic analysis and elaboration and prose segmentation, interpretation, and recall.

Limitations

To explore further how working memory limitations affect linguistic skills, a correlational study was carried out, which investigated the relationship among adults' production of complex syntactic structures, their ability to imitate complex sentences, and measures of their working-memory capacity.

A group of 60 adults, 30 men and 30 women, between the ages of 50 and 89 years were recruited as participants. Each adult was interviewed to verify age and educational history. During each interview, the adults were asked to relate personal narratives about significant events in their lives: a 20-minute sample of spontaneous speech was obtained from these narratives. In addition, each adult was tested with

Table 4.5. *Means and results of the ANOVA*

	Age group				ANOVA
	50–59	60–69	70–79	80–89	F (3.56)
Education	13.2	12.8	12.1	12.2	.73
Vocabulary	73.1	73.2	71.6	75.2	.81
Forward span	7.2	6.5	6.0	5.7	7.38**
Backward span	5.7	5.2	4.8	4.8	1.99
Mean clause length	2.8	2.3	1.9	1.7	22.22**
Right branch	1.6	1.6	1.5	1.4	.57
Left branch	1.2	.7	.3	.3	3.86*
Right span	9.1	9.1	8.8	7.6	3.03
Left span	7.2	7.2	6.1	5.6	5.34*

*$p < .05$.
**$p < .01$.

the 80-item vocabulary test from the Wechsler Adult Intelligence Scale (WAIS) and with the forward and backward digit span tests from the WAIS. Finally, each adult was tested for ability to imitate right-branching and left-branching constructions like those in Table 4.4. The longest embedded clause, in terms of the total number of words, which the adults' could imitate verbatim, was recorded.

The speech sample was analyzed by first computing the mean number of clauses per sentence for the entire sample. Second, the mean number of right-branching clauses and the mean number of left-branching clauses were also computed for the sample. Left-branching clauses included gerunds used as sentential subjects, relative clauses modifying the subjects, and that-clauses and wh-clauses used as subjects. Right-branching clauses included infinitive complements, relative clauses modifying predicate objects, and that-clause and wh-clause complements.

Thus, for each adult, there were nine measures: the number of years of formal education completed, WAIS vocabulary, forward digit span, backward digit span, the mean number of clauses per sentence (MCL), the mean number of left-branching embeddings per sentence (left-branches), the mean number of right-branching embeddings per sentence (right-branches), imitative span for right-branching sentences (right-branching span), and imitative span for left-branching sentences (left-branching span). Forward and backward digit span were assumed to measure working-memory capacity; MCL and predicate and subject embeddings are indices of the syntactic complexity of speech; left- and right-branching span assess imitative ability.

The results of these tests are given in Table 4.5. A series of one-way ANOVAs with age as a between-subjects factor were used to analyze the results. As Table 4.5 also indicates, significant age-group differences were obtained for the measures of forward digit span, MCL, subject embeddings, and left-branching span.

Two correlation matrices were also obtained so as to investigate the interrelationships among these measures of working-memory capacity, the complexity of spontaneous speech, and imitation ability. The matrix of correlations presented in

Table 4.6. *Matrix of correlations*

	Age	Education	Vocabulary	Forward	Backward	MCL	Right branch	Left branch	Right span	Left span
Age	—									
Education	−.20	—								
Vocabulary	+.08	+.58**	—							
Forward span	−.53**	+.10	+.07	—						
Backward span	−.52**	−.06	−.09	+.47**	—					
Mean clause length (MCL)	−.75**	+.22	+.10	+.61**	+.35**	—				
Right branch	−.00	+.08	+.00	+.08	+.01	+.70**	—			
Left branch	−.59**	−.03	−.06	+.63**	+.57**	+.62**	+.60**	—		
Right span	−.36**	+.29*	+.03	+.26	+.25	+.30*	+.24	+.19	—	
Left span	−.44**	+.12	+.09	+.34*	+.34*	+.36**	+.17	+.38**	+.47**	—

*$p < .05$, two-tailed.
**$p < .01$, two-tailed.

Table 4.6 indicates that age was significantly correlated with both digit span measures and with MCL, right branches, and right- and left-branching span. Although education was correlated with performance on the WAIS vocabulary test, neither education nor WAIS vocabulary was significantly correlated with any of the other measures. Three of the four span measures (forward and backward digit span, left-branching span) were significantly intercorrelated. Finally, MCL and left branches in spontaneous speech correlated significantly with these three span measures.

When the linear effects of age were removed, the resulting matrix of partial correlations, Table 4.7, conveys the same pattern. Education was correlated with performance on the WAIS vocabulary test, but these two measures did not correlate with the others. Forward and backward digit span were significantly correlated with left-branching span, and these three span measures were correlated with MCL and left branches.

These results clearly indicate that age group as well as individual differences in working-memory capacity, as indexed by forward and backward digit span, are linked with adults' ability to produce complex syntactic constructions involving multiclause sentences, especially those with left-branching structures, and their ability to imitate left-branching structures. Of interest is the finding that right-branching span and predicate embeddings were not correlated with the other measures of working-memory capacity or the complexity of spontaneous speech. It appears that simpler right-branching constructions do not impose sufficient processing demands on working memory to index adults' capacity limitations.

These results suggest that verbal ability, as indexed by vocabulary scores, is not significantly correlated with measures of syntactic processing ability as indexed by MCL, left branches, or left-branching span. It may be that semantic knowledge of lexical items and syntactic processing ability are distinct. Indeed, individual differences in patterns of first language acquisition (Nelson, 1985; Peters, 1983) and

Table 4.7. *Matrix of partial correlations after removing the linear effects of age*

	Educa- tion	Vocabu- lary	For- ward	Back- ward	MCL	Right branch	Left branch	Right span	Left span
Education	—								
Vocabulary	+.61**	—							
Forward span	−.00	+.13	—						
Backward span	−.11	−.07	+.43**	—					
Mean clause length (MCL)	+.11	+.24	+.38**	+.29*	—				
Right branch	+.09	+.00	+.10	+.01	+.25	—			
Left branch	+.01	−.08	+.41**	−.63**	+.37**	+.61**	—		
Right span	+.24	+.06	+.09	−.04	−.06	+.34*	+.20	—	
Left span	+.03	+.14	+.34*	+.47**	+.35**	+.30*	+.38**	+.38**	—

$*p < .05$, two-tailed.
$**p < .01$, two-tailed.

second language acquisition (Carroll, 1979; Wong Fillmore, 1979) provide partial support for this conclusion.

Written production

The differences between the syntax of middle-aged and elderly adults reported by Kynette and Kemper (1986) are reminiscent of reported differences between informal, spoken, and formal written language (Beaman, 1984; Hildyard & Olson, 1978, 1982). Chafe (1982) has argued that written texts are characterized by the frequent use of nominalizations, gerunds, participles, complement clauses, relative clauses, and passive sentences. Consequently, the syntax of written texts is assumed to be more complex than the syntax of oral texts. However, this difference in the complexity of oral and written language may be disappearing. Ong (1967, 1980) has argued that oral language is becoming increasingly "literal" as it takes on the characteristics and complexities of written language. Thus, it may be that a generational difference results, such that the speech of younger adults is more "literal," hence syntactically more complex, than the speech of older adults, whereas the written language of young and old adults is equally complex. If so, age-related differences in syntactic complexity might not be obtained if written language were analyzed.

In order to examine changes in adults' written language, I analyzed a collection of diaries, kept by the same individuals over many decades (Kemper, 1987). Previous studies of adults' diaries and letters have been limited to measures of word and sentence length and word frequency (Dennis, 1960; Smith, 1955, 1957). In this study, 12 different measures of syntactic complexity were computed. Both a longitudinal sample spanning seven decades and a cohort-sequential sample across four decades were examined, although only the longitudinal sample is discussed in this chapter. Similar results were obtained from the two samples (see Kemper, 1987, for details).

Eight sets of diaries, kept by the same individuals for seven or more decades,

Table 4.8. *Examples of complex syntactic constructions (target constructions are underscored)*

Relative clauses

Subject position: The mare that I bought over to Wilson's Corners foaled last night.

Predicate position: We planted the pasture that Pa rented from old man Silas.

That-clauses

Subject position: That the stallion would never be a good sire never occurred to me.

Predicate position: We didn't realize that we had a hard life.

Wh-clauses

Subject position: Whoever put in the most wheat fixed harvest meals.

Predicate position: I remember when we first heard about the new mechanical planters.

Infinitives

Subject position: To go to the Chicago Exposition was a grand undertaking.

Predicate position: For five cents, my father rented me out with a team of horses to pull gravel out of the riverbed.

Subordinates

Sentence-initial: Since we had to pay the taxes with cash money, Dickie and I always planted some tobacco.

Sentence-final: The Irishmen are building a new railroad, so we will soon ship our pigs to Chicago.

Gerunds

Subject position: Losing your children makes you old.

Predicate position: We had counted on getting a better crop.

Double embeddings

Subject position: The interurban that ran to Springfield which I took to see the President's funeral train now goes all the way to Chicago.

Predicate position: He always said he married Essie because she could get a hen from barnyard to supper table in an hour.

Triple embeddings

Subject position: What the rains left and the 'hoppers missed and the dust didn't blow away weren't enough.

Predicate position: He always claimed he lost the farm because he decided to feed the corn to the hogs for the slaughter house.

Coordinates

Subjects: Henry and I would race across the meadows.

Predicates: We lost two babies to the typhoid and lost two to the cough.

Fragments

Noun phrases: Those needless deaths.

Verb phrases: Plowed all day.

Source: Kemper (1987), by permission of the *Journal of Gerontology*, published by the Gerontological Society of America.

were analyzed. The diaries were written by six men and two women, all of whom were native speakers of English. These men and women were born between 1856 and 1876; they died between 1943 and 1967.

Many diary entries could not be analyzed: water spots, insect damage, and faded inks rendered some entries unusable; many consisted of short, abbreviated remarks about the weather, crops, or other topics; illegible handwriting further limited the analyzable entries. To control partially for variation in topic and style, only the two longest entries from the half-decade (e.g., 20–24 years, 25–29 years, etc.) were analyzed from each set. No entries were selected from the last 18 months of the diarists' lives so as to avoid any effects of "terminal drop" (Botwinick, West, & Storandt, 1978) in performance foreshadowing death. The entries ranged in length from 150 to 1,300 words, mean = 328 words. The average length of the entries did not vary with the age of the diarists. Most entries were meditations that reviewed personally significant events such as family deaths, crop failures, the loss of valuable farm animals, extensive journeys, or major undertakings.

Ten different syntactic constructions were identified in each entry. The analyzed constructions were (1) relative clauses, (2) that-clauses, (3) wh-clauses, (4) infinitive complements, (5) subordinate phrases, (6) gerunds, (7) double embeddings such as a relative clause modifying the direct object of an infinitive complement, and (8) triple embeddings such as an infinitive occurring in a relative clause that in turn modified the direct object of an infinitive complement, (9) coordinate subjects or predicates, and (10) sentence fragments. In addition, mean sentence length in words and in clauses was also computed for each entry. The examples in Table 4.8 are taken from Kemper (1987).

For 10 of the 12 measures, there was a significant effect of age; as they became older, the adults used fewer relative clauses, that-clauses, wh-clauses, infinitives, subordinates, gerunds, double and triple embeddings, and coordinates, resulting in fewer clauses per sentence. Although sentence word length did not decline and sentence fragments did not increase, sentence complexity deteriorated with age.

The analysis also examined the position of the embedded or subordinate clause with respect to the main clause. Relative clauses, that-clauses, wh-clauses, infinitives, gerunds, and double and triple embeddings occurred as part of the sentential subject or as part of the sentential predicate. Subordinates preceded the sentential subject or followed the predicate. Fragments were either noun phrases or verb phrases. As Figures 4.1, 4.2, and 4.3 show, there was a decline in the use of these complex syntactic constructions with age. Further, the position of the embedded clause or subordinate phrase did interact with the age decline. Predicate or right-branching relative clauses, that-clauses, wh-clauses, and infinitives, as well as sentence-final subordinates and coordinate predicates, were more common than subject or left-branching embedded clauses or sentence-initial constructions.

The results of the longitudinal sample are consistent with the hypothesis that adults' ability to produce complex syntactic structures declines with age. Age-related declines in the adults' use of relative clauses, that-clauses, wh-clauses, infinitives, subordinates, double and triple embeddings, and coordinates were observed.

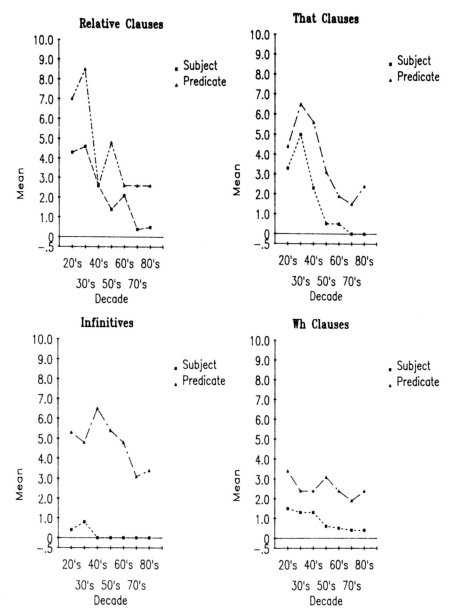

Figure 4.1. Frequency of relative clauses, that-clauses, infinitives, and wh-clauses, in subjects (S) or predicates (P). (Adapted from Kemper, 1987.)

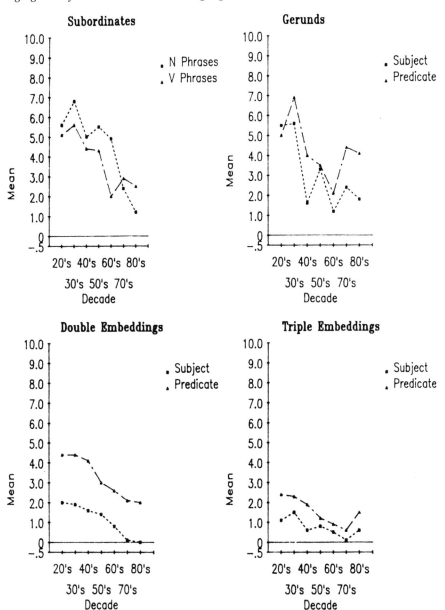

Figure 4.2. Frequency of subordinates, gerunds, double embeddings, and triple embeddings in subjects (S) or predicates (P). (Adapted from Kemper, 1987.)

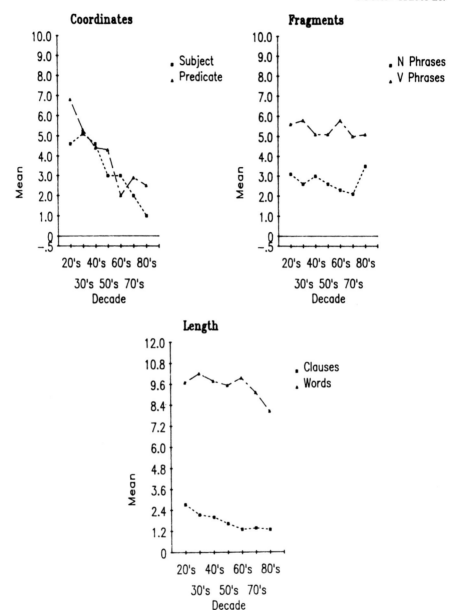

Figure 4.3. Frequency of subject (S) or predicate (P) coordinates, noun phrase (NP) or verb phrase (VP) fragments, and mean clause length and mean sentence length. (Adapted from Kemper, 1987.)

Left-branching constructions showed a somewhat greater decline with age than did right-branching constructions. These results are consistent with the hypothesis that production limitations are due to reductions of working-memory capacity.

Conclusions

The overall pattern of results in these studies of elderly adults' production and imitation of complex syntactic constructions is that there is an asymmetry in their production and imitation of right- and left-branching structures. There is an overall decline in adults' production and imitation of complex, multiply-embedded sentences with age, and this age-related decline appears to be more precipitous for left-branching constructions than for right-branching ones. I have taken this asymmetry as evidence for the hypothesis that limitations of working memory affect elderly adults' production and imitation of left-branching structures because these structures impose high processing demands. Working-memory limitations do not affect elderly adults' production and imitation of right-branching structures because these structures impose lower processing demands.

An alternative explanation could be that language structure undergoes a process of differentiation in adulthood, resulting in the separation of linguistic rules governing subject (left-branching) and object (right-branching) embeddings. Phrase structure grammars generally assume that categories such as noun phrase (NP) subjects and objects are most economically and productively represented by a single set of phrase structure rules. Thus, for example, relative clauses can be produced as modifiers of both subject and object noun phrases by one rule applying to the general category of NPs (Pinker, 1984). Similar considerations would postulate general categories for gerunds, that-clauses, wh-clauses, and other constructions which can optionally occur as subjects or objects producing either left- or right-branching constructions. Under this view, "performance" mechanisms such as working-memory limitations restrict the production or comprehension of left- versus right-branching structures (cf. Berwick & Weinberg, 1984; Church, 1982; Frazier & Fodor, 1978; Kimball, 1973).

Alternatively, some have assumed that children initially learn distinct rules for producing subjects and objects and that their grammar is later reorganized around economical phrase structure categories like NP (Bowerman, 1973, 1982; Brown, 1973; but see Pinker, 1984). This argument could be extended to account for the observed asymmetry in elderly adults' production of left- and right-branching constructions by proposing that a second reorganizational process occurs in late adulthood. Whereas the first reorganization results in a parsimonious grammar with general categories, this second reorganization results in a grammar with distinct subject and object categories and separate embedding rules for subjects and objects. The subject embedding rules restrict or prohibit left-branching embeddings, whereas the object embedding rules still permit right-branching embeddings. Thus, in this view, processing considerations are directly incorporated in the grammar rather than being accounted for by separate "performance" mechanisms such as working-memory limitations.

Two arguments weigh against this account: First, elderly adults do produce and imitate some left-branching constructions. It appears that the length of the left-branching construction is an important consideration. Short constructions were produced by the elderly adults in my studies of oral and written production. Additionally, the tests of adults' imitative span revealed an average left-branching span of 5.6 words for adults in their 80s (compared to an average right-branching span of 7.6 words).

Second, as Pinker (1984) points out, even young adults show a preference for right-branching structures rather than left-branching structures for both production and comprehension (Bever, 1970; Cooper & Paccia-Cooper, 1980; Slobin, 1973). Further, subjects typically refer to "old," "given," or "topic" information, whereas objects refer to "new" or "comment" information (Clark & Haviland, 1977; MacWhinney, 1982). Consequently, subjects typically are shorter and grammatically less complex than predicates because subjects are more often lexicalized and pronominalized whereas objects are more likely to be expanded and elaborated (Bates & MacWhinney, 1979, 1982).

Thus, it appears that the asymmetries observed in elderly adults' production and imitation of left- and right-branching constructions are extensions of those observed in young adults. The asymmetries are most naturally explained by "performance" mechanisms such as working-memory limitations rather than by positing distinct grammatical rules for subjects and objects. Such working-memory limitations also may affect elderly adults' comprehension and recall of complex syntactic constructions and so affect their performance in other psycholinguistic tasks.

References

Albert, M. L. (1981). Changes in language with aging. *Seminars in Neurology, 1*, 43–46.

Baddeley, A. D., & Hitch, G. (1974). Working memory. In G. H. Bower (Ed.), *The psychology of learning and motivation* (Vol. 8, pp. 67–89). New York: Academic Press.

Bates, E., & MacWhinney, B. (1979). A functionalist approach to the acquisition of grammar. In E. Ochs & B. B. Schieffelin (Eds.), *Developmental pragmatics* (pp. 175–214). New York: Academic Press.

Bates, E., & MacWhinney, B. (1982). Functionalist approaches to grammar. In E. Wanner & L. R. Gleitman (Eds.), *Language acquisition: The state of the art* (pp. 173–218). Cambridge: Cambridge University Press.

Beaman, K. (1984). Coordination and subordination revisited: Syntactic complexity in spoken and written narrative discourse. In D. Tannen (Ed.), *Coherence in spoken and written discourse* (pp 45–80). Norwood, NJ: Ablex.

Berwick, R. C., & Weinberg, A. S. (1984). *The grammatical basis of linguistic performance: Language use and acquisition.* Cambridge, MA: MIT Press.

Bever, T. G. (1970). The cognitive basis for linguistic structures. In J. R. Hayes (Ed.), *Cognition and the development of language* (pp. 279–352). New York: Wiley.

Blumenthal, A. L. (1966). Observations with self-embedded sentences. *Psychonomic Science, 6*, 453–454.

Bock, K. (1982). Toward a cognitive psychology of syntax: Information processing contributions to sentence formulation. *Psychological Review, 89*, 1–47.

Borod, J. C., Goodglass, H., & Kaplan, E. (1980). Normative data on the Boston Diagnostic Aphasia Examination, Parietal Lobe Battery, and the Boston Naming Test. *Journal of Clinical Neuropsychology, 2*, 209–215.

Botwinick, J., West, R., & Storandt, M. (1978). Predicting death from behavior test performance. *Journal of Gerontology, 33,* 755–762.

Bowerman, M. (1973). *Early syntactic development: A cross-linguistic study with special reference to Finnish.* Cambridge: Cambridge University Press.

Bowerman, M. (1982). Reorganizational processes in lexical and syntactic development. In E. Wanner & L. R. Gleitman (Eds.), *Language acquisition: The state of the art* (pp. 319–346). Cambridge: Cambridge University Press.

Brown, R. (1973). *A first language: The early stages.* Cambridge, MA: Harvard University Press.

Carroll, J. B. (1979). Psychometric approaches to the study of language ability. In C. J. Fillmore, D. Kempler, & W. S-Y. Wang (Eds.), *Individual differences in language ability and language behavior* (pp. 13–32). New York: Academic Press.

Chafe, W. L. (1982). Integration and involvement in speaking, writing, and oral literature. In D. Tannen (Ed.), *Spoken and written language: Exploring orality and literacy* (pp. 35–54). Norwood, NJ: Ablex.

Church, K. W. (1982). *On memory limitations in natural language processing.* Bloomington, IN: Indiana University Linguistics Club.

Clark, H. H., & Clark, E. V. (1977). *Psychology and language.* New York: Harcourt Brace Jovanovich.

Clark, H. H., & Haviland, S. E. (1977). Comprehension and the given-new contract. In R. O. Freedle (Ed.), *Discourse production and comprehension* (pp. 1–40). Norwood, NJ: Ablex.

Cooper, W. E., & Paccia-Cooper, J. (1980). *Syntax and speech.* Cambridge, MA: Harvard University Press.

Craik, F. I. M., & Simon, E. (1980). Age differences in memory: The roles of attention and depth of processing. In L. W. Poon, J. L. Fozard, L. S. Cermak, D. Arenberg, & L. W. Thompson (Eds.), *New directions in memory and aging: Proceedings of the George A. Talland Memorial Conference* (pp. 95–112). Hillsdale, NJ: Erlbaum.

Daneman, M., & Carpenter, P. A. (1980). Individual differences in working memory and reading. *Journal of Verbal Learning and Verbal Behavior, 19,* 450–466.

Dempster, F. N. (1980). Memory span: Sources of individual and developmental differences. *Psychological Bulletin, 19,* 450–466.

Dennis, W. (1960). The long-term constancy of behavior: Sentence length. *Journal of Gerontology, 15,* 195–196.

Duffy, J. R., Keith, R. L., Shane, H., & Podraza, B. L. (1976). Performance of normal (non-brain-injured) adults on the Porch Index of Communicative Ability. In R. H. Brookshire (Ed.), *Clinical Aphasiology Conference Proceedings* (pp. 32–42). Minneapolis: BRK Press.

Emery, O. (1985). Language and aging. *Experimental Aging Research, 11,* 3–60.

Emery, O. (1986). Linguistic decrement in normal aging. *Language & Communication, 6,* 47–64.

Frazier, L., & Fodor, J. D. (1978). The sausage machine: A new two-stage parsing model. *Cognition, 6,* 291–325.

Gleason, J. B., Goodglass, H., Obler, L., Green, E., Hyde, M. R., & Weintraub, S. (1980). Narrative strategies of aphasic and normal-speaking subjects. *Journal of Speech and Hearing Research, 23,* 370–382.

Hildyard, A., & Olson, D. R. (1978). Memory and inference in the comprehension of oral and written discourse. *Discourse Processes, 1,* 91–117.

Hildyard, A., & Olson, D. R. (1982). On the comprehension and memory of oral vs. written language. In D. Tannen (Ed.), *Spoken and written language: Exploring orality and literacy* (pp. 19–34). Norwood, NJ: Ablex.

Hunt, E. (1978). The mechanics of verbal ability. *Psychological Review, 85,* 109–130.

Hunt, E. (1985). Verbal ability. In R. J. Sternberg (Ed.), *Human abilities: An information-processing approach* (pp. 31–58). San Francisco: Freeman.

Hunt, K. (1970). Syntactic maturity in school children and adults. *Monographs of the Society for Research in Child Development, 35,* Serial No. 134.

Kemper, S. (1986). Imitation of complex syntactic constructions by elderly adults. *Applied Psycholinguistics, 7,* 277–287.

Kemper, S. (1987). Life-span changes in syntactic complexity. *Journal of Gerontology, 42,* 323–328.

Kimball, J. (1973). Seven principles of surface structure parsing in natural language. *Cognition, 2,* 15–47.

Kynette, D., & Kemper, S. (1986). Aging and the loss of grammatical forms: A cross-sectional study of language performance. *Language & Communication, 6,* 65–72.

Light, L. L., & Anderson, P. A. (1985). Working-memory capacity, age, and memory for discourse. *Journal of Gerontology, 40,* 737–747.

MacWhinney, B. (1982). Basic processes in syntactic acquisition. In S. A. Kuczaj (Ed.), *Language development* (Vol. 1, pp. 73–136). Hillsdale, NJ: Erlbaum.

McNeill, D. (1966). Developmental psycholinguistics. In F. Smith & G. A. Miller (Eds.), *The genesis of language: A psycholinguistic approach* (pp. 15–84). Cambridge, MA: MIT Press.

Menyuk, P. (1977). *Language and maturation.* Cambridge, MA: MIT Press.

Nelson, K. (1985). *Making sense: The acquisition of shared meaning.* New York: Academic Press.

Obler, L. K. (1980). Narrative discourse style in the elderly. In L. K. Obler & M. L. Albert (Eds.), *Language and communication in the elderly* (pp. 75–90). Lexington, MA: Heath.

Obler, L. K. (1985). Language through the life-span. In J. Berko Gleason (Ed.), *The development of language* (pp. 277–306). Columbus, OH: Merrill.

Obler, L. K., & Albert, M. L. (1985). Language skills across adulthood. In J. Birren & K. W. Schaie (Eds.), *Handbook of the psychology of aging* (2nd ed., pp. 463–473). New York: Van Nostrand Reinhold.

Ong, W. (1967). *The presence of the word.* New Haven, CT: Yale University Press.

Ong, W. (1980). Literacy and orality in our times. *Journal of Communication, 30,* 197–204.

Owens, R. R. (1984). *Language development.* Columbus, OH: Merrill.

Peters, A. M. (1983). *The units of language acquisition.* Cambridge: Cambridge University Press.

Pinker, S. (1984). *Language learnability and language development.* Cambridge, MA: Harvard University Press.

Salthouse, T. A. (1982). *Adult cognition: An experimental psychology of human aging.* New York: Springer-Verlag.

Schuell, H. M. (1965). *Minnesota Test for Differential Diagnosis of Aphasia.* Minneapolis, MN: University of Minnesota Press.

Slobin, D. I. (1973). Cognitive prerequisites for the development of grammar. In C. Ferguson & D. I. Slobin (Eds.), *Studies in child language development* (pp. 175–276). New York: Holt, Rinehart and Winston.

Slobin, D. I. (1981). *Psycholinguistics.* Glenview, IL: Scott Foresman.

Smith, A. D. (1980). Age differences in encoding, storage, and retrieval. In L. W. Poon, J. L. Fozard, L. S. Cermak, D. Arenberg, & L. W. Thompson (Eds.), *New directions in memory and aging: Proceedings of the George A. Talland Memorial Conference* (pp. 23–45). Hillsdale, NJ: Erlbaum.

Smith, M. E. (1955). Linguistic constancy in individuals when long periods of time are covered and different types of material are sampled. *Journal of General Psychology, 53,* 109–143.

Smith, M. E. (1957). Relation between word variety and mean letter length of words with chronological and mental ages. *Journal of General Psychology, 56,* 27–43.

Spilich, G. J. (1985). Discourse comprehension across the span of life. In N. Charness (Ed.), *Aging and human performance* (pp. 143–190). New York: Wiley.

Stine, E. L., Wingfield, A., & Poon, L. W. (in press). Speech comprehension and memory through adulthood: The roles of time and strategy. In L. W. Poon, D. C. Rubin, & B. A. Wilson (Eds.), *Everyday cognition in adulthood and late life.* Cambridge: Cambridge University Press.

Walker, V. G., Hardiman, C. J., Hedrick, D. L., & Holbrook, A. (1981). Speech and language characteristics of an aging population. In J. J. Lass (Ed.), *Advances in basic research and practice* (Vol. 6, pp. 143–202). New York: Academic Press.

Wechsler, D. (1945). *The measurement and appraisal of adult intelligence.* Baltimore: Williams & Wilkins.

Wong Fillmore, L. (1979). Individual differences in second language acquisition. In C. J. Fillmore, D. Kempler, & W. S-Y. Wang (Eds.), *Individual differences in language ability and language behavior* (pp. 203–228). New York: Academic Press.

5 Aging and memory activation: The priming of semantic and episodic memories

Darlene V. Howard

According to their own reports and to clinical and laboratory tests, as people grow older they often experience difficulties in understanding and remembering spoken and written language. Some of these communication problems are due to sensory deficits, but some complaints that are attributed to sensory loss are likely due to cognitive deficits. Even when people of different ages are equated on peripheral sensory loss (via an audiometric examination), elderly people are still poorer than the young at identifying spoken speech (Hayes, 1981). Furthermore, self-assessments of hearing impairment are not predicted well by the degree of peripheral hearing loss. For example, Weinstein and Ventry (1983) found that an audiometric evaluation accounted for less than 50% of the variance in self-assessed hearing handicap. This discrepancy may be due in part to the fact that the self-assessment of hearing handicap is sensitive to cognitive difficulties, whereas the audiometric evaluation is not. One of the goals of this chapter is to suggest specific cognitive deficits that might underlie these age-related communication difficulties.

Despite the increase in communication and memory problems, normal aging does not bring with it a complete deterioration of memory and language. The losses, although annoying and sometimes frightening, are only rarely debilitating. Therefore, clinicians and researchers need to determine not only what is lost, but also what is saved. Differentiating age-sensitive from age-constant components of cognition provides a more accurate theoretical account of cognitive aging. Furthermore, knowing what is saved may make it possible to help elderly people learn to tap such components so that they can compensate for what is lost. And knowing what is saved in normal aging provides a baseline for distinguishing it from pathological aging, such as senile dementia.

This research was supported by Grants R23 AG00713 and RO1 AG02751 awarded by the National Institute on Aging. I have been fortunate to have been assisted by a number of fine undergraduate students over the years. The contributions of some of these people are reflected by the fact of their joint authorship on several of the studies cited in this chapter. In addition, I am happy to acknowledge the excellent work of Maria Acosta, Jeff Amerman, Stephen Burns, Margie DelGreco, Martha Farmelo, Wendy Eicholzer, Holly Gomes, Peter Gordon, Marijean Hosking, Carolyn Marfizo, Michelle Millis, Mitch Sommers, Cathy Stanger, Tom Steif, Lisa Swartz, Anne Watson, Ed Wisniewski, and Bob Zozus. I am also grateful to Jim Howard for his advice on all of my research and for his comments on a draft of this manuscript.

This chapter reviews and integrates research we have been conducting on the activation of long-term memory. Some of the studies discussed have already been published, whereas others have yet to be reported in detail. The purposes of this review are (1) to identify possible sources of the communication and memory difficulties suffered by the elderly, (2) to specify components of cognition that do not decline in normal aging, and (3) to consider the implications of our findings for certain theoretical distinctions, including automatic versus effortful processes, episodic versus semantic memory, and implicit versus explicit memory.

Theoretical perspective

The research described here was suggested by *network theories of long-term memory* (e.g., Anderson, 1983, 1984; Collins & Loftus, 1975). Such theories assume that our knowledge of concepts (i.e., our semantic memory according to Tulving, 1972) consists of a semantically organized network of concept *nodes* interconnected by labeled, directed *associations* (i.e., *relations* or *links*). On the basis of empirical evidence (e.g., Neely, 1977), it is assumed that when a word (or a picture or idea) is encountered, the corresponding memory node becomes activated temporarily (i.e., more accessible), and this activation spreads along the node's associations, thereby activating nearby semantically related nodes. This spreading activation is automatic in that it occurs rapidly, is independent of the person's intentions and expectations, and is unlimited in capacity (i.e., there is no limit to the number of nodes that can be activated simultaneously in this fashion). In addition to this *automatic spreading activation*, there is assumed to be a *controlled* or *effortful activation*, in which the person focuses attention on (and thereby activates) nodes corresponding to concepts that are likely in context. Because this latter form of activation calls upon the individual's limited capacity attention, it has a longer latency, and there is a limit on how many nodes can be activated in this fashion at once.

Network theories assume that the patterns of activation of long-term memory underlie memory retrieval, language comprehension and production, and thinking. For example, research indicates that as people listen to a speaker or read, they use the linguistic and nonlinguistic context to anticipate what is likely to occur next (cf. the review by Howard, 1983b, chap. 9). The context is used immediately such that the characteristics of a given word are used to help identify the word that follows. For example, Cole and Jakimik (1978) asked young adults to detect mispronunciations in sentences such as *He noticed that a green_____garpet covered the hallway*. The mispronunciation of the word *carpet* was detected more rapidly when the blank contained the word *shag* (which renders *carpet* highly predictable) than when it contained the word *rag*. According to network models, patterns of semantic activation underlie this use of context. In the example sentence above, processing the word *shag* results in automatic activation spreading from the node for *shag* to the closely related word for *carpet*, thus making it easier to identify. Under at least some conditions, effortful activation would also be used if the person has time to direct attention to nodes that are particularly likely in context.

Viewing memory and language comprehension from the perspective of network theories has led us to phrase questions about cognitive aging in terms of changes and/or constancies in long-term memory activation. In order to make inferences about patterns of activation, the research described here measures *priming,* that is, the extent to which processing a given word facilitates processing of a related word. According to network theory, if activation spreads from the *animal* node to the *dog* node, then making a decision about the word *animal* should speed decisions for *dog* relative to a control condition in which *dog* follows an unrelated word, for example, *building.* Thus, subtracting response time on related trials from response time on unrelated control trials yields a measure of the *prime effect.*

In the research that follows, then, we will be concerned with whether and how prime effects vary with adult age. In all of the studies, we compare the performance of young and elderly adults. The elderly people are community-dwelling volunteers who judge themselves to be in good health. In some of the studies the young people are college students, and in others they are young adults who have already graduated. The young group usually ranges in age from 20 to 35 years of age and the elderly from 65 to 80 years. The age groups are always similar in Wechsler Adult Intelligence Scale (WAIS) vocabulary score and in years of education.

So far our research has examined four general questions concerning aging and memory activation. Each of the following sections focuses on one of these, and then the final section summarizes our findings and their theoretical implications.

Patterns of semantic activation

It has been argued that the relatively poor memory of elderly adults is due to a deficit in semantic processing (e.g., Craik & Byrd, 1982; Eysenck, 1974). For example, Eysenck (1974) proposed the processing-deficit hypothesis which states, "young subjects are able to process to-be-remembered information to a greater depth than old subjects." Exactly what is meant by "semantic processing" is typically left unspecified, a state of affairs that has made such theoretical notions very difficult to test. Network theory suggests that one way to define a processing deficit more precisely would be to hypothesize that there is an age-related decline in the spread of activation in the semantic network. Thus, there might be a decline in the likelihood that seeing a dog or the word *dog* results in activation of the node for *animal.* We conducted a series of studies to test this hypothesis.

In the first of these (Howard, Lasaga, & McAndrews, 1980), we presented young and elderly people with a modification of the Stroop task introduced by Warren (1972). On each of a series of trials, people were given a memory set of three category members (e.g., *dog, cat, horse*) followed by a base item printed in colored ink. They were instructed to name the ink color in which the base item was printed as quickly as possible, ignoring the base item itself. Warren had shown that college students took longer to say the color when the base item was the category name of the words in the memory set (e.g., *animal*) than when it was an unrelated control name (e.g., *building*). This suggested that holding the category members in memory had resulted in activation spreading to their category name, making it more difficult to suppress when they attempted to name the ink color. In this case then, *semantic*

Table 5.1. *Prime effects (msec) and percentage prime effects in studies of semantic priming*

Reference	Task	Other details		Prime effect[a]		Percentage prime effect[b]	
				Young	Elderly	Young	Elderly
Howard et al. (1980)	Modified Stroop	Category	(a)	34	38	4	4
Howard et al. (1981)	Simultaneous lexical decision	Category	(b)	63	166	6	11
		Property	(c)	75	116	8	7
Howard (1983c)	Simultaneous lexical decision	High-dom.	(d)	155	87	11	6
		Low-dom.	(e)	125	105	9	7
Bowles & Poon (1985), Study 1	Prime-target lexical decision	Category	(f)	81	93	9	10
Cerella & Fozard (1984)	Naming	Free associates	(g)	28	27	5	5
Howard, Shaw, & Heisey (1986)	Prime-target lexical decision	150 msec	(h)	34	9*	6	1*
		450 msec	(i)	47	45	9	6
		1000 msec	(j)	34	47	7	7

[a]Prime effect = Control RT − Primed RT.
[b]Percentage prime effect = Prime effect ÷ Control RT.
*Nonsignificant ($p > .10$) prime effect.

interference is measured by subtracting response time on unrelated trials from response time on related trials. Row (a) of Table 5.1 shows the absolute magnitude of this interference effect for young and elderly subjects in the next-to-last pair of columns. The extreme-right pair of columns show the percentage interference effect, which is the interference effect expressed as a percentage of that group's control response time. The findings were unambiguous; young and elderly people showed nearly identical interference effects. Thus, when people hold three members of a category in memory, activation spreads to the category node for young and elderly people alike.

It seemed possible that this age similarity in activation of the category name node holds only when several members of a category are encountered, thus producing cumulative effects. In addition, we were concerned because the modified Stroop procedure had resulted in a great deal of between-subjects variability in the magnitude of the interference effect. Therefore, we conducted a second experiment (Howard, McAndrews, & Lasaga, 1981) in which we presented people with a simultaneous lexical decision task. Each trial consisted of a pair of letter-strings. The person was to say "yes" if both letter-strings were words and "no" otherwise. On control trials the words were unrelated to each other (e.g., *rain–bright*), whereas on related trials the words were either category-member associates (e.g., *rain–snow*) or descriptive-property associates (e.g., *rain–wet*) drawn from age-appropriate norms (Howard, 1980b). We included these two different kinds of relatedness in order to find out whether there were age differences in the kind of relation along which activation spreads. This seemed possible because some studies have revealed small but significant age differences in semantic structure (e.g., Botwinick, West, & Storandt, 1975; Howard, 1983a; Riegel & Riegel, 1964).

The prime effects (unrelated minus related response times) and percentage prime effects (prime effect divided by that group's unrelated response times) we obtained are shown in rows (b) and (c) of Table 5.1. It is clear that the elderly reveal at least as much priming as the young, and that this is true for both kinds of semantic relation. In fact, prime effects are in the direction of being greater for the elderly than the young, but the age difference is not significant (and is likely due to age differences in overall response time and strategy, as discussed in Howard, McAndrews, & Lasaga, 1981). Thus, when combined with the findings of the Stroop study, this experiment demonstrates that there are age similarities in semantic activation even when only one related word has been processed, when two different measures of activation are used (facilitation of lexical decisions and interference with color naming), and when either of two different kinds of relations is employed. Furthermore, the lexical decision task yielded prime effects that were reliable across individuals; of the 24 subjects in each age group, 20 of the young and 18 of the elderly showed the prime effect.

In both of the previous studies, the items on related trials were highly associated with each other. For example, in the lexical decision study the second item was either the first or the second most frequent associate of the first. In order to determine whether age constancy in activation would occur for less highly associated nodes, we conducted another simultaneous lexical decision experiment (Howard, 1983c) in which category name–category member pairs (drawn from the age-appropriate norms of Howard, 1980a) occurred on related trials. On half of these, the category member was a high-dominance instance of the category, for example, *bird–robin*, whereas on the other half the category name was a low-dominance member, for example, *bird–duck* (though of equal overall frequency in the English language). The results of this experiment are shown in rows (d) and (e) of Table 5.1. Once again there was age similarity in priming, and in this case for both high-dominance and low-dominance pairs.

Age similarity in semantic activation has also been demonstrated in other laboratories using other tasks. Bowles and Poon (1985, Study 1) used a prime-target version of the lexical decision task in which a prime, to which the person need make no overt response, is followed by a target for a lexical decision. In their experiment the related pairs consisted of words from the same category. The prime effects and percentage prime effects they obtained are shown in row (f) of Table 5.1. Again young and elderly alike revealed percentage prime effects on the order of 10%. Cerella and Fozard (1984) used a prime-target naming task in which the subject was asked to name a target item following either an unassociated or an associated prime (the latter drawn from the Palermo and Jenkins, 1964, norms). Their results are shown in row (g) of Table 5.1. As is typical of the naming task, Cerella and Fozard found smaller percentage priming effects than we or Bowles and Poon (1985) did. Once again, however, the magnitude of the effect was identical for young and elderly participants. Still other researchers have shown that there is age similarity in priming for naming (Cohen & Faulkner, 1983) and for lexical decisions (Burke & Yee, 1984; Burke & Harrold, this volume), even when the prime is a semantically related sentence context, instead of an individual word.

Several of the above studies have ruled out the possibility that we are simply testing elderly people who show no cognitive declines at all. These same people are significantly poorer than the young in intentional memory and categorical clustering of a separate free-recall list (Howard, McAndrews, & Lasaga, 1981). They are also significantly poorer than young people at incidental recognition and recall of the words presented in the lexical decision task (Howard, 1983c; Howard, Shaw, & Heisey, 1986). In addition, Burke and Yee (1984) have shown that the elderly participants are significantly poorer than the young at recognizing the sentences that yielded age equivalence in priming. Thus, even among people who are experiencing typical age-related deficits in memory for the occurrence of individual words and sentences, there is no evidence of a decline in semantic activation.

This constancy of semantic priming holds even among individuals who have been diagnosed as suffering from mild to moderate dementia of the Alzheimer's type. Nebes and his colleagues (Nebes, Martin, & Horn, 1984) found that when such patients are given a naming task, they reveal as much priming among semantic associates as do age-matched controls. Thus, this is one aspect of semantic processing that is saved not only in normal aging, but also in at least one form of pathological aging.

In summary, the above studies have isolated one component of long-term memory that remains constant. There is no change with age in either the likelihood that activation will spread to semantically related nodes or in the types of relations along which activation spreads. These findings place constraints on any theories that would attribute memory deficits in the elderly to a decline in semantic processing, and they challenge theoreticians to specify more clearly what such a processing deficit might entail. This topic is considered again in the next section.

Time course of semantic activation

There is a slowing with age in a wide range of cognitive processes (e.g., Birren, Woods, & Williams, 1980; Salthouse, 1982), and thus it seemed likely that the rate at which semantic activation occurs might decline in old age. The above studies would not have been sensitive to any such slowing because they did not place a severe limit on the time allowed for activation to occur. Several of the studies used simultaneous presentation of the prime and target so that participants themselves controlled the time between processing of the first and second items. In the others the experimenter did control the stimulus onset asynchrony (SOA) between onset of the prime and target, but with values that would have been long enough to allow considerable time for activation to spread to the target node.

If there is any slowing in the rate of semantic activation, it would be one potential source of age differences in language comprehension and speech understanding. Language is potentially ambiguous at many levels. Not only can a given string of words be parsed differently to yield different interpretations (e.g., Chomsky's *They are eating apples* or *Visiting relatives can be a nuisance*), but individual words can have more than one meaning (e.g., the color vs. the mood interpretation of *blue*). At an even more elementary level, handwriting and spoken speech sounds are potentially ambiguous. For example, the acoustic stream itself is not segmented into words; thus listeners must do this themselves (Cole & Jakimik, 1980). The same acoustic string that can be heard as "more rice" can also be heard as "more ice," and which interpretation will be adopted depends on the linguistic and nonlinguistic context in which the speech stream occurs. Network models suggest that spreading activation normally helps people to disambiguate language. If there is a slowing in semantic activation in the course of normal aging, this might make it difficult for older people to comprehend rapid speech. Indeed, it is clear that elderly individuals do have particular difficulty in perceiving speech when it is speeded (Wingfield, Poon, Lombardi, & Lowe, 1985), yet it is under exactly such conditions that speech is often experienced in everyday life.

In order to investigate the time course of semantic activation, we used a prime-target version of the lexical decision task, and we varied the SOA across subjects, using SOAs of 150, 450, and 1000 msec. In this way, we hoped to influence the time allowed for activation to spread to the target item. If there is a slowing with age in the rate of semantic activation, then older people should require a longer SOA than young in order to reveal priming. The prime effects obtained for each of the SOAs are shown in rows (h), (i), and (j) of Table 5.1. At the two longer SOAs, we once again found age similarity in semantic priming. At the 150-msec SOA, however, the young showed significant priming, but the elderly participants did not. Thus, as the slowing hypothesis would predict, there is an age difference in the minimum SOA at which priming is obtained. Evidence for this conclusion can also be seen when correlations between age and magnitude of the percentage prime effect are examined. This correlation is negative and significant at the 150-msec SOA ($r = -.34$, $p < .05$), negative but not significant at the 450-msec SOA ($r = -.16$, $p > .10$), and near zero at the 1000-msec SOA ($r = -.03$, $p > .10$).

This lack of priming at the low SOA among the elderly cannot be attributed to the target's having backward-masked the prime at this low SOA, because subsequent tests revealed that these same elderly individuals showed above-chance incidental recognition of the primes in the 150-msec condition. In general, the age differences in incidental recall and recognition of the primes were no greater at the 150-msec SOA than they were at the two longer SOAs. It appears that the elderly people perceived the prime at all SOAs but that at the shortest there was not sufficient time for activation to spread to the target node to influence the speed of its processing.

Several questions suggested by these findings indicate the need for further research. First, this experiment does not make it possible to determine the exact locus of slowing. Network models suggest that the age difference in the onset of priming could be due to an age-related slowing in one or both of two stages: (1) the rate at which an external stimulus activates the appropriate concept node, and/or (2) the rate at which activation spreads from node to node in the semantic network. Our research to date cannot distinguish between these two forms of slowing.

A second question raised by the present findings concerns the reason for the high between-subjects variability among the elderly people at the 150-msec SOA. Although the majority of elderly people in the 150-msec condition did not show a prime effect, some of them did. (This variability is in sharp contrast to the consistent prime effects that are seen for young subjects at all SOAs and for elderly subjects at the two longer SOAs.) We hypothesize that this variability reflects differences among individuals in mental speed, with some having suffered a slowing and thus failing to reveal priming, but others not. This hypothesis must rest only upon speculation, however, until studies are conducted in which SOA is varied across a wide range of values for each individual, making it possible to ascertain the minimal SOA at which priming occurs for each participant. Ideally, some independent measure of mental speed also should be obtained for each individual, such as the slope in a Sternberg (1966) memory search task or the latency of the P300 component of the evoked potential (Woodruff, 1982). Then it would be possible to determine whether there is a correlation between the minimal SOA at which a person exhibits priming and some other measure of mental speed.

Finally, it must be noted that it would be inherently difficult to detect any age differences in the time course of semantic activation using the SOA technique, because it is not possible to control precisely the time allowed for activation to spread. Activation can spread (and influence response time) not only until onset of the target, but until initiation of the subject's response (Fischler & Goodman, 1978). Because elderly people usually take longer to respond than young, at a given SOA there is a longer time for activation to spread for the elderly than for the young. Thus, the SOA technique underestimates the effect of any mental slowing.

Despite the difficulties of isolating any age-related change in the time course of semantic activation, the task seems worth the effort because of the effect any such change would have on the communication difficulties encountered by the elderly. We are proposing that a decrease in the speed of semantic activation would make it difficult for elderly people to use expectations and context to help them disambiguate the speech signal – a particularly debilitating problem for people who are likely to be experiencing peripheral sensory losses which would render expectations more useful than ever before.

The findings reported in two recent papers might at first appear to contradict the above argument. Cohen and Faulkner (1983) described two relevant experiments. In one (Experiment 2), people made speeded lexical decisions about individual words following either a visually presented sentence or a series of *X*'s. In the other (Experiment 3), comparisons were made between the accuracy of identification of a spoken word in isolation versus in the context of a previously spoken related sentence. In both experiments, Cohen found that the elderly actually showed a larger effect of context (i.e., a larger prime effect) than did the young participants. Burke and Yee (1984) had participants read sentences that were presented a word at a time on a screen and then make a lexical decision about a visually presented target. They found that word targets that were instruments implied by the sentence were identified more rapidly than unrelated targets, and that this pattern occurred just as much for elderly as for young adults.

The Burke and Yee (1984) and Cohen and Faulkner (1983) experiments demonstrate that elderly individuals can and do use contextual constraints efficiently under some conditions. Nonetheless, there was no time pressure in any of these experiments. In Cohen and Faulkner's Experiment 2, the sentence context was displayed for 5 seconds prior to the lexical decision target. In Experiment 3, the speed with which the sentences were presented was not specified, but it appears to have been slow because it is stated (p. 246) that "maximum clarity of diction" was attempted. In Burke and Yee's study, the sentences were presented visually at the relatively comfortable rate of 250 msec per word. We hypothesize that if speeded presentation of sentences were to be used (rates typical of those often experienced in daily life), then the elderly would find it relatively more difficult than the young to use context. Thus, at rapid rates of sentence presentation, elderly people would be expected to show less priming than younger individuals.

Our research on the time course of semantic activation also has implications for two other theoretical issues. The first is that it suggests one possible reformulation of processing-deficit theory. Elderly people may suffer from a deficit in the rate of semantic processing, which under speeded conditions results in a decreased spread of semantic activation in the network.

The second theoretical issue concerns the distinction between automatic and effortful forms of activation. Hasher and Zacks (1979) had proposed the hypothesis that effortful processes change with age, but automatic do not. The results of previous research (e.g., Neely, 1977) indicate that our short SOA value of 150 msec is tapping automatic processes, whereas our longer SOAs are tapping primarily effortful processes. Contrary to the predictions of Hasher and Zacks, however, we are finding age differences in priming only at the short SOA, and hence in automatic processes. (See Howard, Shaw, & Heisey, 1986, for a fuller discussion.) Other evidence inconsistent with the Hasher and Zacks hypothesis comes from recent studies (e.g., Burke & Harrold, this volume; Burke, White, & Diaz, 1987; Chiarello, Church, & Hoyer, 1985; Cohen & Faulkner, 1983) that have failed to find the predicted age differences in the effortful components of priming. Thus, research on priming suggests that this influential theory will require modification.

Activation of episodic memory: Implicit associative memory

So far we have discussed only the priming of highly practiced "old" memories for general concepts – that is, what Tulving (1972) called semantic memory. However, network theories assume that newly learned time- and place-specific episodic memories are also stored in the network when they are learned, resulting in new connections. Research with college student subjects (e.g., McKoon & Ratcliff, 1979; Ratcliff & McKoon, 1978, 1981) indicates that activation spreads along these new pathways as well. For example, if young people study a set of sentences, the nouns within a sentence come to prime each other even though they were unassociated previously.

Having found age constancy in the patterns of semantic priming, we wondered whether the priming of episodic memories would be saved as well. Older adults show poorer memory than young in most tests of episodic memory (see reviews by Burke & Light, 1981; Kausler, 1982), and "new" memories seem to decline more in old age than do "old" memories (e.g., Botwinick & Storandt, 1980); thus it seemed possible that the priming of newly learned episodic associations would decline in old age even though semantic priming does not.

We have been conducting a series of studies of aging and episodic priming, using an item recognition task developed by McKoon and Ratcliff (1979; Ratcliff & McKoon, 1978). In each experiment, people are presented with a list of 36 unrelated sentences for study. Each sentence (e.g., *The dragon sniffed the fudge* or *The ocean washed away the trash*) contains nouns that are unassociated with each other according to norms. Then participants see a series of item recognition trials, each containing an individual noun to which the person is to respond "yes" if it had occurred in the sentences studied and "no" otherwise. Response time and accuracy are recorded. On primed trials, the noun tested on the immediately preceding trial had been in the same sentence as the test noun (e.g., a test of *fudge* after a test of *dragon*). On control trials, the noun tested on the preceding trial had been in a different study sentence (e.g., a test of *fudge* after a test of *ocean*). The magnitude of the prime effect is determined by subtracting response time on correct primed trials from response time on correct control trials.[1]

It seemed likely that the degree of study of the sentences would influence the magnitude of priming; therefore, in our initial experiments (Howard, Heisey, & Shaw, 1986), some people had extended study of the sentences (up to a total of 40 seconds and three separate studies of each sentence), others had two presentations (a total of 25 seconds of study per sentence), and still others had only one presentation

(15 seconds of study per sentence). Our results are shown in rows (a), (b), and (c) of Table 5.2. We found that after either extended study (row a) or two presentations (row b), both young and elderly people showed significant priming, and there was no significant age difference in the magnitude of the prime effect. After only one study (row c), however, the young showed significant priming, but the elderly did not. In these experiments, we also included a cued-recall test after the item recognition series. On each trial, a verb was presented and the participant was asked to recall the sentence in which the verb had occurred. We found that elderly people showed significantly poorer recall than the young for all three degrees of study, even those that had yielded age equivalence in priming. These findings indicate, then, that priming among the nouns within a recently studied sentence provides a sensitive measure of what is stored in memory, revealing age constancy of episodic memory even under some conditions that yield significant age differences in cued recall of the same sentences.

Our results also suggest that priming is tapping a kind of memory that is qualitatively different from that tapped by the more frequently used tests of recall and recognition accuracy. This conclusion is based on several kinds of evidence. One comes from individual item analyses we conducted to determine whether the sentences that a given individual recalled well yielded more priming than those he or she recalled poorly. We found that for moderate (i.e., two presentations) and extended degrees of study, people of both ages showed just as much priming for sentences they recalled poorly as for those they recalled well. At the lowest level of study, however, sentences that were recalled well yielded significantly more priming than those that were recalled poorly. This suggests that some minimal degree of study is required to yield either priming or recall, but once that level has been reached, priming and recall tap different forms of memory.

Another kind of evidence for a qualitative difference comes from examing correlations across subjects within an age group to determine whether people who are relatively good at recall also show relatively large prime effects. We found that at all levels of study, cued-recall accuracy correlated significantly with item recognition accuracy (the latter being how accurate the person was at judging whether a word had occurred in the set of studied sentences). In contrast, the magnitude of an individual's prime effect did not correlate with either item recognition accuracy or cued recall at either the moderate or extended degrees of study. After the single study, there was a significant correlation between item recognition accuracy and priming. Thus, as in the case of the item analyses, we found independence of priming and the other memory measures after moderate degrees of study, but some relation at a lower degree of study.

We have replicated and extended the latter findings in another item recognition priming experiment in which people studied 36 more complex two-propositional sentences, for example: *The oatmeal turned to mold so the monk added sugar*. People received two presentations of each sentence for a total of 30 seconds of study. As in the earlier experiments, the item recognition series consisted of individual nouns from the studied sentences and distractors. In order to facilitate comparisons of priming and the other memory measures, we added a cued-recall test in which the

Table 5.2. *Overall prime effects (msec) and percentage prime effects in studies of episodic priming*

Reference	Sentence type	Test delay (days)	Number of presentations		Prime effect[a] Young	Prime effect[a] Elderly	Percentage prime effect[b] Young	Percentage prime effect[b] Elderly
Howard, Heisey, & Shaw (1986)	1 Proposition	0	Several	(a)	88	101	12	10
	1 Proposition	0	2	(b)	86	61	13	7
	1 Proposition	0	1	(c)	122	2*	15	0*
Howard (1985)	2 Proposition	0	2	(d)	96	74	11	6
Unpublished data	1 Proposition	0	3	(e)	63	96	8	9
	1 Proposition	3	3	(f)	153		18	
Unpublished data	1 Proposition	0	3	(g)	121	73	14	7
	1 Proposition	7	3	(h)	120		14	

[a] Prime effect = Control RT − Primed RT.

[b] Percentage prime effect = Prime effect ÷ Control RT.

*Nonsignificant ($p > .10$) prime effect.

cue on each trial was one of the nouns from each sentence, and the task was to produce the other three nouns from that sentence. We also gave paired recognition tests in which each trial consisted of two nouns from the studied sentences, and the subject was to respond "yes" if both nouns had been in the same sentence and "no" otherwise. Thus the priming, recall, and paired recognition tests all assess the extent to which the person has stored away the associations among the nouns in the sentences.

The overall prime effects we obtained in this study are shown in row (d) of Table 5.2. Once again both young and elderly showed significant prime effects, and there were no significant age differences in their magnitude. There were, however, significant age differences favoring the young in cued recall, with the young recalling an average of 1.54 nouns per sentence (of a maximum of 3) and the elderly recalling only .83. There were also significant age differences in paired recognition accuracy, with the young correct on 94% of the trials and the elderly on only 84%.

When correlations across subjects were examined, we found that people who were good at paired recognition were also good at recall, with a correlation between these two measures of .69 among the young and .85 among the elderly (in both cases, $n = 36$, $p < .0001$). This suggests that these measures are tapping a common component of memory. In contrast, when we correlated the magnitude of the prime effect with percentage correct paired recognition and with cued recall, we found correlations of near zero among the elderly, suggesting that priming is independent of the other memory measures for this group. Among the young there is some evidence of a correlation between priming and the other memory measures, however, with an r of .28 for paired recognition and the prime effect, and of .35 for cued recall and the prime effect ($n = 36$, $p < .05$ in both cases). Nonetheless, the most important point is that once again priming has revealed relative constancy across age when compared with more commonly used measures of associative memory; furthermore, under at least some conditions, whether or not a person is good at these more commonly used tests is unrelated to that person's relative degree of priming.

There is yet another kind of evidence for qualitative differences between priming on the one hand and recall and recognition accuracy on the other; they are influenced differently by certain variables. One example of this is the effect of degree of study on the magnitude of age differences in memory. If priming taps the same component of memory as recall and recognition accuracy, then age differences on all three measures should be influenced by degree of study in the same way. However, the results of our first studies of episodic priming (Howard, Heisey & Shaw, 1986) suggested that they are not. As rows (a), (b), and (c) of Table 5.2 show, when degree of study is increased, age differences in priming *decrease* (indeed disappear). In contrast, for these same subjects, age differences in both item recognition accuracy and cued recall *increase* as the amount of study is increased (with the age difference in mean recall, for example, being .23 after one presentation, .45 after two presentations, and .67 after extended study).

Other evidence that a given variable can have different effects on priming as opposed to the other memory tests comes from a study we have just completed in which people study one-propositional sentences (three presentations each, for a total of 30 seconds of study per sentence) and then are tested for priming between the sentence nouns both on the same day (as in the studies described above) and after a retention interval of 3 days. We predicted that the delay would influence the memory measures differently, and that is what we found. As the results in rows (e) and (f) of Table 5.2 show, these findings replicate those above in revealing equal priming for the young and elderly on the first day of testing. This result was obtained despite the fact that there were significant age differences favoring the young on a cued-recall test in which the cue was one of the nouns from each sentence, and the subject was to produce the other; the mean number of nouns recalled per sentence was .83 for the young and .57 for the elderly. Furthermore, although the elderly showed significant forgetting across the 3-day retention interval when recall was measured (recalling an average of only .36 nouns per sentence after the delay), they showed no significant decline in the magnitude of the prime effect. Thus among the elderly, the delay is influencing recall but not priming.

The data from the young subjects were less clear-cut. They too failed to show a decline in priming across the delay (indeed they were in the direction of showing *more* priming on the second day than on the first), but they did not show any significant forgetting by the recall measure either. To find out whether there would be a dissociation between priming and recall among the young people, we tested a group of young people in a 7-day delay condition. The pattern obtained was similar to the one described above for the elderly; the young showed significant forgetting over the delay by the recall measure, obtaining an average of .82 words correct on the immediate, but only .59 correct on the delayed test. Nonetheless, as rows (g) and (h) of Table 5.2 show, there was no decline in the magnitude of priming over days, confirming the conclusion that retention interval influences recall and priming in different ways, with the former showing more forgetting than the latter.

The comparisons we have just outlined between recall and recognition accuracy on the one hand, and episodic priming on the other, fit with a distinction between two different forms of memory that has been postulated by researchers from diverse fields of study. The dichotomy has been given various names including explicit versus implicit memory (e.g., Graf & Schacter, 1985), memories versus habits (e.g., Mishkin & Petri, 1984), memory with versus memory without awareness (Jacoby & Witherspoon, 1982), autobiographical memory versus perceptual learning (Jacoby & Dallas, 1981), knowing *that* versus knowing *how* (e.g., Cohen & Squire, 1980). What all of these dichotomies have in common is that in each the first form of memory requires an introspective report of remembering on the part of the rememberer. The usual tests of recognition and recall accuracy are of this *explicit* sort. In contrast, the second form of memory in each dichotomy is *implicit* because memory is inferred from some other aspect of performance and so does not require an introspective awareness of remembering on the part of the person. In these terms, then, in our studies of sentence memory above, the recall and recognition accuracy measures tapped explicit memory, because subjects were asked, on paired recognition tests, for example: *Do you remember having seen "dragon" and "fudge" in the same sentence?* In contrast, the prime effect tapped implicit memory, because we inferred from facilitation in response times that the person remembered that *dragon* and *fudge* had occurred in the same sentence. No conscious judgment of remembering the connection was required.

Researchers have been led to propose that there are qualitative differences between explicit and implicit memory, because there are notable dissociations between them. Whereas amnesics are very poor at explicit memory, they often are not different from normals on implicit memory tests (e.g., see the review by Schacter, 1985). We saw a similar dissociation in the episodic priming studies above, in that age differences were often nonexistent by the implicit priming measure, even though they were large according to the explicit measures. Furthermore, several researchers (e.g., Graf & Mandler, 1984; Jacoby & Dallas, 1981; Tulving, 1984) have reported that the two kinds of memory are sometimes influenced differently by the same variables. As described above, we also found such dissociations in our episodic priming studies when we varied both degree of study and delay. Finally, it has been reported (e.g., Eich, 1984; Jacoby & Witherspoon, 1982; Tulving, 1984) that the two kinds of memory can be independent, such that whether or not an individual reveals explicit memory for an item is independent of whether that individual shows implicit memory for the same item. The item analyses described above (reported more fully in Howard, Heisey, & Shaw, 1986) revealed this sort of dissociation in our episodic priming studies as well.

For present purposes, it is important to note, too, the distinction between implicit memory for individual well-known items (*implicit item memory*) versus implicit memory for new associations among items (*implicit associative memory*). For example, in the typical study of implicit item memory, people might first be given a list of individual words to study (including, for example, the word *bread*). Then implicit memory for the words would be tested by asking the person to complete a series of word fragments. If people are better at completing fragments that correspond to words they had just studied (e.g., *bre_*) than fragments corresponding to words they had not studied (e.g., *app_*), then they have demonstrated implicit item memory. In contrast, tests of implicit associative memory test for implicit memory of newly formed associations, as we have done in our studies of episodic priming. If our subjects had retained a memory only that the word *dragon* had occurred in the studied set, then there is no reason they would have responded more rapidly to *dragon* following another noun from the same sentence (e.g., *fudge*) than following another studied noun from a different sentence (e.g., *ocean*). Thus, priming among the nouns in a sentence taps implicit associative memory.

So far most previous studies of implicit memory have examined item memory rather than associative memory. However, Graf and Schacter (1985; Schacter, 1985) have conducted some studies comparing these two kinds of implicit memory (using a different measure of associative memory than we have reported here). They found that both implicit item memory and implicit associative memory are saved in amnesic patients, but that the two types of implicit memory are influenced differently by at least one variable (i.e., degree of elaborative processing).

Our episodic priming results above suggest the hypothesis that implicit associative memory declines less in the course of normal aging than does explicit associative memory. There is already some evidence that the same is true for item memory. Light, Singh, and Capps (1986) had people study a list of individual words, and then later tested explicit memory (via a yes/no recognition memory test) and implicit memory (via a word fragment completion test). They found that after a 7-day delay, there were age differences favoring the young on the explicit but not the implicit memory test. We have also collected some evidence for age constancy of implicit item memory using a procedure based on work by Jacoby and Witherspoon (1982) and Eich (1984). We asked people to listen to a study list consisting of pairs of related words. Embedded in the list were a number of pairs containing a homophone that was paired with a word biasing the infrequent spelling of the homophone, for example, *prison–cell*. We tested implicit memory by observing the extent to which people gave the biased spelling in a later spelling test in which they were asked simply to write down isolated words presented on a tape recording. We found that the elderly people (39% correct cued recall) were significantly poorer than the young (60% correct) at an explicit cued-recall test (e.g., *what word was paired with "prison"?*). However, they showed an equal spelling bias (spelling bias scores of 30% and 34% for the young and elderly, respectively), suggesting that the two age groups have equivalent implicit memory for the items (Howard, 1986; Howard, in press). This particular age constancy in implicit memory is interesting because it relies upon semantic processing at the time of presentation. This suggests again that, in contrast to the predictions of processing-deficit theory, elderly people were just as likely as young to use the stimulus word to affect their interpretation of the response member of each pair.

In summary, our studies of episodic priming suggest two general conclusions. First, priming offers a sensitive measure of what is stored in memory; we frequently found older people showing as much priming as young, even though there were significant (and often large) age differences in recall and recognition accuracy. This is in keeping with the argument (e.g., Burke & Light, 1981) that the memory difficulties of elderly people are due at least in part to retrieval, as opposed to storage problems. Our findings suggest that this is even true of the age deficits that often appear on recognition tests, which are thought to be less susceptible to retrieval problems than are recall measures. Of course, this leaves unanswered an important question: What underlies the lack of priming among the elderly people when they received only one presentation of the sentences? The findings discussed in the next section will prove relevant to this question, suggesting that the elderly are indeed showing priming even after a single study, but only under certain conditions.

A second general conclusion is that priming of new associations offers a measure of implicit associative memory that is, under some conditions at least, qualitatively different from the memory tapped by explicit tests. It is likely that the conclusions that we have come to accept regarding age changes in memory, being based almost exclusively on tests of explicit memory, will not hold true when implicit memory is tested. Until we investigate implicit memory and aging more fully, we will have an incomplete picture of the ways in which memory does and does not change over the life-span.

Table 5.3. *Within-proposition versus between-proposition prime effects (msec) and percentage prime effects in a study of episodic priming among the nouns in two-propositional sentences*

Age group	Prime effect[a]		Percentage prime effect[b]	
	Within-proposition	Between-proposition	Within-proposition	Between-proposition
Young	114	78	13	9
Elderly	61	86	5	7

[a]Prime effect = Control RT − Primed RT.
[b]Percentage prime effect = Prime effect ÷ Control RT.

Priming and the structure of sentence memory

Research in which the subjects are college students has indicated that patterns of priming are useful indices of the structure of information stored in memory (e.g., Guindon & Kintsch, 1984; McKoon & Ratcliff, 1980; Ratcliff & McKoon, 1978). The logic underlying this measure is that if two concepts or words prime each other, then their nodes must be related in memory, and the more they prime each other, the more closely related they must be. This method should be particularly useful for studying the structure of what people of different ages store in memory. Unlike the typically used explicit tests of memory for text, it is an implicit test and is less likely to be influenced by age differences in cautiousness or response criterion.

So far, we have examined two possible kinds of age differences and similarities in memory structure for sentences. The first concerns the extent to which people of different ages are sensitive to the propositional structure of sentences. Ratcliff and McKoon (1978) gave college students two-propositional sentences of the form $noun_1$–$verb_1$–$noun_2$–$conj$–$noun_3$–$verb_2$–$noun_4$. They found that after a 20-minute delay, there was more priming between nouns from the same proposition (within-proposition priming), than between nouns from different propositions in the same sentence (between-propositions priming). For example, if college students studied the sentence *Geese crossed the horizon as wind swept away the clouds, geese* primed *horizon* more than *wind* primed *horizon*. The fact that within-proposition priming was greater than between-propositions priming indicates that the young people had stored the underlying propositional structure of the sentences. In order to determine whether this is equally true for the elderly, we broke down the prime effects in our two-propositional study mentioned above into within- and between-proposition effects. The results are displayed in Table 5.3. Although the relevant interaction with age was not significant, these data are suggestive of an age difference in sensitivity to underlying propositional structure. The young people showed the pattern of greater within- than between-proposition priming reported by Ratcliff and McKoon, but the elderly did not.

Another possible age difference in memory structure concerns the directional symmetry of priming. In their work with college students, Ratcliff and McKoon

Table 5.4. *Forward versus backward prime effects (msec) and percentage prime effects in studies of episodic priming*

Reference	Test delay (days)	Number of presentations		Prime effect[a]				Percentage prime effect[b]			
				Young		Elderly		Young		Elderly	
				For.	Back.	For.	Back.	For.	Back.	For.	Back.
Howard et al. (1986)	0	Several	(a)	82	95	86	116	11	13	9	12
	0	2	(b)	114	59	60	62	16	9	7	7
	0	1	(c)	133	112	69	−64	16	14	7	−7
Unpublished data	0	3	(d)	65	60	85	107	8	8	8	11
	3	3	(e)	155	151	164	−19	18	18	14	−2
Howard (1985)	0	2	(f)	93	103	73	73	10	11	6	6

Note: For. = forward; Back. = backward.
[a]Prime effect = Control RT − Primed RT.
[b]Percentage prime effect = Prime effect ÷ Control RT.

(1978) found that priming of the words within a sentence is symmetrical in that backward priming (in which a later word in the sentence primes an earlier one) is just as great as forward priming (in which an earlier word primes a later one). For example, after study of the sentence *The dragon sniffed the fudge, fudge* primes *dragon* just as much as *dragon* primes *fudge*. Ratcliff and McKoon argued that this demonstrates that the sentences have been stored in an abstract form, rather than as a string of words. We have examined the relative magnitude of forward and backward priming in the studies of episodic priming described above, and the patterns we obtained are summarized in Table 5.4.

In general, statistical analyses revealed similar structure in the two age groups, since the relevant interactions with age were not significant in any of the individual studies. Nonetheless, when these data are compared across experiments, there is the suggestion of an age difference, but only under certain conditions. The pattern of equal forward and backward priming holds consistently for the young people across all of the conditions we have tested, in keeping with Ratcliff and McKoon's findings. This pattern also holds for the elderly, but with two notable exceptions. For both the single-presentation condition with same-day testing (row c) and the three-presentation condition with 3-day-delayed testing (row e), the elderly people revealed forward but not backward priming. In fact, for the 3-day-delay study, the relevant interaction with age was marginally significant ($p = .10$), and a separate matched t test on the 3-day-delay data for the elderly alone revealed a significant difference between the magnitude of forward and backward priming ($t[15] = 3.59$, $p < .01$). Thus these data suggest the hypothesis that under conditions in which the sentences are relatively well learned (e.g., several studies and immediate test) both young and old retain a similar abstract representation of the sentences. However, under difficult memory conditions (either a single study or an extended retention interval), the elderly retain a mental representation that is functionally closer to a surface string.

In summary, then, analyses of the data we have collected so far indicate that under many conditions the patterns of priming – and by inference the underlying memory structure of sentences – is similar for young and elderly individuals. However, comparisons across experiments suggest that age differences may be present either when only minimal study has occurred or when there is a delay between study and test. It is, of course, exactly the latter conditions that occur most often in daily life, so these possible age differences warrant further study.

Conclusions

Summary of findings

We have used priming as a way of examining the patterns of memory activation that occur when people encounter and make decisions about words. We have found that in the case of well-learned semantic associations, there is age constancy in the patterns and likelihood of activation, at least for the kinds and degrees of relation that have been investigated so far. This age constancy occurs even among elderly individuals who do show deficits in comparison to the young when memory for the same material is measured later via recall or recognition accuracy. There is, however, evidence for a decline with age in the speed of semantic activation, a conclusion based on age differences in the minimum stimulus onset asynchrony at which priming is observed. This decline would be likely to have important consequences for the elderly person's ability to use context to assist in communication, at least under conditions of rapid presentation of speech.

When we examined newly learned episodic associations presented in sentences, we again found surprising age constancy in the degree to which episodic priming occurs; at only moderate levels of study that yield consistent age differences on explicit memory measures such as recall and recognition, there are no age differences in the degree to which newly associated words prime each other. At lower levels of study, there are age differences in priming, although the exact nature and cause of these are yet to be determined. There is some tentative evidence that at such low levels of study there are age differences in the structure of what is stored.

Summary of theoretical implications

The results described here have implications for a number of theoretical attempts to describe what changes and what does not in the course of normal aging. First, the theory that effortful processes change with age whereas automatic processes do not (Hasher & Zacks, 1979) is called into question. We have found no age differences in the effortful components of semantic priming (in agreement with Burke & Harrold, this volume; Burke, White, & Diaz, 1987; and Chiarello, Church, & Hoyer, 1985), yet we have found age differences in the rate of what appears to be automatic semantic activation.

Second, the notion that semantic processes are age constant but episodic memory is not also receives little support from our findings. On the one hand, we have found evidence of a change in at least one aspect of semantic processing – the speed of semantic activation. On the other, we have found that after only moderate degrees of study there is age constancy in the degree of priming among newly learned episodic associations. This is not to say that the above distinctions are of no help in considering cognitive aging, but it is to stress that any statements about the age constancy of automatic or semantic processes, and the age differences observed in effortful or episodic processes, must be qualified in important ways.

Third, our data on episodic priming provide a new kind of evidence for the ubiquity of retrieval difficulties for newly learned materials among the elderly. The fact that we could find age constancy in priming among the nouns in a sentence when other measures such as cued recall and paired recognition revealed age differences indicates that a great deal more of new material is stored by elderly people, and indeed influencing their performance, than is usually appreciated.

Fourth, our findings place constraints on notions concerning any processing deficits of the elderly. It is quite possible that elderly people are indeed less likely than young to generate extensive elaborations among words, for example, when asked to commit them to memory. However, the notable age constancy we have observed for both semantic and episodic priming indicates that there is no decline in the likelihood that activation will spread from among either semantically or episodically related nodes in memory. The one sort of processing deficit that we do find is in the time course of semantic activation. Thus, we join those theorists (e.g., Salthouse & Kail, 1983; Waugh & Barr, 1982) who stress the importance of the slowing of cognitive processes in causing many of the cognitive deficits seen in old age.

Finally, our studies of episodic priming suggest that we must begin to examine more carefully the aging of implicit memory, both implicit memory for individual items and implicit memory for new associations (Howard, in press). The results of studies conducted so far suggest that the aging of implicit memory will look quite different from the aging of explicit memory, revealing that more of memory is saved with aging than we had been led to believe. This presents the empirical challenge of comparing implicit and explicit memory more fully, the theoretical challenge of determining how this distinction can be built into models of memory and aging, and the practical challenge of determining whether there is any way in which people can learn to tap these unconscious memories to help compensate for their failing explicit memory.

Note

1 This restriction to correct trials means that we are examining priming only for sentences in which the individual nouns were recognized correctly. This should not present problems for age comparisons, because item recognition error rates in the experiments to be described are low, ranging across experiments from 3% to 15%, and are similar for both age groups. The one exception occurs in the delay studies described later in this section: For the 3-day-delay test, the elderly group had an error rate of 20%, which is significantly greater than the 14% error rate of the young participants.

References

Anderson, J. R. (1983). A spreading activation theory of memory. *Journal of Verbal Learning and Verbal Behavior, 22,* 261–295.

Anderson, J. R. (1984). Spreading activation. In J. R. Anderson & S. M. Kosslyn (Eds.), *Tutorials in learning and memory*. San Francisco: Freeman.

Birren, J. E., Woods, A. M., & Williams, M. V. (1980). Behavioral slowing with age: Causes, organization, and consequences. In L. W. Poon (Ed.), *Aging in the 1980s* (pp. 293–308). Washington, DC: American Psychological Association.

Botwinick, J., & Storandt, M. (1980). Recall and recognition of old information in relation to age and sex. *Journal of Gerontology, 35,* 70–76.

Botwinick, J., West, R., & Storandt, M. (1975). Qualitative vocabulary test responses and age. *Journal of Gerontology, 30,* 574–577.

Bowles, N. L., & Poon, L. W. (1985). Aging and retrieval of words in semantic memory. *Journal of Gerontology, 40,* 71–77.

Burke, D. M., & Light, L. L. (1981). Memory and aging: The role of retrieval processes. *Psychological Bulletin, 90,* 513–546.

Burke, D. M., White, H., & Diaz, D. L. (1987). Semantic priming in young and older adults: Evidence for age-constancy in automatic and attentional processes. *Journal of Experimental Psychology: Human Perception and Performance, 13,* 79–88.

Burke, D. M., & Yee, P. L. (1984). Semantic priming during sentence processing by young and older adults. *Developmental Psychology, 20,* 903–910.

Cerella, J., & Fozard, J. L. (1984). Lexical access and age. *Developmental Psychology, 20,* 235–243.

Chiarello, C., Church, K. L., & Hoyer, W. J. (1985). Automatic and controlled semantic priming: Accuracy, response bias, and aging. *Journal of Gerontology, 40,* 593–600.

Cohen, G., & Faulkner, D. (1983). Word recognition: Age differences in contextual facilitation effects. *British Journal of Psychology, 74,* 239–251.

Cohen, N. J., & Squire, L. R. (1980). Preserved learning and retention of pattern-analyzing skill in amnesia: Dissociation of "knowing how" and "knowing that." *Science, 210,* 207–209.

Cole, R. A., & Jakimik, J. (1978). Understanding speech: How words are heard. In G. Underwood (Ed.), *Strategies of information processing* (pp. 67–116). London: Academic Press.

Cole, R. A., & Jakimik, J. (1980). A model of speech perception. In R. A. Cole (Ed.), *Perception and production of fluent speech* (pp. 133–163). Hillsdale, NJ: Erlbaum.

Collins, A. M., & Loftus, E. F. (1975). A spreading-activation theory of semantic processing. *Psychological Review, 82,* 407–428.

Craik, F. I. M., & Byrd, M. (1982). Aging and cognitive deficits: The role of attentional resources. In F. I. M. Craik & S. Trehub (Eds.), *Aging and cognitive processes* (pp. 191–211). New York: Plenum.

Eich, E. (1984). Memory for unattended events: Remembering with and without awareness. *Memory & Cognition, 12,* 105–111.

Eysenck, M. W. (1974). Age differences in incidental learning. *Developmental Psychology, 10,* 936–941.

Fischler, I., & Goodman, G. O. (1978). Latency of associative activation in memory. *Journal of Experimental Psychology: Human Perception and Performance, 4,* 455–470.

Graf, P., & Mandler, G. (1984). Activation makes words more accessible but not necessarily more retrievable. *Journal of Verbal Learning and Verbal Behavior, 23,* 553–568.

Graf, P., & Schacter, D. L. (1985). Implicit and explicit memory for new associations in normal and amnesic subjects. *Journal of Experimental Psychology: Learning, Memory, and Cognition, 11,* 501–518.

Guindon, R., & Kintsch, W. (1984). Priming macropropositions: Evidence for the primacy of macropropositions in the memory for text. *Journal of Verbal Learning and Verbal Behavior, 23,* 508–518.

Hasher, L., & Zacks, R. T. (1979). Automatic and effortful processes in memory. *Journal of Experimental Psychology: General, 108,* 356–388.

Hayes, D. (1981). Central auditory problems and the aging process. In D. S. Beasley & G. A. Davis (Eds.), *Aging: Communication processes and disorders* (pp. 257–266). New York: Grune & Stratton.

Howard, D. V. (1980a). Category norms: A comparison of the Battig and Montague (1969) norms with the responses of adults between the ages of 20 and 80. *Journal of Gerontology, 35,* 225–231.

Howard, D. V. (1980b). Restricted word association norms for adults between the ages of 20 and 80. *JSAS Catalog of Selected Documents in Psychology, 10*, 6. (Ms. No. 1991)

Howard, D. V. (1983a). A multidimensional scaling analysis of aging and the semantic structure of animal names. *Experimental Aging Research, 9*, 27–30.

Howard, D. V. (1983b). *Cognitive psychology: Memory, language, and thought.* New York: Macmillan.

Howard, D. V. (1983c). The effects of aging and degree of association on the semantic priming of lexical decisions. *Experimental Aging Research, 9*, 145–151.

Howard, D. V. (1985, August). *Aging and episodic priming: The propositional structure of sentences.* Presented at the meetings of the American Psychological Association, Los Angeles.

Howard, D. V. (1986, August). *Implicit memory and aging: Effects of delay on spelling bias.* Presented at the meetings of the American Psychological Association, Washington, D.C.

Howard, D. V. (in press). Implicit and explicit assessment of age differences in cognition. In C. J. Brainerd & M. L. Howe (Eds.), *Cognitive development in adulthood.* New York: Springer-Verlag.

Howard, D. V., Heisey, J. G., & Shaw, R. J. (1986). Aging and the priming of newly learned associations. *Developmental Psychology, 22*, 78–85.

Howard, D. V., Lasaga, M. I., & McAndrews, M. P. (1980). Semantic activation during memory encoding across the adult lifespan. *Journal of Gerontology, 35*, 884–890.

Howard, D. V., McAndrews, M. P., & Lasaga, M. I. (1981). Semantic priming of lexical decisions in young and old adults. *Journal of Gerontology, 36*, 707–714.

Howard, D. V., Shaw, R. J., & Heisey, J. G. (1986). Aging and the time course of semantic activation. *Journal of Gerontology, 41*, 195–203.

Jacoby, L. L., & Dallas, M. (1981). On the relationship between autobiographical memory and perceptual learning. *Journal of Experimental Psychology: General, 110*, 306–340.

Jacoby, L. L., & Witherspoon, D. (1982). Remembering without awareness. *Canadian Journal of Psychology, 36*, 300–324.

Kausler, D. H. (1982). *Experimental psychology and human aging.* New York: Wiley.

Light, L. L., Singh, A., & Capps, J. L. (1986). Dissociation of memory and awareness in young and older adults. *Journal of Clinical and Experimental Neuropsychology, 8*, 62–74.

McKoon, G., & Ratcliff, R. (1979). Priming in episodic and semantic memory. *Journal of Verbal Learning and Verbal Behavior, 18*, 463–480.

McKoon, G., & Ratcliff, R. (1980). Priming in item recognition: The organization of propositions in memory for text. *Journal of Verbal Learning and Verbal Behavior, 19*, 369–386.

Mishkin, M., & Petri, H. L. (1984). Memories and habits: Some implications for the analysis of learning and retention. In L. R. Squire & N. Butters (Eds.), *Neuropsychology of memory* (pp. 287–296). New York: Guilford Press.

Nebes, R. D., Martin, D. C., & Horn, L. C. (1984). Sparing of semantic memory in Alzheimer's disease. *Journal of Abnormal Psychology, 93*, 321–330.

Neely, J. H. (1977). Semantic priming and retrieval from lexical memory: Roles of inhibitionless spreading activation and limited capacity attention. *Journal of Experimental Psychology: General, 106*, 226–254.

Palermo, D. S., & Jenkins, J. J. (1964). *Word association norms: Grade school through college.* Minneapolis: University of Minnesota Press.

Ratcliff, R., & McKoon, G. (1978). Priming in item recognition: Evidence for the propositional structure of sentences. *Journal of Verbal Learning and Verbal Behavior, 17*, 403–417.

Ratcliff, R., & McKoon, G. (1981). Automatic and strategic priming in recognition. *Journal of Verbal Learning and Verbal Behavior, 20*, 204–215.

Riegel, K. F., & Riegel, R. M. (1964). Changes in associative behavior during later years of life: A cross-sectional analysis. *Vita Humana, 7*, 1–32.

Salthouse, T. A. (1982). *Adult cognition: An experimental psychology of human aging.* New York: Springer-Verlag.

Salthouse, T. A., & Kail, R. (1983). Memory development throughout the life span: The role of processing rate. In P. B. Baltes & O. G. Brim (Eds.), *Life-span development and behavior* (Vol. 5, pp.89–116). New York: Academic Press.

Schacter, D. L. (1985). Multiple forms of memory in humans and animals. In N. M. Weinberger, J. L. McGaugh, & G. Lynch (Eds.), *Memory systems of the brain: Animal and human cognitive processes* (pp. 351–379). New York: Guilford Press.

Sternberg, S. (1966). High-speed scanning in human memory. *Science, 153,* 652–654.

Tulving, E. (1972). Episodic and semantic memory. In E. Tulving & W. Donaldson (Eds.), *Organization of memory* (pp. 381–403). New York: Academic Press.

Tulving, E. (1984). How many memory systems are there? *American Psychologist, 40,* 385–398.

Warren, R. E. (1972). Stimulus encoding and memory. *Journal of Experimental Psychology, 94,* 90–100.

Waugh, N. C., & Barr, R. A. (1982). Encoding deficits in aging. In F. I. M. Craik & S. Trehub (Eds.), *Aging and cognitive processes* (pp. 183–190). New York: Plenum.

Weinstein, B. E., & Ventry, I. M. (1983). Audiometric correlates of the Hearing Handicap Inventory for the Elderly. *Journal of Speech and Hearing Disorders, 48,* 379–384.

Wingfield, A., Poon, L. W., Lombardi, L., & Lowe, D. (1985). Speed of processing in normal aging: Effects of speech rate, linguistic structure, and processing time. *Journal of Gerontology, 40,* 579–585.

Woodruff, D. S. (1982). Advances in the psychophysiology of aging. In F. I. M. Craik & S. Trehub (Eds.), *Aging and cognitive processes* (pp. 29–54). New York: Plenum.

6 Automatic and effortful semantic processes in old age: Experimental and naturalistic approaches

Deborah M. Burke and Rose Marie Harrold

The study of aging and cognition has, not surprisingly, relied on experimental paradigms and theoretical frameworks developed within experimental psychology. Thus much of the research on aging, particularly aging and memory, follows an experimental psychology tradition that has been called "*general principles memory research,* by which is meant a search for principles or generalizations and their underlying mechanisms and processes" (Bruce, 1985, p. 78). The general principles approach in memory research has been questioned recently by critics who contend that it has yielded accounts of performance on artificial, laboratory tasks designed to test theories, but little insight into memory functioning in everyday life (Hirst & Levine, 1985; Neisser, 1976, 1978, 1982, 1985). Neisser suggests, "If X is an interesting or socially significant aspect of memory, then psychologists have hardly ever studied X" (Neisser, 1978, p. 4).

Memory decline in old age is unquestionably an "interesting" and "socially significant aspect of memory." The approach of general-principles memory research to this problem has yielded an impressive progression of methodologically rigorous studies that attempt to identify mechanisms underlying memory decline. However, testing of proposed mechanisms has occurred primarily within the laboratory. Further, the starting point for this research is generally a specific principle identified in young adults and tested within a particular experimental paradigm. As a result, this approach has yielded aging research that tends to involve a limited repertoire of experimental tasks (see Kausler, 1985, for a discussion of this problem). Further, laboratory findings seem to have little relation to older adults' reports of their everyday memory abilities (Sunderland, Watts, Baddeley, & Harris, 1986; Zelinski, Gilewski, & Thompson, 1980).

Here we examine the popular view derived from the levels of processing framework that impaired semantic encoding is a mechanism contributing to memory decline in old age, and to impaired language comprehension as well (e.g., Cohen,

The research reported in this chapter was supported by grant AG02452 from the National Institute on Aging. This chapter benefited considerably from stimulating discussions with Alan Baddeley, Lorraine Tyler, and Karalyn Patterson while the first author was a visitor at the MRC Applied Psychology Unit, Cambridge, England.

1979; Craik & Rabinowitz, 1984). This view starts with the principle that the nature of encoding affects the level of retention and thus can be inferred from retention. Consequently, the research has tended to use memory paradigms to study semantic encoding and comprehension. Such paradigms, however, may not reflect the semantic representations that are initially derived during language comprehension (Marslen-Wilson & Tyler, 1981), especially in older adults (Burke & Yee, 1984). In addition, older adults' self reports of cognitive difficulties do not seem to indicate semantic encoding or comprehension difficulties (Sunderland et al., 1986). Indeed, we have been impressed with the absence of spontaneous complaints about comprehension difficulties from our older subjects (see Stine, Wingfield, & Poon, in press, for a similar informal observation).

In this chapter we present evidence that "on-line" tasks, which measure comprehension processes as they occur, are more appropriate than memory paradigms for investigation of semantic encoding in the laboratory. We report a series of studies involving on-line techniques that has led us to quite different conclusions about semantic encoding in old age which are more compatible with informal observations of older adults' comprehension abilities. Finally, we report a study of naturally occurring memory failures in young and older adults. We argue that research strategies for identifying the nature and origins of cognitive decline in old age should combine a general-principles approach with consideration of naturalistic behavior.

The levels of processing approach

One of the most popular frameworks for the study of memory and aging is the levels of processing framework (see Zacks & Hasher, this volume). This framework was developed to account for young adults' memory for word lists in laboratory tasks, and in particular, for the effects of variables thought to influence the nature of information encoded in memory (Craik & Lockhart, 1972; Craik & Tulving, 1975). It has as its basis the general principle that there are different ways of encoding incoming information and that these vary from shallow to deep encoding; deeper or more semantic encoding produces a richer or more elaborated memory trace than nonsemantic encoding, which is more resistant to forgetting. There are also differences in the level of elaboration of encoding within the semantic domain (e.g., Craik & Tulving, 1975). *Elaboration* refers to the extensiveness of encoding, which some investigators have suggested is the number of encoded features within the semantic domain (Johnson-Laird, Gibbs, & deMowbray, 1978).

Applied to aging research, these principles translate into the hypothesis that older adults have poorer episodic memory performance because they encode information less deeply, that is, because they have a deficit in semantic encoding (e.g., Craik & Byrd, 1982; Craik & Simon, 1980; Eysenck, 1974; Hess, 1984; see Burke & Light, 1981, for a review of the empirical basis for this conclusion). Craik and his colleagues argue, for example, that older adults encode semantic information, but the encoding is less "elaborated" and less sensitive to the semantic context (Craik & Rabinowitz, 1984). The mechanism underlying this deficit in semantic processing is a hypothesized age-related reduction in the attentional resources available for mental operations. Semantic processes are believed to require more attentional capacity and thus to be more impaired than nonsemantic processes requiring little attention, and to show greater impairment as the attention required increases (Cohen, this volume).

The levels of processing explanation also predicts deficits in language comprehension as well as memory (Craik & Rabinowitz, 1984). That is, memory impairment is the result of a deficit in a stage of processing prior to retention, namely, in the initial representation of linguistic meaning. Such a deficit would be expected to affect the immediate understanding of language before retention. And indeed, on the basis of older adults' ability to remember what they have read or heard, it has been proposed that they have impairments in such basic comprehension processes as elaboration of word meaning, drawing of inferences, or integration of elements in a discourse (Cohen, 1979, 1981; Craik & Rabinowitz, 1984; Till & Walsh, 1980).

On-line studies of semantic processes

There is considerable evidence that semantic analysis of language occurs as it is being heard (Marslen-Wilson & Tyler, 1980, 1981) or read (Stanovich & West, 1983); construction of a meaningful interpretation is initiated at the beginning of the language input and affects subsequent linguistic processing. Evidence for this view comes from studies in which comprehension processes are evaluated "on-line" as they occur. These studies usually use reaction time tasks that require a response during the process being examined. For example, Marslen-Wilson & Tyler (1980) measured the latency to detect a target word that was presented in normal prose, semantically anomalous but syntactically correct prose, or a string of scrambled words. Detection was faster in the normal prose than in the anomalous prose, and both of these were faster than in the scrambled words. These effects were obtained even when the target appeared in the first few words of a sentence, but the size of the effect increased for targets later in the sentence. This result suggests that the listener developed a semantic and syntactic interpretation at the very beginning of the utterance and that this interpretation facilitated subsequent processing.

The representation that is the output of these "on-line" comprehension processes would comprise the memory code, which is then also available for "off-line" analyses. However, Marslen-Wilson & Tyler (1981) suggest, "These later analyses are idiosyncratic and variable, and not, we believe, central to the normal process of speech understanding" (p. 322). To locate a deficit at the stage in which language is semantically encoded or interpreted, one must use an experimental paradigm that requires a response close in time to these processes. In this way, one can distinguish age-related problems that occur in comprehension – that is, in the construction of a meaningful representation – from problems that occur after the representation has been constructed, such as decay of the stored representation, or inability to retrieve it. The ability to make this distinction is especially important in aging research because older adults have demonstrated problems in "off-line" processing – for example, retention – even when attempts are made to control encoding (Burke & Light, 1981). Further, Tyler's (1985) work with aphasics demonstrates that on-line tasks may be more sensitive to deficits in interpretive processes than off-line tasks.

In our studies we have focused on one mechanism involved in semantic encoding, namely activation of word meaning. Current models of information processing postulate that activation is the mechanism underlying retrieval of semantic information (Anderson, 1983; Collins & Loftus, 1975; Posner & Snyder, 1975). Identification of a word activates corresponding semantic information in memory that becomes available to the person. Activation also spreads through the semantic network to related concepts, priming them so that this information is easier to retrieve. During language comprehension, priming can occur from two sources: Lexical-level priming effects are based on the semantic relatedness of individual words in the sentence, whereas sentence-level priming effects are based on interpretation of the sentence as a whole, independent of associations of individual words (e.g., Forster, 1979). Our studies examine semantic priming at both the lexical level and the sentence level.

Activation processes establish semantic encoding and thus would play a key role in the construction of a meaningful interpretation of language. As Foss (1982) has pointed out, "While it is unlikely that the phenomenon exists to help us to do experiments on the structure of the lexicon, it is likely that priming has to do with the processing of natural language" (p. 593). Further, inasmuch as the interpreted representation of the language forms the basis for the memory representation, we would expect activation processes to be involved in episodic memory as well (Anderson, 1983). Indeed, they appear to be the link between semantic and episodic knowledge. For example, manipulation of depth of processing through an orienting task has a parallel effect on semantic priming and retention. Orienting tasks that require "shallow" nonsemantic analysis of a prime word reduce both retention and semantic priming effects, as compared to a naming or semantic orienting task (e.g., Parkin, 1979; Smith, Theodore, & Franklin, 1983). Smith et al. (1983) have suggested that the link between level of processing and semantic priming is in the number of semantic features that are activated during encoding (i.e., deeper tasks activate more semantic features), and that this increases the magnitude of priming. Thus if older adults process information less deeply and extensively and if this is the source of their memory problems, then we should find that they have reduced semantic priming associated with reduced memory.

Semantic priming by single words

In the first study in this series (Burke, White, & Diaz, 1987), we examined semantic processes that occur immediately after recognition of a single word and that are believed to facilitiate language perception and comprehension (e.g., Foss, 1982). Both young and older adults make faster lexical decisions for word targets following a semantically related rather than an unrelated word, and this facilitation is attributed to semantic priming from the preceding word (e.g., Bowles & Poon, 1985; Howard, 1983, this volume; Howard, McAndrews, & Lasaga, 1981). The priming in these previous studies could result from subjects' expectation of related words, an attentional process, as well as from automatic processes involving a spread of activation through the semantic network to related words independent of expectancy (but see Howard, Shaw, & Heisey, 1986, for isolation of automatic priming). It is hypothesized that older adults' deficit in semantic processes is a result of diminished attentional resources, and thus a deficiency would be expected in attentional, not automatic, priming (Hasher & Zacks, 1979; Zacks & Hasher, this volume). In the present study, subjects made a lexical decision for a target following a prime word. We manipulated three variables – namely, processing time, expectancy, and prime–target relatedness – in order to isolate attentional and automatic priming effects (cf. Neely, 1977).

First, automatic priming occurs rapidly whereas attentional processes require more time. We used prime–target stimulus onset asynchronies (SOA) of 410 msec and 1550 msec. The shorter SOA seems to be the minimum interval in which shifting of attention can occur; our expectation was that attentional processes would be just beginning to have an effect at this interval whereas automatic priming would have a strong effect. At the longer SOA, priming should result from attentional rather than automatic processes because the latter will have decayed (Neely, 1977).

Second, we varied the subjects' expectation orthogonally with prime–target relatedness. Our subjects worked with only two prime words at a time, and both were category names (e.g., *weather; fruit*). They were instructed to expect target words in the same category with one prime word (e.g., *weather–fog*) and target words in a different but specified category (e.g., *insect*) with the other prime word (e.g., *fruit–ant*). Expected targets occurred on 80% of the word trials, whereas unexpected targets occurred on 20% of the word trials. The unexpected targets were from a different category than the prime when a same-category target was expected (e.g., *weather–elm*), and were from the same category as the prime when a different-category target was expected (e.g., *fruit–lemon*).

Speeding of lexical decision responses to expected targets would reflect attentional processes, whereas speeding of responses to same-category targets would reflect automatic processes. If older adults had impaired attentional processes because they required more time to shift or focus attention, then we might see small expectancy effects for young adults at the 410-msec SOA, and none for older adults. If older adults simply had reduced attentional resources overall, then expectancy effects should be smaller for older adults at both SOAs.

The subjects in this and the following study were primarily young and older graduates of Pomona and Pitzer colleges with comparable education and vocabulary scores, but the older adults generally had slightly smaller digit spans. The results from 32 young and 32 older adults showed that although overall latency was slower for older adults, the magnitude of both attentional and automatic priming effects was the same across age. Table 6.1 shows the absolute and percentage priming effects at each SOA. The automatic effect, in milliseconds, was obtained by combining unexpected and expected conditions and subtracting latency for same-category targets from latency for different-category targets. The attentional effect, in milliseconds, was obtained by combining same- and different-category conditions and subtracting latency for expected targets from latency for unexpected targets. These differences are expressed as percentages of the baseline in the percentage effect column.

As predicted, same-category targets were significantly faster than different-category targets (the automatic effect), but only at the shorter SOA. Expected tar-

Table 6.1. *Automatic and attentional effects on lexical decision latency by age and SOA*

	Automatic effect				Attentional effect			
	410 SOA		1550 SOA		410 SOA		1550 SOA	
	msec	%	msec	%	msec	%	msec	%
Young	43*	5.7	17	2.2	68*	8.8	113*	13.9
Old	92*	9.5	31	2.6	83*	8.9	162*	14.3

*p < .01.
Source: D. M. Burke, H. White, & D. L. Diaz (1987). Semantic priming in young and older adults: Evidence for age constancy in automatic and attentional processes. *Journal of Experimental Psychology: Human Perception and Performance, 13,* 84. Copyright 1987 by the American Psychological Association, Inc.

gets were significantly faster than unexpected targets (the attentional effect) at both SOAs, but the magnitude of the effect increased at the longer SOA. These patterns of an interaction of SOA with the expectancy effect, and with the semantic relatedness effect, were obtained for both young and older adults. There was no evidence that older adults required more time to shift attention to the expected targets because expectancy (the attentional effect) decreased latency by about 9% at the short SOA, and by about 14% at the long SOA for both age groups.

Although there was no evidence of age differences in the priming of semantic information by single words when either automatic or attentional processes were involved, older adults did recall fewer categories and target words in a surprise free-recall test. Both expectancy and relatedness improved recall of target words. These variables also increased priming, and together these results suggest that the semantic processing induced by these variables facilitated recall. There was also some evidence that expectancy had a greater effect on recall than relatedness, which is consistent with previous findings suggesting that attentional semantic activation has a stronger effect on episodic memory (Balota, 1983). Correlations of each subject's prime effect with recall showed a significant correlation for attentional but not automatic priming, and only in the longer SOA for young adults. This correlation was in the right direction for older adults but did not reach significance (p < .14). Clearly, further work is needed to clarify the mechanism common to semantic priming and episodic memory and to identify the factor that disrupts this relation in older adults.

In sum, the results show that older adults have a deficit in episodic memory but not in either automatic or attentional semantic priming. This suggests that the source of their memory problem lies in a mental process other than semantic encoding. On the other hand, it is possible that the attentional requirements of the present task (i.e., expecting a particular category of words and then making a lexical decision) were too small to show an age deficit in attentional resources. Craik and his colleagues (e.g., Rabinowitz, Craik, & Ackerman, 1982) have suggested that older adults may be capable of encoding dominant "general" aspects of meaning but not more subtle meaning. Presumably this means that attentional resources are insufficient to prime associated concepts that are too great a semantic distance from the prime word. In our study, however, many of the category instances were not dominant members of their category according to category norms and, in fact, about one third of the instances were produced by 10% or fewer of the older adults in the norming sample (Howard, 1980).

Further, it is important to note that deficits in semantic processing have been postulated as the cause of older adults' poorer memory for single words in studies where the attentional requirements seem comparable to those of the present task. That is, experiments using the levels of processing paradigm typically require subjects to answer a question involving semantic or phonemic information about the target. Older adults' poorer incidental memory for targets under these conditions is attributed to deficient semantic encoding.

Nonetheless, we pursued the possibility that older adults might reveal a deficit in semantic processing during the more demanding task of reading a sentence. Further, one mechanism not measured in the first study that could produce semantic deficits is an age-related increase in the rate of decay of semantic activation. Thus, in the next study we examined on-line semantic processing of sentences by measuring semantic priming immediately after presentation of a prime word in the sentence, or several words downstream from the prime. Subjects read aloud a sentence presented one word at a time on a computer screen at a rate of about two words per second. A lexical decision was made for a target immediately following the sentence.

In each sentence there was a prime word which was either semantically related or unrelated to the target. Half the sentences were presented in a short version in which the prime word was the last word in the sentence, as with "book" in (1), and half were presented in a long version in which a three- or four-word prepositional phrase intervened between the prime and target, as in (2). If older adults have a deficit in semantic processing especially when attentional demands are high as in reading, then we would expect less priming of related targets and thus less reduction of related latency relative to unrelated latency. Further, the study allowed comparison of the duration of priming in young and older subjects in the long condition where three or four words intervened between prime and target.

(1)　The little girl begged her mother to read the book.
　　　Related target: *story*; unrelated target: *nose*
(2)　The little girl begged her mother to read the book before her bedtime.
　　　Related target: *story*; unrelated target: *nose*

The results from 32 young and 32 older adults are shown in Table 6.2. Older adults had slower latencies overall, and semantic relatedness speeded lexical decision for both age groups. However, semantic priming effects depended on sentence length and age. Priming was obtained for young adults in the short condition but not in the long condition. Older adults showed semantic priming in the long condition but not in the short. Further, sentence length had different effects on young and older adults' latency overall; the longer sentences consistently produced faster response times for older but not young adults.

We think that this pattern of results suggests that older adults were slower to

Table 6.2. *Mean latency and priming effects for prime words in sentences by age and prime–target interval*

Sentence length	Young adults			Old adults		
	Related	Unrelated	Priming effect	Related	Unrelated	Priming effect
Short	577	615	38*	1032	1045	13
Long	610	605	−5	966	1010	44*

*$p < .01$.

process the words in the sentence and that they caught up with processing during the final three-word phrase which tended to be highly redundant. This catching-up reduced the interference between the sentence reading task and the lexical decision task, so that both related and unrelated lexical decision targets could be processed more quickly in long than short sentences. Further, if older adults are slower to process sentence words, processing of the prime word would be delayed and hence its priming effects as well. Thus priming effects for older adults are observed further downstream in the sentence (three words after the prime word), when compared to priming effects for young adults which are observed for the word following the prime.

This suggests that older adults are slower in the on-line processing of words in a sentence. This is consistent with Stine et al.'s (in press) report that older adults' immediate recall of sentences was more disrupted by fast speech rates than was the recall of young adults. Their results also indicate that despite the decline in recall at fast speech rates, older adults showed no deficit in semantic and syntactic analysis of the sentences. That is, variations in the propositional complexity of the sentences or in their semantic and syntactic coherence, had similar effects on young and older adults, although older adults showed, if anything, more benefit from semantic and syntactic constraints. The Stine et al. study measured recall, and thus the locus of the observed effects cannot be located in on-line comprehension rather than off-line memory processes. Further, in both their study and the present one, the observed slowing could be the result of age-related slowing at the sensory level rather than at a more central level. However, these studies are consistent with the view that although older adults may be slower to process language, they engage in the same types of linguistic analysis and the interpretative representation appears to be the same across age.

The results discussed so far would not be incompatible with the view that older adults are able to encode "general" meanings of words but are unable to encode context-specific interpretations. This idea is nicely expressed by Rabinowitz, Craik, and Ackerman (1982) who suggested

that such a reduction [in attentional resources] is associated with poor integration of the encoded item with its context, so that the context is a poor cue for the target item in a subsequent retention test . . . Finally, it is postulated that whereas specific relational information is difficult to encode when resources are reduced, the general semantic features of an item are still encoded under such circumstances. (p. 342)

Comprehension clearly involves going beyond dictionary meanings of words and also using semantic and pragmatic knowledge to construct interpretations of word meaning relevant in a linguistic context. Indeed, there is evidence that the process of encoding word meaning involves selection, elaboration, and integration of the word meaning based on the sentential context (e.g., Seidenberg, Waters, Sanders, & Langer, 1984; Stanovich & West, 1983). One source of this evidence is research using priming paradigms to evaluate the effects of sentence context on semantic encoding of word meaning. Tabossi and Johnson-Laird (1980) demonstrated that a property biased by the sentential context is primed and irrelevant properties are inhibited. For example, verification that "a diamond is hard" was faster after a sentence implying this property (3) than after a neutral sentence that did not imply any specific property (4) and slower after a sentence that implied another property (5).

(3)   The goldsmith cut the glass with the diamond.
(4)   The film showed the person with the diamond.
(5)   The mirror dispersed the light from the diamond.

The measurement of the effect of sentence context on the encoding of word meaning provides a sensitive instrument for evaluating the interpretation of sentences and the use of this interpretation in specifying word meanings. If these abilities were impaired, we would expect to see less effect of context on word meaning. Indeed, in a study in which elementary school children read a sentence and then performed a Stroop task, children having poor reading comprehension showed color-naming interference with properties as the Stroop words, regardless of whether the latter were relevant or irrelevant to a preceding sentence. Children with good comprehension showed interference for contextually relevant but not irrelevant properties (Merrill, Sperber, & McCauley, 1981). Thus if older adults have deficits in constructing an interpretation of a sentence or in using this interpretation to specify word meaning, we would expect them to show reduced effects of sentential context on the encoding of word meaning.

We used a noun–property verification task to examine whether there are age-related changes in the extent to which linguistic context primes relevant properties of nouns and suppresses irrelevant properties. We asked 30 young and 30 older adults to read a sentence at their own pace and, when finished, to press a key on the computer that would cause a question about a noun–property relation to be displayed. The task was to verify the relation as true or false by depression of the appropriate button on the computer, and on half the trials the correct response was true and on half it was false.

There were three types of sentences on true trials, as can be seen in Table 6.3. In *biased* sentences, a property of the target noun is suggested by the sentence as a whole, but not by any individual word. In *verb-augmented bias* sentences, a property was suggested by the verb as well as by the whole sentence. In *neutral* sentences, no particular property of the target noun was suggested by the sentence. We confirmed our intuitions about the bias of the sentences by asking young and older adults to

Table 6.3. *Sample sentences and targets for property verification task*

Sentence condition example	Sentence example	Question condition	Question
Biased	The oranges fell off the uneven table.	Appropriate	Oranges–Round?
		Inappropriate	Oranges–Juicy?
Verb-augmented bias	The oranges rolled off the uneven table.	Appropriate	Oranges–Round?
		Inappropriate	Oranges–Juicy?
Neutral	The oranges remained in the basket.	Neutral	Oranges–Round?
			Oranges–Juicy?
Biased	The oranges satisfied the thirst of the hot children.	Appropriate	Oranges–Juicy?
		Inappropriate	Oranges–Round?
Verb-augmented bias	The oranges quenched the thirst of the hot children.	Appropriate	Oranges–Juicy?
		Inappropriate	Oranges–Round?

Table 6.4. *Mean response time (msec) and error percentages for appropriate, inappropriate, and neutral sentence–question conditions*

	Condition				
	Appropriate	Inappropriate	Neutral	Facilitation	Inhibition
Young	1082 (3.6%)	1207 (6.4%)	1098 (5.0%)	16	109*
Old	1656 (0.6%)	1952 (3.1%)	1807 (5.0%)	151*	145*

*$p < .01$.

rate how much the sentences made them think of the target properties. We used only those sentences that yielded ratings consistent with the intended bias and that had similar ratings across age. Each sentence type was followed equally often by the appropriate (i.e., the biased) property or by the inappropriate (i.e., the nonbiased) property in the noun–property verification question.

The verification latencies are shown in Table 6.4 for appropriate, inappropriate, and neutral conditions. The biased and verb-augmented bias conditions are combined because there was no difference in latencies in these conditions. Older adults had slower latencies in all conditions, but both young and older adults had faster latencies for properties that were appropriate to the preceding sentence than for properties that were inappropriate, and the size of this effect was statistically the same across age. These results demonstrate clearly that both young and older adults use sentential context to specify word meaning. There was, however, a different pattern of results for the two age groups when the appropriate and inappropriate conditions were compared to the neutral condition in which the sentence biased no specific property of the noun. The young had slower verifications in the inappropriate than in the neutral condition, but no difference between appropriate and neutral conditions. For older adults, verification was also slower in the inappropriate than in the neutral condition, but verification was faster in the appropriate than in the neutral as well.

There are several possible explanations for the age differences in the pattern of latencies across sentence conditions. First, there may have been age differences in the extent to which sentences biased the target properties. However, a separate sample of young and older adults had given comparable ratings of how much the sentences biased the properties in a pretest of the materials. We confirmed this by asking subjects in a subsequent study to produce the first property that came to mind for a noun target that followed a biased or neutral sentence. The noun targets and sentences were the same as in the verification study. If young adults were less likely to produce appropriate properties after biased sentences and more likely to produce properties after neutral sentences, the age differences in the pattern of latencies would be explained. However, 30 young and 30 older adults both produced the relevant property or a synonym on 50% of the trials with biased sentences. In no cases were these properties given after the neutral sentences. These data confirm that the sentences have equivalent effects across age in implying properties of nouns.

It seems more likely that older adults had larger facilitation from appropriate sentences because they were slower to make property verifications. Stanovich and West (1983) presented substantial evidence that factors that increase the difficulty of word recognition also increase the facilitatory effects of sentence contexts on recognition. They argue that the spreading activation resulting from interpretation of a sentence can compensate for a deficit in lexical access. Extending their logic to the property verification task, the larger facilitation effects for older adults result because older adults are slower to access target-property information. Stanovich and West also argued that inhibitory effects of sentences occur at a later stage of processing, namely response selection. Incompatibility between a sentence and a target biases the subject to respond "no," thus slowing the correct positive response. The finding of comparable inhibitory effects in young and older adults suggests that this bias is unaffected in old age.

The important point here, however, is that semantic context clearly influenced the encoding of word meaning for older adults. This effect depends on the formation of an interpreted representation of the sentence as it is read and on the selection of meaning for successive words that is consistent with this interpretation. Finally, despite this evidence that older adults encoded these sentences semantically and in a contextually distinct manner, they had poorer recognition of the sentences in an incidental memory test.

Conclusions about semantic processing during language comprehension

Our investigations of semantic processing in old age using on-line experimental techniques have led us to conclusions quite different from those based on studies using memory paradigms within the levels of processing framework. In particular, in our experiments we consistently find similarity across age in the semantic processing of material for which older adults have poorer subsequent retention. In our first study, we examined semantic encoding of single words by isolating automatic and attentional processes involved in semantic activation. The results indicate age constancy in the time course and the strength of priming resulting from each type of process. In the second study, we examined semantic encoding of words during sentence processing. Here older adults appeared to be slower to interpret words in a sentence semantically, but there was no evidence that the interpretation was any different across age. The third study demonstrated that older adults construct interpretations of sentences and use them to specify word meaning.

The results of our studies invite the conclusion that semantic processes involved in interpretation of a sentence are well preserved in old age. Our studies focus on semantic activation processes within a single word or sentence, but there is converging evidence for this conclusion from studies of comprehension using other tasks. Light and her colleagues have demonstrated that young and older adults do not differ in the use of semantic and pragmatic constraints in completing a sentence fragment or in identifying the correct referent for an ambiguous pronoun (Light & Albertson, this volume; Light & Capps, 1986). Similarly, Zelinski (this volume) demonstrated that older adults were just as accurate as young adults in answering questions that required matching coreferential terms across sentences. Further, there is evidence that in perceptual processing older adults rely at least as much as younger adults on semantic and syntactic interpretation of the linguistic context rather than the sensory input (Cohen & Faulkner, 1983; Stine et al., in press).

Thus we are left with the question of the role of comprehension processes in older adults' memory declines. We think that this should be rephrased to the question of the role of memory declines in older adults' comprehension processes (see Light & Albertson, this volume, for a similar view). That is, evidence is accumulating from our own and other studies with independent measures of semantic processing and retention, that older adults show memory deficits for material that they have semantically encoded in a manner similar to young adults (Burke, White, & Diaz, 1987; Burke & Yee, 1984; Howard, 1983; Howard, Shaw, & Heisey, 1986). This indicates that older adults have a memory impairment that is unrelated to semantic processing. However, although young and older adults appear to have similar off-line semantic representations of sentences immediately after interpretation, older adults lose this representation more rapidly over a delay (Cohen & Faulkner, 1981). Thus when the interpretive representation of prior discourse must be preserved for subsequent on-line comprehension processes, age differences may occur in on-line processes. Indeed, Light has demonstrated that older adults have difficulty resolving ambiguous pronouns under such conditions (Light & Albertson, this volume; Light & Capps, 1986).

Everyday memory and aging

Research resulting from the application of the levels of processing framework to age-related memory decline started from the principle that semantic encoding deficits produce memory deficits. An alternative to this general-principles memory approach starts with observations of everyday behavior of a particular age group and from that derives principles and mechanisms. This latter approach can be characterized as "bottom-up" research because it starts with naturalistic data or observations, whereas the general-principles memory approach is more "top-down" because it starts with principles. The "bottom-up" research approach has been more visible in the study of child development than in the study of adult development. For example, children's spontaneous utterances in everyday life provide the basis for derivation of principles of development and basic cognitive mechanisms. Piaget's developmental theory provides a model for this approach as it is derived from naturalistic observations of infants and children. Thus, the observation of everyday performance does more than validate experimental paradigms. It can provide the basis for theories concerning the nature of cognition as well as developmental change.

We will report some preliminary findings from a study of naturally occurring memory problems which we think provides a promising direction for future research (Burke, Worthley, & Martin, 1988). Contrary to the levels of processing approach, our "bottom-up" analysis of these data identifies retrieval deficits as a cause of some of older adults' memory problems. The motivation for this research came from the frequent complaints of our older subjects about the frustration of being unable to retrieve a well-known word, even though they felt it was imminent. Further, they said such "tip of the tongue" (TOT) experiences seemed to be getting more frequent. Our sense that this was a significant memory problem in old age was confirmed by Sunderland et al. (1986). They found that TOT experiences were the most frequent everyday memory problem reported by older adults. And yet, we could find only one published study of TOT experiences in older adults, and this study examined only proper names (Cohen & Faulkner, 1986). There have been studies of TOT states in the laboratory (e.g., Brown & McNeill, 1966; Rubin, 1975) or in everyday life (e.g., Reason & Lucas, 1984), but they have involved young adults.

We asked young and older adults to keep a record of their spontaneous TOT experiences for 1 month using a diary with a standardized set of questions. The results from 30 subjects in each age group show that older adults reported more TOTs over the month than young adults, with means of 6.1 and 3.9 TOTs, respectively. In order to understand better the nature of these experiences, we examined the characteristics of the TOT words and factors associated with resolution.

Most of the TOTs were resolved: Older adults resolved 97.3%, and young adults 91.5%. A variety of strategies were used to retrieve the desired word, but older adults used each type of strategy less often and they used no strategy more often. However, the probability that a strategy would produce the sought-after word was the same for young and old; young adults just used more strategies. The high resolution rate of the older adults was due to spontaneous recovery in which the target word popped into mind with no conscious retrieval effort. These "pop-ups" accounted for 41.2% of the young adults resolutions and 57.8% of the older adults. Previous laboratory studies have concluded that such automatic, nonconscious processing which results in sought-after information popping into mind, is relatively rare (e.g., Read & Bruce, 1982). The present results, however, suggest that pop-ups occur frequently with TOTs, especially for older adults. Further, on a confidence rating scale, older adults were significantly more confident that they would be able to retrieve the TOT word eventually. We suspect that they have learned to rely on the word popping into mind, and this may account for their confidence and their reduced use of strategies for searching memory.

The TOT words tended to be multisyllabic words that were rated as familiar by the subjects. What was most surprising and perhaps most important, was that young and older adults had TOTs for quite different types of words. The majority of TOTs for both young (55.9%) and old (68.2%) were proper names of people or places. Most of the other TOTs for older adults were common names of objects (e.g., *silo, frisbee, blender, azalea*). Young adults almost never had TOTs for object names. Their remaining TOTs were for intangibles, namely procedures (e.g., *amniocentesis*), abstract nouns (e.g., *typicality*), and adjectives and verbs (e.g., *ambitious, exude*).

The TOT experience is consistent with the view that there are separate memory domains for semantic information about concepts and for lexical information about the sounds and orthography of words. Within these domains there is a network of connections, and the two domains are connected with each other (Baddeley, 1982). TOT states would arise when semantic information has been accessed but the corresponding information in the lexical domain about the appropriate word is temporarily inaccessible (cf. Bowles & Poon, 1985). Thus TOTs result from retrieval failures within the lexicon when the retrieval is driven by semantic information. Word-finding problems in aphasia or in Alzheimer's disease have been related to deviant or incomplete semantic representations (see Huff, this volume), but there is no evidence for such deterioration in old age (e.g., Burke & Peters, 1986). Further, the disruption of retrieval is temporary and seems to recover spontaneously which would not be expected if the underlying representation were permanently damaged.

In sum, this study of spontaneous memory failures points us in a quite different direction from the levels of processing approach. First, the increase in TOT experiences during adulthood suggests that failure of retrieval processes may be a source of memory problems in old age. Some of the TOTs in our study were for recently learned names, suggesting that such retrieval failures may be a factor in memory for new information as well as for well-known vocabulary words. Furthermore, these retrieval failures do not seem to be related to impoverished semantic information, because older adults in our study had higher performance than young adults on a vocabulary test requiring definitions of words. Second, TOT experiences seem to involve failure of a process that is effortless. Thus, limiting the search for age deficits to mental operations that require effort would seem to be premature.

It is important to combine naturalistic studies such as this one with laboratory research because they are susceptible to reporting biases on the part of the participants. Thus we are in the process of attempting to replicate our results in the laboratory with induced TOTs. Nonetheless, we think that the "bottom-up" approach of such naturalistic studies provides a foundation for developing general principles which will increase our understanding of the nature of cognitive changes in old age.

References

Anderson, J. R. (1983). A spreading activation theory of memory. *Journal of Verbal Learning and Verbal Behavior, 22,* 261–295.

Baddeley, A. D. (1982). Domains of recollection. *Psychological Review*, *85*, 139–152.

Balota, D. A. (1983). Automatic semantic activation and episodic memory encoding. *Journal of Verbal Learning and Verbal Behavior*, *22*, 88–104.

Bowles, N. L., & Poon, L. W. (1985). Aging and retrieval of words in semantic memory. *Journal of Gerontology*, *40*, 71–77.

Brown, R., & McNeill, D. (1966). The "tip of the tongue" phenomenon. *Journal of Verbal Learning and Verbal Behavior*, *5*, 325–337.

Bruce, D. (1985). The how and why of ecological memory. *Journal of Experimental Psychology: General*, *114*, 78–90.

Burke, D. M., & Light, L. L. (1981). Memory and aging: The role of retrieval processes. *Psychological Bulletin*, *90*, 513–546.

Burke, D. M., & Peters, L. J. (1986). Word associations in old age: Evidence for consistency in semantic encoding during adulthood. *Psychology and Aging*, *1*, 283–292.

Burke, D. M., White, H., & Diaz, D. L. (1987). Semantic priming in young and older adults: Evidence for age-constancy in automatic and attentional processes. *Journal of Experimental Psychology: Human Perception and Performance*, *13*, 79–88.

Burke, D. M., Worthley, J., & Martin, J. (1988). I'll never forget what's-her-name: Aging and the tip of the tongue experience. In M. M. Gruneberg, P. Morris, & R. N. Sykes (Eds.), *Practical aspects of memory: Current research and issues* (Vol. 2, pp. 113–118). Chichester: Wiley.

Burke, D. M., & Yee, P. L. (1984). Semantic priming during sentence processing by young and older adults. *Developmental Psychology*, *20*, 903–910.

Cohen, G. (1979). Language comprehension in old age. *Cognitive Psychology*, *11*, 412–429.

Cohen, G. (1981). Inferential reasoning in old age. *Cognition*, *9*, 59–72.

Cohen, G., & Faulkner, D. (1981). Memory for discourse in old age. *Discourse Processes*, *4*, 253–265.

Cohen, G., & Faulkner, D. (1983). Word recognition: Age differences in contextual facilitation effects. *British Journal of Psychology*, *74*, 239–251.

Cohen, G. & Faulkner, D. (1986). Memory for proper names: Age differences in retrieval. *British Journal of Developmental Psychology*, *4*, 187–197.

Collins, A. M., & Loftus, E. F. (1975). A spreading-activation theory of semantic processing. *Psychological Review*, *82*, 407–428.

Craik, F. I. M., & Byrd, M. (1982). Aging and cognitive deficits: The role of attentional resources. In F. I. M. Craik & S. Trehub (Eds.), *Aging and cognitive processes*. New York: Plenum.

Craik, F. I. M., & Lockhart, R. S. (1972). Levels of processing: A framework for memory research. *Journal of Verbal Learning and Verbal Behavior*, *11*, 671–684.

Craik, F. I. M., & Rabinowitz, J. C. (1984). Age differences in the acquisition and use of verbal information: A tutorial review. In H. Bouma & D. G. Bouwhuis (Eds.), *Attention and performance X: Control of language processes* (pp. 471–499). Hillsdale, NJ: Erlbaum.

Craik, F. I. M., & Simon, E. (1980). Age differences in memory: The roles of attention and depth of processing. In L. W. Poon, J. L. Fozard, L. S. Cermak, D. Arenberg, & L. W. Thompson (Eds.), *New directions in memory and aging: Proceedings of the George A. Talland Memorial Conference* (pp. 95–112). Hillsdale, NJ: Erlbaum.

Craik, F. I. M., & Tulving, E. (1975). Depth of processing and the retention of words in episodic memory. *Journal of Experimental Psychology: General*, *104*, 268–294.

Eysenck, M. W. (1974). Age differences in incidental learning. *Developmental Psychology*, *10*, 936–941.

Forster, K. I. (1979). Levels of processing and the structure of the language processor. In W. E. Cooper & E. C. T. Walker (Eds.), *Sentence processing: Psycholinguistic studies presented to Merrill Garrett* (pp. 27–85). Hillsdale, NJ: Erlbaum.

Foss, D. J. (1982). A discourse on semantic priming. *Cognitive Psychology*, *14*, 590–607.

Hasher, L., & Zacks, R. T. (1979). Automatic and effortful processes in memory. *Journal of Experimental Psychology: General*, *108*, 356–388.

Hess, T. M. (1984). Effects of semantically related and unrelated contexts on recognition memory of different-aged adults. *Journal of Gerontology*, *39*, 444–451.

Hirst, W., & Levine, E. (1985). Ecological memory reconsidered: A comment on Bruce's "The how and why of ecological memory." *Journal of Experimental Psychology: General*, *114*, 269–271.

Howard, D. V. (1980). Category norms: A comparison of the Battig and Montague (1968) norms with the responses of adults between the ages of 20 and 80. *Journal of Gerontology, 35,* 225–231.

Howard, D. V. (1983). The effect of aging and degree of association on the semantic priming of lexical decisions. *Experimental Aging Research, 9,* 145–151.

Howard, D. V., McAndrews, M. P., & Lasaga, M. I. (1981). Semantic priming of lexical decisions in young and old adults. *Journal of Gerontology, 36,* 707–714.

Howard, D. V., Shaw, R. J., & Heisey, J. G. (1986). Aging and the time course of semantic activation. *Journal of Gerontology, 41,* 195–203.

Johnson-Laird, P. N., Gibbs, G., & deMowbray, J. (1978). Meaning, amount of processing, and memory for words. *Memory & Cognition, 6,* 372–375.

Kausler, D. H. (1985). Episodic memory: Memorizing performance. In N. Charness (Ed.), *Aging and human performance.* (pp. 101–141). New York: Wiley.

Light, L. L., & Capps, J. L. (1986). Comprehension of pronouns in young and older adults. *Developmental Psychology, 22,* 580–585.

Marslen-Wilson, W. D., & Tyler, L. K. (1980). The temporal structure of spoken language understanding. *Cognition, 8,* 1–71.

Marslen-Wilson, W. D., & Tyler, L. K. (1981). Central processes in speech understanding. *Philosophical Transactions of the Royal Society London, 295,* 317–332.

Merrill, E. C., Sperber, R. D., & McCauley, C. (1981). Differences in semantic encoding as a function of reading comprehension skill. *Memory & Cognition, 9,* 618–624.

Neely, J. H. (1977). Semantic priming and retrieval from lexical memory: Roles of inhibitionless spreading activation and limited capacity attention. *Journal of Experimental Psychology: General, 106,* 226–254.

Neisser, U. (1976). *Cognition and reality.* San Francisco: Freeman.

Neisser, U. (1978). Memory: What are the important questions? In M. M. Gruneberg, P. M. Morris, & R. N. Sykes (Eds.), *Practical applications of memory* (pp. 3–24). London: Academic Press.

Neisser, U. (Ed.). (1982). *Memory observed: Remembering in natural contexts.* San Francisco: Freeman.

Neisser, U. (1985). The role of theory in the ecological study of memory: Comment on Bruce. *Journal of Experimental Psychology: General, 114,* 272–276.

Parkin, A. J. (1979). Specifying levels of processing. *Quarterly Journal of Experimental Psychology, 31,* 175–195.

Posner, M. I., & Snyder, C. R. R. (1975). Attention and cognitive control. In R. Solso (Ed.), *Information processing and cognition* (pp. 55–85). Hillsdale, NJ: Erlbaum.

Rabinowitz, J. C., Craik, F. I. M., & Ackerman, B. P. (1982). A processing resource account of age differences in recall. *Canadian Journal of Psychology, 36,* 325–344.

Read, J. D., & Bruce, D. (1982). Longitudinal tracking of difficult memory retrievals. *Cognitive Psychology, 14,* 280–300.

Reason, J. T., & Lucas, D. (1984). Using cognitive diaries to investigate naturally occuring memory blocks. In J. E. Harris & P. E. Morris (Eds.), *Everyday memory: Actions and absent-mindedness* (pp. 53–70). London: Academic Press.

Rubin, D. C. (1975). Within word structure in the tip-of-the-tongue phenomenon. *Journal of Verbal Learning and Verbal Behavior, 14,* 392–397.

Seidenberg, M. S., Waters, G. S., Sanders, M., & Langer, P. (1984). Pre- and postlexical loci of contextual effects on word recognition. *Memory & Cognition, 12,* 315–328.

Smith, M. C., Theodore, L., & Franklin, P. E. (1983). The relationship between contextual facilitation and depth of processing. *Journal of Experimental Psychology: Learning, Memory, and Cognition, 9,* 697–712.

Stanovich, K. E., & West, R. F. (1983). On priming by a sentence context. *Journal of Experimental Psychology: General, 112,* 1–36.

Stine, E. L., Wingfield, A., & Poon, L. W. (in press). In L. W. Poon, D. C. Rubin, & B. A. Wilson (Eds.), *Everyday cognition in adulthood and late life.* Cambridge: Cambridge University Press.

Sunderland, A., Watts, K., Baddeley, A. D., & Harris, J. E. (1986). Subjective memory assessment and test performance in the elderly. *Journal of Gerontology, 41,* 376–384.

Tabossi, P., & Johnson-Laird, P. N. (1980). Linguistic context and the priming of semantic information. *Quarterly Journal of Experimental Psychology, 32,* 605–624.

Till, R. E., & Walsh, D. A. (1980). Encoding and retrieval factors in adult memory for implicational sentences. *Journal of Verbal Learning and Verbal Behavior, 19,* 1–16.

Tyler, L. K. (1985). Real-time comprehension processes in agrammatism: A case study. *Brain and Language, 26,* 259–275.

Zelinski, E. M., Gilewski, M. J., & Thompson, L. W. (1980). Do laboratory tests relate to self-assessment of memory ability in the young and old? In L. W. Poon, J. L. Fozard, L. S. Cermak, D. Arenberg, & L. W. Thompson (Eds.), *New directions in memory and aging: Proceedings of the George A. Talland Memorial Conference* (pp. 95–112). Hillsdale, NJ: Erlbaum.

7 Integrating information from discourse: Do older adults show deficits?

Elizabeth M. Zelinski

There are currently two major routes of explanation for age-related deficits in discourse memory. The first, more empirical approach, seeks complex interactions among subject, task, and text characteristics (Hultsch & Dixon, 1984; Meyer, in press; Meyer & Rice, 1983, in press). Meyer and Rice have argued that age differences are heightened when people low in verbal ability are compared, relative to when those high in verbal ability are tested, when narratives rather than expository passages are presented, and when short rather than long texts are studied. In a meta-analysis of the extant literature, we verified that the first two suggested factors – high verbal ability and expository passages – reduced the effect size of age differences in prose recall, but the third did not (Zelinski & Gilewski, in press): Age differences were reliably smaller in studies in which subjects high in verbal ability were tested and in which expository texts were used, but the differences remained highly significant across studies. Thus, the interaction of certain factors with age does account for some variance in discourse recall, but the age differences are not fully explained by this approach.

The second, more theoretically based, class of explanations for age deficits in discourse recall is that there are fundamental differences in how adequately older adults process text information as compared to younger ones. The working-memory capacity deficit model, which is reviewed in the chapters by Hasher and Zacks and by Cohen in this volume, suggests that older adults have insufficient working-memory capacity to process complex relationships among concepts in discourse and that this deficit impairs their language comprehension. Higher-order processing used in understanding language – for example, the use of inference to fill gaps when implications are left to the comprehender – is less likely to be invoked by the elderly. As a result, older people have difficulty comprehending and remembering prose when the processes underlying comprehension place an excessive burden on working memory. This means that they may have difficulties in developing an accurate representation of what they have read because they do not engage in the higher-order processes that link information from a discourse into a unitary whole. Because the basis of discourse comprehension is integration of information (e.g., Kintsch & van Dijk, 1978), and because accuracy of memory is contingent on comprehension

Preparation of this chapter was funded in part by grant R01 AG4114 from the National Institute on Aging to the author.

117

(e.g., Bransford & Johnson, 1972), it is important to determine whether older adults have difficulty in integrating information in discourse and whether this accounts for their poorer recall of texts.

In this chapter, we evaluate this issue in a review of the literature on age differences in the integration of information in discourse and present new findings from our laboratory. Two aspects of integration are examined. The first is the integration of generic knowledge with text information, which represents discourse macroprocesses in comprehension (cf. Kintsch & van Dijk, 1978). These processes are observed in research on the effects of domain knowledge on text recall, on patterns of recognition to different types of foils in script memory, and on effects of story organization on recall. The second aspect of integration to be examined is comprehension of related terms in pairs of sentences. We report a series of our own studies that use sentence reading times to measure local integration processes involved in representing the microstructure of texts (Kintsch & van Dijk, 1978). Our discussion begins with an overview of a model of reading comprehension to illustrate the role of integration at both levels in understanding what has been read.

The development of theory explaining how people understand discourse is still in its preliminary stages. Although there are many flaws in existing theories, largely because they are too broad and/or do not provide adequate parameters for empirical tests (cf. Reiser & Black, 1982), there is a consensus about the major processes in discourse comprehension and memory. Essentially, the comprehender constructs a representation or knowledge structure of the discourse as it is being comprehended. The basic ideas or propositions in the discourse are processed and stored in the representation. As new information is presented, the model of the discourse is updated to include it. The relationships between propositions are determined, and connections between them are also included in the representation. The mental model of a discourse involves the integration of the propositions and their relationships into a unitary whole, which can later be retrieved and remembered (e.g., Kintsch & van Dijk, 1978).

On the basis of a synthesis of models of comprehension devised by a number of authors (Abbott, Black, & Smith, 1985; Kintsch & van Dijk, 1978; Lorch, Lorch, & Matthews, 1985; Malt, 1985; Morrow, 1985; Sanford & Garrod, 1981; Schank & Abelson, 1977), we assume that knowledge-based and text-based processes are used to devise the representation of a discourse. Knowledge-based processes are important in comprehension because they provide the background that the individual needs in order to understand what he or she is reading on a global level. Text-based processes analyze the specific information that is being read on a local level. For example, when reading a story about a couple going to dinner at a restaurant, the reader accesses generic information about social relationships and about the typical actions people engage in at a restaurant, and uses this information, known as a script, to generate expectations about the character's actions in the story as well as to make inferences about the actions of the characters which are not articulated in the text (Schank & Abelson, 1977). The reader incorporates the new information being read into a knowledge structure that integrates it with the information accessed from generic memory.

At the same time, relationships between propositions in the text are being evaluated on a local level so that they can be integrated into a microstructural representation of the discourse (Kintsch & van Dijk, 1978). One basic process here is in determining coreference. Comprehension of propositions as being coreferential involves multiple steps: (1) holding recently processed information in working memory, (2) using that information to predict what will be presented next, (3) processing new material for meaning, (4) searching for terms in the new material which match those currently in working memory, (5) matching the new terms with those already in working memory, and (6) integrating both terms when they match into the knowledge structure (e.g., Garrod & Sanford, 1977). Once a proposition has been incorporated into the mental representation, it is considered "old" or given information, and propositions that have not yet been integrated will be comprehended as "new" until they, too, are integrated. Thus integration of old and new information also occurs at the propositional level.

Working memory, as has been implied here, plays a crucial role in integration and therefore comprehension. It is thus important to determine whether the proposed deficits in working-memory capacity affect older adults' ability to perform the basic processes of integrating generic and new information on a global level and integrating related ideas across sentences at a local level. As the reader will see, these aspects of integration do not seem to show much qualitative impairment with age, although memory for specific material may be deficient.

Integration of generic knowledge with text information

The model of reading comprehension outlined here suggests that, on a global level, comprehension is based on the integration of stored world knowledge with specific text information. This has been shown in studies evaluating the role of expertise in particular knowledge domains and those investigating memory for scripts, which are more general domains.

Studies examining differences between how experts deal with texts in their areas of expertise and how novices deal with the same information show that experts recall more from such passages (e.g., Spilich, Vesonder, Chiesi, & Voss, 1979). They also expend more processing capacity while reading such passages because they activate their knowledge and use it to compare to the information they are currently acquiring (Britton & Tesser, 1982). Britton and Tesser also suggest that the activation of large amounts of knowledge occupies a relatively large amount of working-memory capacity, and the integration of that knowledge with new information helps reinforce the memorability of that information.

Scripts involve general areas of world knowledge. Scripts are generic representations of stereotypical series of actions, props, and roles used in activities engaged in frequently, such as eating out at a restaurant or going to the doctor (Schank & Abelson, 1977). When the comprehender hears or reads about a character going to a restaurant, the restaurant script is activated from long-term memory and entered into working memory. The comprehender uses the activated generic representation in understanding and predicting what particular actions are engaged in by the characters. In normal texts, not every action involved in a particular scripted activity is mentioned. It is therefore a requirement of comprehension that the comprehender make inferences about the occurrence of those actions. Apparently because of the generation of such inferences, readers often incorrectly "recall," or recognize falsely, scripted actions that are typical for a script but were never mentioned in a passage. They are also likely to remember actions that would be unusual for a script because of their novelty (Graesser, Gordon, & Sawyer, 1979). People utilize their knowledge in comprehension of and memory for a text by appending its specific new information to the generic knowledge structure evoked by the passage, creating a new knowledge structure which integrates new and old information.

If older adults have difficulties in integrating generic information with text information, we would expect age to interact with degree of prior knowledge in some domain. We assume that because accessing generic knowledge structures is automatic, older people should have no difficulty in retrieving what they already know. However, because they have less available processing capacity, they will be limited in how much they can integrate with the new information being studied. As a result, they may rely to a greater extent than younger adults on the generic representation. In experiments investigating knowledge domain, their recall should be especially poor in areas where they are more knowledgeable because of this reliance. In script memory studies, they should show higher false recognition rates for typical but new foils and poorer recognition rates for atypical script actions. They would also be expected to have more script-relevant intrusions in recall.

One study has examined knowledge domains and text memory in the elderly. Hultsch and Dixon (1983) examined recall of biographical sketches of figures rated to be well known to subjects of different ages, and to figures rated to be more familiar to particular cohorts of individuals. They found that younger adults recalled about the same number of propositions as older adults from the biography of the individual known to people of all ages. There were also no age differences in recall of the text about the "old" cohort-relevant figure, but young people recalled more from the passage about the "young" figure than did the old. This study suggests that older people benefit from world knowledge when text memory is tested. They had apparently been able to integrate what they knew with the specific text information they had read; otherwise they would have shown memory deficits under the conditions in which they could have applied their knowledge.

Other experiments have evaluated memory for scripts in young and older adults. Light and Anderson (1983, Experiment 2) tested memory for typical and atypical actions in a scripted narrative and found older adults to be less accurate overall, but not to differ from the young in terms of false recognitions of typical but new script actions, in recall intrusions of typical actions, or in recall of atypical actions. This pattern of findings suggests that older adults were no more likely than younger ones to utilize their generic knowledge when their memory of the scripts were tested. We therefore infer that they integrated their representation of the scripts with their knowledge of the basic scripts.

In an experiment from our laboratory, Zelinski and Miura (in press) examined the effects of a theme on script memory. We presented young and old subjects in one

Table 7.1. *Mean proportion correct recognitions of test items as "new" in the script memory study*

	Item types	
	Theme-consistent	Theme-inconsistent
No thematic background		
Young	.82	.65
Old	.48	.32
Marginal	.65	.49
Thematic background		
Young	.67	.91
Old	.44	.74
Marginal	.56	.83

Source: Zelinski and Miura (in press).

group with a thematic statement that could be used to infer motives of the protagonist in undergoing scripted actions. This statement had to do with the protagonist's suspicion that she was pregnant by one of her professors, and the scripts in which she engaged included going to the doctor, attending a lecture given by a professor, and going to a cocktail party at which the professor was present. Previous work by Owens, Bower, and Black (1979) had shown that subjects exposed to this thematic statement were more likely to recognize falsely statements that were consistent with the theme and less likely to recognize falsely statements that were inconsistent with the theme than those not presented with the theme. We found that young and older adults showed the same pattern of recognition of consistent and inconsistent theme statements as a function of experimental condition when memory was tested 24 hours after the material was studied, as seen in Table 7.1. We also found that older people did not differ from the young in false recognition of typical but new script actions. Cohen and Faulkner (1984) also reported that older adults did not differ from younger ones in the likelihood of erroneously selecting theme-relevant foils in a recognition test following the study of passages.

The results of both our own and Cohen and Faulkner's studies, like those of Light and Anderson, suggest that older adults integrate generic knowledge with specific text information in memory for prose similarly to younger adults. On the other hand, Hess and his colleagues (Hess, 1985; Hess, Donley, & Vandermas, 1986) found that older adults were less likely than young adults to correctly recognize old atypical than typical script actions. Older adults were also more likely to falsely recognize new typical and atypical script actions. The discrepancy in findings here may be due to the number of recognition items tested. In the studies showing no age differences in patterns of recognition, fewer items were tested than in Hess's studies. It is possible that older people made more errors in recognizing old and new statements because of interference among items, forcing them to rely to a greater extent on generic knowledge to respond to test items.

Another means of determining whether people use generic knowledge structures in comprehension and memory of discourse is to disrupt the organization of information in a story by ordering the story's statements randomly and to examine the extent to which recall is affected. There is evidence that stories generally follow a schema, which links statements according to their specific roles in the narrative (e.g., Mandler & Johnson, 1977). Narratives typically include causal sequences and information on the temporal ordering of events (e.g., Smith, 1985); such cues make narratives memorable (Nezworski, Stein, & Trabasso, 1982). When sequences are disrupted, memory for the story should be poor because people normally integrate their knowledge of story schemata with the specifics of the story studied. Thorndyke (1977) presented passages to young subjects with the sentences in normal or scrambled order. He found that recall was better with normal ordering and that subjects attempted to reconstitute correct ordering in their recall of the scrambled texts. This suggests that story schemata are so important to the creation of organized knowledge structures from passages that subjects attempt to integrate what they know about schemata with text information, even when there is no basis for it in the original material.

If older adults have difficulty integrating their generic knowledge of story organization with specific information from narratives, we would expect them to show no effects of organization on their recall. Smith, Rebok, Smith, Hall, and Alvin (1983) presented stories in several experimental conditions, including a normal story, and a scrambled story, where the sentences were randomly ordered. Recall was better in the normal story than scrambled story condition. There were no age differences in overall recall, and there were no age differences in the amount recalled or in the pattern of recall as a function of the roles or nodes of propositions in the story structure. This suggests that older adults benefit from organization in a story, just as younger ones do.

Mandel and Johnson (1984) used a similar approach to that of Smith et al. They presented normal and scrambled stories to young and old subjects, but preserved temporal ordering of information in the scrambled stories by inserting temporal phrases (e.g., Before this, ...) when the order of an event in the story was disrupted. There were no age differences in the number of nodes correctly recalled, and subjects were more accurate in the normal than scrambled story conditions. Age did not interact with organizational context. The inclusion of temporal information to assist subjects in organizing the order of events benefited the older adults in this study. In addition, subjects of all ages in the scrambled condition were likely to show distortions in recall, which suggested that they were attempting to reorder the events in a canonical fashion.

Thus, when story organization is disrupted, older adults show the same kinds of difficulties in recall as younger ones, indicating that they integrate story schemata with the particular material studied, just as younger adults do.

Taken together, research examining utilization of generic knowledge structures in memory for prose shows that older people can and do use existing knowledge structures in remembering discourse. They appear to have little difficulty in utilizing generic knowledge and integrating it with text information under a variety of memory paradigms, ranging from studies examining utilization of specific knowledge domains, memory for scripts, and the effects of disrupting the organization of stories.

Comprehension of discourse

As we have seen, older adults do not appear to be impaired at the global level of integrating generic knowledge with specific text information, which suggests that, contrary to the working-memory capacity deficit hypothesis, they do not have major comprehension problems in dealing with complex aspects of discourse. It would also suggest that older people do not have problems in the early aspects of integration, specifically, with local comprehension processes or text microprocesses.

However, this has not been clearly established. The studies that we have cited cannot localize to any extent where, in the course of comprehension, integration takes place, that is, whether it occurs during encoding or at retrieval. It is thus possible that the studies involving memory measures, which have inferred integration of newly acquired information with existing or newly created knowledge structures, were evaluating integration at retrieval only. The other problem is that memory studies confound remembering with comprehension, and memory deficits under particular conditions are assumed to reflect problems during integration. If older adults' basic problem in discourse memory is one of comprehension, we need to isolate comprehension processes as much as possible from memory. In order to approximate more closely whether older adults might be deficient in integration during input, we examined age differences in the relative speed of comprehending (and therefore integrating) pairs of coreferential sentences, a process that involves the local aspects of integration.

The experiments reported here examine age-related differences in the processes of matching new information with old information already in working memory. According to many theorists, the matching process is crucial to discourse comprehension (Garrod & Sanford, 1977) because it is the mechanism by which coreferential relationships between propositions are determined. Concepts based on words are stored in long-term memory in the form of networks of associations (e.g., Collins & Loftus, 1975). When words are read, there is an automatic activation of semantic information associated with those words. (Models of semantic activation and aging are discussed in greater detail in the chapters by Burke & Harrold and by Howard, this volume.) To determine whether the sentence being currently processed is related to material that has already been processed, its semantic representation is matched with previously processed information already in working memory, which may include anticipated information. When sufficient commonalities in representations are found for particular terms across sentences, they are comprehended as coreferential, and integration of the sentences or propositions containing those terms transforms them into a single representation of the information in working memory.

The time course of comprehension of propositions as coreferential varies as a function of the extensiveness of the search for common associations. Readers take less time to comprehend pairs of sentences as referring to each other if the antecedent term and its coreferent term are identical, as in (1a) and (1b),

(1a)   Ed was given an alligator for his birthday.
(1b)   The alligator was his favorite present.

than if the antecedent is a general term and the coreferent term is an exemplar for that term, as in (2a) and (2b),

(2a)   Ed was given lots of things for his birthday.
(2b)   The alligator was his favorite present.

(Haviland & Clark, 1974). Matching identical terms in coreferential sentence pairs is faster than matching category names with exemplars presumably because semantic activation is identical for identical terms when the sentence context indicates that they are coreferential. Matching is slower for related nonidentical terms such as category names and exemplars because semantic activation differs across terms, and this requires searching through activated nodes and finding common associations before the terms are matched in working memory and comprehended to be coreferents.

If older adults have less available working memory capacity, we would expect age to interact with condition on reading time, with greater slowing for older adults occurring when matching becomes more complex, because the greater demands of matching information burden working memory.

The work we describe here evaluates comprehension rather than memory (although comprehension presumes memory operations). The experimental paradigm used involves examining reading times of sentences with various matching requirements by young (age 20–37), young-old (age 55–69), and old-old (age 70–87) subjects, all of whom have had at least some college education. In all the experiments we describe here, the sentences remained on the screen of a microcomputer during the reading and question-answering phases of each trial, to reduce the likelihood that older adults would show differences in reading times and error rates in question-answering because of memory deficits. We do not present error data in this chapter because, in general, error rates did not vary with age.

In our first experiment (Zelinski & Miura, 1986), we studied the effects of matching identical or related antecedent and coreferent terms in sentence pairs. Half of the 64 sentence pairs were presented with category-exemplar terms, half with identical terms. To ensure that subjects were actually reading the sentence pairs, they were given a yes/no question about material in either or both of the sentences to answer. Examples of the stimuli follow:

(3a)   The zoo bought an alligator for its collection.
(3b)   The alligator was shipped from the swamps last week. (Identical)

(4a)   We donated an appliance to our church.
(4b)   The refrigerator will be much appreciated there. (Related)

Subjects read each sentence on a microcomputer at their own pace by pressing keys to summon each sentence and the test question. Both sentences in the pair and the question were visible until after the question was answered with a key press, when the computer screen was cleared. Reading times for each sentence were measured.

Table 7.2. *Mean target sentence reading times (msec) in the first comprehension study*

Age group	Identical terms	Related terms
Young	2762 (900)[a]	2893 (1242)
Young-old	3018 (836)	3255 (966)
Old-old	3184 (1189)	3621 (1426)
Marginal	2958 (996)	3256 (1245)

[a]Standard deviations in parentheses.

Results showed no reliable age differences in reading times for the target (second sentence). As seen in Table 7.2, targets of identical-term sentence pairs were read more quickly than those of related-term pairs. There was no reliable interaction of age with condition.

The findings of this experiment indicate that older adults had no difficulty in performing the matching of coreferential terms from the two sentences. All subjects needed more time to comprehend the sentences with related terms, suggesting that the matching process was relatively more difficult in that condition than in the identical-terms condition. The fact that age did not interact with condition indicates further that older people had no difficulty matching either the identical or the related terms in working memory.

These results therefore suggest that older adults had no difficulty comprehending the sentence pairs in either condition relative to the young, which is contrary to the working-memory deficit hypothesis. However, it can be argued that the related-term condition did not burden working memory in the older adults, and hence it did not differentially increase their reading times relative to the identical-term condition. We conducted a second experiment involving more complex matching requirements to determine if this was true.

In our second experiment (Zelinski & Miura, submitted), we examined effects of the generality of the antecedent term and of the typicality of information on comprehension. Readers have more difficulty comprehending coreferential sentences if the antecedent term is general, such as a category name, and its coreferent term is specific, such as a category exemplar, as in (5a) and (5b),

(5a)   Some money lay in the middle of the sidewalk.
(5b)   The dollar was picked up by the elderly man.

than if the terms are presented in the reverse order, as in (6a) and (6b),

(6a)   A dollar lay in the middle of the sidewalk.
(6b)   The money was picked up by the elderly man.

(Garrod & Sanford, 1977). Matching a specific coreferent exemplar term to a general antecedent that is its category name is relatively slow because it is more difficult to predict what the exemplar will be, given the generality of the antecedent; prediction of the particular category in a sentence pair is easy when the antecedent is an exemplar of that category. Within the context of the antecedent sentence, matching is slower when the antecedent is general because it has many more potential associations with exemplars activated in working memory than does the coreferent, and thus a more thorough search for overlapping associations must be conducted than when mapping a general coreferent term onto a specific antecedent.

Matching of strongly related coreferents should be easier than matching of weakly related ones because the associative networks of strongly related referents are more similar and therefore rapidly matched. They are also more predictable because of their strong associations. Garrod and Sanford (1977) found that highly typical category-exemplar referents in sentence pairs were comprehended faster than relatively atypical referents.

The paradigm used in the first experiment was repeated here. Conditions for the 64 sentence pairs were crossed with generality of the antecedent and typicality of the exemplar. Fact and inference comprehension questions were equally distributed within sentence conditions. An example of a specific-typical sentence pair is given in (7a) and (7b). An example of a general-typical pair follows in (8a) and (8b).

(7a)   A spoon fell to the floor with a clatter.
(7b)   The utensil was slightly nicked in several places.

(8a)   A flower won first prize in its category.
(8b)   The daffodil was the biggest of its kind.

Analysis of target sentence reading times revealed reliable age differences, as seen in Table 7.3, with the young reading more quickly than the young-old and the old-old, who did not differ from each other. Targets of general antecedent sentences were read more slowly than targets of specific antecedents. However, the typicality effect was not reliable, and no interactions were significant. Roth and Shoben (1983) also found no effects of the typicality of antecedent–anaphor terms and have suggested that the context of the antecedent sentence has a much stronger effect than typicality per se on reading times because context serves to limit the spread of activation to plausible associations in semantic memory.

The major finding of this experiment is that although older people apparently needed more time to process the target sentence than the young, the matching processes in working memory tested here appeared to be unimpaired with age. All age groups were sensitive to the treatment, and all showed that the sentences were integrated in working memory before the question was answered. This experiment thus replicates the findings of the first one: Older adults had no difficulty in comprehending the antecedent-coreferent relations presented.

Our first two experiments indicate that older adults are not impaired in comprehension of coreferential sentences under two sets of conditions that require increasingly more complex matching. This does not support the working-memory deficit hypothesis predictions of age interaction with matching requirements. We made a third test of this hypothesis by increasing the number of sentences between the antecedent and target, to determine whether this increase would burden working memory in older adults and produce an interaction of age with the number of intervening sentences.

Table 7.3. *Mean target sentence reading times (msec) in the second comprehension study*

Age group	Specific term		General term	
	Typical	Atypical	Typical	Atypical
Young	2552 (785)[a]	2521 (720)	2578 (730)	2675 (810)
Young-old	3242 (788)	3233 (929)	3388 (970)	3478 (1093)
Old-old	3512 (1352)	3623 (1384)	3670 (1354)	3951 (1548)
Marginal	3102 (1077)	3126 (1131)	3212 (1135)	3368 (1287)

[a]Standard deviations in parentheses.

In the third experiment (Zelinski & Anthony, 1987), we examined the effects of interpolating sentences that foreground the antecedent terms in coreferent sentence pairs on comprehension. *Foregrounding* presupposes that information in a currently read sentence refers to something already in working memory, as in a story where all sentences refer to the same theme (e.g., Lesgold, Roth, & Curtis, 1979). Glanzer and his colleagues (Glanzer, Fischer, & Dorfman, 1984) found a decrease in the reading time of targets with an increasing number of interpolated foregrounded sentences. This suggests that the number of references to the antecedent increases anticipation of the target coreferent material, thereby reducing target reading time. In this experiment, we varied the number of interpolated sentences so that there were zero, two, or four intervening statements between the antecedent and anaphor. All interpolated sentences foregrounded the antecedent. There were 20 antecedent-anaphor pairs in which an exemplar served as antecedent and the category name as the anaphor in each of the interpolated sentences conditions. Examples of the sentence sets follow:

(9a) A dollar lay in the middle of the sidewalk.
(9b) The money was picked up by the elderly man.

(10a) A dollar lay in the middle of the sidewalk.
(10b) It had fallen from a woman's change purse.
(10c) It was finally noticed by someone walking by.
(10d) The money was picked up by the elderly man.

(11a) A dollar lay in the middle of the sidewalk.
(11b) It had fallen from a woman's change purse.
(11c) It was blown by a gust of wind.
(11d) It landed on the pavement by a newsstand.
(11e) It was finally noticed by someone walking by.
(11f) The money was picked up by the elderly man.

As in the previous experiments, subjects read the sentences, which were presented individually, at their own pace. All sentences in a set were visible on the screen until a comprehension question requiring a fact or inference response had been answered.

Results showed no reliable age differences in reading times for the target sentence. As seen in Table 7.4, the condition effect was reliable, with reductions in reading

Table 7.4. *Mean target sentence reading times (msec) in the third comprehension study*

Age group	Number of sentences between the antecedent and target		
	Zero	Two	Four
Young	2609 (724)[a]	2410 (574)	2397 (608)
Young-old	3019 (1249)	2858 (981)	2829 (1117)
Old-old	2777 (888)	2952 (881)	2659 (816)
Marginal	2802 (977)	2740 (851)	2629 (876)

[a]Standard deviations in parentheses.

times occurring as a function of an increase in the number of interpolated sentences. There was no interaction of age and condition.

This experiment shows that the older people read the target sentences somewhat more slowly than younger ones, but not reliably so. This finding suggests that they had no difficulty in performing the matching of coreferential terms under the conditions studied. All subjects showed facilitation effects in reading the targets as a function of the number of intervening sentences. The fact that age did not interact with condition indicates further that older people were as likely to be primed by the foregrounding of the antecedent as younger ones were.

The three experiments on reading times reported here show no age differences in the pattern of reading times as a function of manipulations used to vary the requirements for matching information in working memory, regardless of whether matches were based on identical versus related terms, whether antecedents were general or specific, or whether two or four sentences foregrounding the antecedent intervened. This indicates that even the very elderly do not appear to be deficient in the processes of integration required for comprehension, as measured in these experiments. Work by Light and Capps (1986) also corroborates these findings: As long as the topics of sentences were foregrounded, older adults were as adept as younger ones in correctly assigning ambiguous pronouns as the coreferential terms. However, when the topics were not foregrounded because of a topic change, older adults had more difficulty. It is therefore likely that as long as the relevant coreferential terms are available in working memory, integration occurs in old adults.

Another finding of these experiments is that in the first and third experiments, the two elderly groups were slower than the young group in reading times, but not reliably so. It is likely that the absence of age differences in target reading times is due to the wide range of variability on this measure. Nevertheless, it suggests that older people do not need significantly more time than younger ones to comprehend what they are reading, at least with the syntactically simple sentences used here. We must also keep in mind that the older subjects in our experiments are all highly educated as compared to their peers, and very likely active readers, thus maintaining their skills; thus these findings may not generalize to other populations of older people.

Do older adults show deficits in integrating information from discourse?

We are now in a position to evaluate whether older people use operations in comprehension and memory for discourse in a way that is similar to or different from what has been inferred about younger adults. The literature reviewed here suggests that older people behave very much like young adults when they are required to access existing knowledge structures. At the level of determining relationships between individual propositions, older people show no impairment in the kinds of on-line processing used to match and integrate coreferential sentences. It is thus clear that older people can and do integrate new information they are encountering in discourse with what they already know. The fact that they do not differ qualitatively from younger adults in dealing with this aspect of language processing is encouraging, as it suggests no serious decline in dealing with the complexities of language, even though there are concomitant age-related deficits after age 67 in many aspects of intellectual functioning (Schaie, 1979).

There are several implications of our findings for theories of working-memory capacity deficits in older adults. We found no evidence that capacity problems cause difficulties in integration of generic knowledge with text material, or in integration of coreferential sentences. This suggests two possibilities: The first is that older adults do not have a deficit in capacity. On this argument, we observe that there is growing evidence that despite individual differences, there are no across-the-board age deficits in capacity, as measured by Daneman and Carpenter's (1980) reading span index (Hartley, 1986; but see Light & Anderson, 1985). There is also some discontent with the circularity with which the capacity deficit model has been invoked, as it has been argued that memory deficits are due to capacity deficits, and that capacity deficits can be measured by memory deficits (cf. Salthouse, in press). Despite these problems with the capacity construct, there is evidence from the literature on inferential reasoning (Zacks & Hasher, this volume) and memory for prose (Cohen, this volume) that a capacity deficit is currently the most adequate explanation for age differences in performance.

The second possibility is that older people do have a capacity deficit which may contribute to problems in comprehension and memory (Cohen, this volume; Light & Capps, 1986; Zacks & Hasher, this volume). However, the component processes underlying comprehension and integration of information may rely less on working-memory capacity than previously assumed. If this is the case, the matching processes in coreference when material is foregrounded may require so little capacity that older adults are not burdened excessively. The use of an independent index of on-line capacity would be required to confirm this, and we are currently conducting research along these lines.

Finally, even though we have suggested that older people show no differences in integration processes as compared to the young, there are, nevertheless, differences in how efficiently older adults use language, and the difficulties appear to center around memory problems. For example, in many cases, they recall less even though they are affected by treatment effects in the same way as younger adults, and this finding has been used to suggest the existence of age-related deficits in language comprehension (see the chapters by Emery and by Kemper on this point). Whether comprehension processes other than integration are impaired when the memory requirements of language tasks are reduced as in our experiments, remains to be seen, however.

Where does this leave us? In general, we see that older adults, even when they remember less than younger ones, do not show qualitative differences in the integration of information from discourse. More sophisticated analyses of the components of reading comprehension and their interaction may provide us with further information about how aging affects adults' ability to understand what they read.

References

Abbott, V., Black, J. B., & Smith, E. E. (1985). The representation of scripts in memory. *Journal of Memory and Language*, *24*, 179–199.

Baddeley, A., & Hitch, G. (1974). Working memory. In G. H. Bower (Ed.), *The psychology of learning and motivation* (Vol. 8, pp. 47–89). New York: Academic Press.

Bransford, J. D., & Johnson, M. K. (1972). Contextual prerequisites for understanding: Some investigations of comprehension and recall. *Journal of Verbal Learning and Verbal Behavior*, *11*, 717–726.

Britton, B. K., & Tesser, A. (1982). Effects of prior knowledge on use of cognitive capacity in three complex cognitive tasks. *Journal of Verbal Learning and Verbal Behavior*, *21*, 421–436.

Cohen, G., & Faulkner, D. (1984). Memory for text: Some age differences in the nature of information that is retained after listening to texts. In H. Bouma & D. G. Bowhuis (Eds.), *Attention and performance X: Control of language processes* (pp. 501–514). Hillsdale, NJ: Erlbaum.

Collins, A. M., & Loftus, E. F. (1975). A spreading-activation theory of semantic processing. *Psychological Review*, *82*, 407–429.

Daneman, M., & Carpenter, P. A. (1980). Individual differences in working memory and reading. *Journal of Verbal Learning and Verbal Behavior*, *19*, 450–466.

Garrod, S., & Sanford, A. J. (1977). Interpreting anaphoric relations: The integration of semantic information while reading. *Journal of Verbal Learning and Verbal Behavior*, *16*, 77–90.

Glanzer, M., Fischer, B., & Dorfman, D. (1984). Short-term storage in reading. *Journal of Verbal Learning and Verbal Behavior*, *23*, 467–486.

Graesser, A. C., Gordon, S. E., & Sawyer, J. D. (1979). Memory for typical and atypical actions in scripted activities: Test of a script pointer + tag hypothesis. *Journal of Verbal Learning and Verbal Behavior*, *18*, 319–332.

Hartley, J. T. (1986). Reader and text variables as determinants of discourse memory in adulthood. *Psychology and Aging*, *1*, 150–158.

Haviland, S. E., & Clark, H. H. (1974). What's new? Acquiring new information as a process in comprehension. *Journal of Verbal Learning and Verbal Behavior*, *13*, 512–521.

Hess, T. M. (1985). Aging and context influences on recognition memory for typical and atypical script actions. *Developmental Psychology*, *21*, 1139–1151.

Hess, T. M., Donley, J., & Vandermas, M. O. *Aging-related changes in the processing and retention of script information*. Manuscript submitted for publication.

Hultsch, D. F., & Dixon, R. A. (1983). The role of pre-experimental knowledge in text processing in adulthood. *Experimental Aging Research*, *9*, 17–22.

Hultsch, D. F., & Dixon, R. A. (1984). Memory for text materials in adulthood. In P. B. Baltes & O. G. Brim (Eds.), *Life-span development and behavior* (Vol. 6, pp. 77–108). New York: Academic Press.

Kintsch, W., & van Dijk, T. A. (1978). Toward a model of text comprehension and production. *Psychological Review, 85*, 363–394.

Lesgold, A. M., Roth, S. F., & Curtis, M. E. (1979). Foregrounding effects in discourse comprehension. *Journal of Verbal Learning and Verbal Behavior, 18*, 291–308.

Light, L. L., & Anderson, P. A. (1983). Memory for scripts in young and older adults. *Memory & Cognition, 11*, 435–444.

Light, L. L., & Anderson, P. A. (1985). Working-memory capacity, age, and memory for discourse. *Journal of Gerontology, 40*, 737–747.

Light, L. L., & Capps, J. L. (1986). Comprehension of pronouns in young and older adults. *Developmental Psychology, 22*, 580–585.

Lorch, R. F., Lorch, E. P., & Matthews, P. D. (1985). On-line processing of the topic structure of a text. *Journal of Memory and Language, 24*, 350–362.

Malt, B. C. (1985). The role of discourse structure in understanding anaphora. *Journal of Memory and Language, 24*, 271–289.

Mandel, R. G., & Johnson, N. S. (1984). A developmental analysis of story recall and comprehension in adulthood. *Journal of Verbal Learning and Verbal Behavior, 23*, 643–659.

Mandler, J. M., & Johnson, N. S. (1977). Remembrance of things parsed: Story structure and recall. *Cognitive Psychology, 9*, 111–151.

Meyer, B. J. F. (in press). Reading comprehension and aging. In K. W. Schaie (Ed.), *Annual review of gerontology and geriatrics* (Vol. 7). New York: Springer.

Meyer, B. J. F., & Rice, G. E. (1983). Learning and memory from text across the adult life span. In J. Fine & R. O. Freedle (Eds.), *Developmental issues in discourse* (pp. 294–306). Norwood, NJ: Ablex.

Meyer, B. J. F., & Rice, G. E. (in press). Prose processing in adulthood: The text, the learner, and the task. In L. W. Poon, D. Rubin, & B. Wilson (Eds.), *Everyday cognition in adulthood and old age*. Cambridge: Cambridge University Press.

Morrow, D. G. (1985). Prominent characters and events organize narrative understanding. *Journal of Memory and Language, 24*, 304–319.

Nezworski, T., Stein, N. L., & Trabasso, T. (1982). Story structure versus content in children's recall. *Journal of Verbal Learning and Verbal Behavior, 21*, 196–206.

Owens, J., Bower, G. H., & Black, J. B. (1979). The "soap opera" effect in story recall. *Memory & Cognition, 7*, 185–191.

Reiser, B. J., & Black, J. B. (1982). Processing and structural models of comprehension. *Text, 2*, 225–252.

Roth, E. H., & Shoben, E. J. (1983). The effect of context on the structure of categories. *Cognitive Psychology, 15*, 346–378.

Salthouse, T. A. (in press). The role of processing resources in cognitive aging. In M. L. Howe & C. Brainerd (Eds.), *Cognitive development in adulthood*. New York: Springer-Verlag.

Sanford, A. J., & Garrod, S. C. (1981) *Understanding written language*. New York: Wiley.

Schaie, K. W. (1979). The primary mental abilities in adulthood: An exploration in the development of psychometric intelligence. In P. B. Baltes & O. G. Brim (Eds.), *Life-span development and behavior* (Vol. 3, pp. 68–115). New York: Academic Press.

Schank, R. C., & Abelson, R. P. (1977). *Scripts, plans, goals, and understanding*. Hillsdale, NJ: Erlbaum.

Smith, E. L. (1985). Text type and discourse framework. *Text, 5*, 229–247.

Smith, S. W., Rebok, G. W., Smith, W. R., Hall, S. E., & Alvin, M. (1983). Adult age differences in the use of story structure in delayed free recall. *Experimental Aging Research, 9*, 191–195.

Spilich, G. J., Vesonder, G. T., Chiesi, H. L., & Voss, J. F. (1979). Text processing of domain related information for individuals with high and low domain knowledge. *Journal of Verbal Learning and Verbal Behavior, 18*, 275–290.

Thorndyke, P. (1977). Cognitive structures in comprehension and memory of narrative discourse. *Cognitive Psychology*, *9*, 77–110.

Zelinski, E. M., & Anthony, C. R. (1987). *Foregrounding and backgrounding effects on anaphor comprehension in the elderly*. Manuscript submitted for publication.

Zelinski, E. M., & Gilewski, M. J. (in press). Memory for prose and aging: A meta-analysis. In M. L. Howe & C. Brainerd (Eds.), *Cognitive development in adulthood*. New York: Springer-Verlag.

Zelinski, E. M., & Miura, S. A. (1987). *Anaphor comprehension in young and old adults*. Manuscript submitted for publication.

Zelinski, E. M., & Miura, S. A. (in press). Context effects on script memory in young and old adults. *Psychology and Aging*.

8 Comprehension of pragmatic implications in young and older adults

Leah L. Light and Shirley A. Albertson

It is well known that memory declines with advancing age. However, the reasons for this impairment in memory are not understood (Burke & Light, 1981). One explanation that has gained currency is that older adults do not process the meaning of new information as effectively as young adults because of reduced processing resources or attentional capacity (e.g., Cohen, 1979, 1981; Craik & Byrd, 1982; Craik & Rabinowitz, 1984; Eysenck, 1974; Hasher & Zacks, 1979; Perlmutter, 1978; Simon, 1979; Till & Walsh, 1980). This explanation presupposes that there are age-related differences in comprehension of word meanings. The bulk of the research in this area has not, however, produced results in accordance with this position (see Light, 1988, for a review). For instance, there is little evidence for age-related declines in vocabulary (Schaie, 1980). The organization of meanings in semantic memory, as indexed by responses on word association tasks, appears to be stable in adulthood (e.g., Burke & Peters, 1986; Howard, 1980). Also, studies of semantic priming in lexical decision tasks find no qualitative differences in the nature of activation of meanings in semantic memory (e.g., Burke & Yee, 1984; Howard, this volume).

Despite these negative findings, there has been a recent spate of suggestions that older adults may experience language comprehension problems (see Burke and Light, 1981; Hartley, Harker, and Walsh, 1980; Hultsch and Dixon, 1984; and Salthouse, 1982, for reviews). For instance, in her discussion of language comprehension in old age, Cohen (1979) said that "the popular belief that language ability is well preserved in old age is illfounded and overdue for revision" (p. 413). Craik and Byrd (1982) have offered the hypothesis that the quality of encoding of new material – which certainly constitutes an area of language use – may suffer in old age. More specifically, they suggest that "older subjects' encodings will contain less associative and inferential information" and that "an encoded event is less modified by the specific context in which it occurs for the older person" (p. 208). And, in this volume, Zacks and Hasher argue that older adults are less likely to make inferences, even very simple ones, than young adults.

In this chapter we review evidence, from our own research as well as that of

Preparation of this chapter was supported by National Institute on Aging Grant 2 R01 AG02452. The authors thank Deborah M. Burke and Timothy A. Salthouse for comments on an earlier version.

133

others, that suggests that these claims are too broad and need to be qualified. We present evidence that older adults draw inferences as well as younger adults and that the two age groups are both highly sensitive to context in language comprehension so long as working memory is not strained. However, when working-memory capacity is taxed, older adults exhibit problems in drawing inferences which are due either to forgetting of information essential for making the inference, or to problems in manipulating information in working memory. Finally, we relate these findings to current theories of memory and aging which suggest that problems in language comprehension underlie problems in memory in old age.

Two kinds of implication, logical and pragmatic, have been studied. We speak of logical implication when an utterance necessarily implies some information and of pragmatic implication (or invited inference) when an utterance leads the hearer or reader to expect something that is neither explicitly stated nor logically implied, but which nevertheless seems likely on the basis of prior experience or general world knowledge (Geis & Zwicky, 1971; Harris & Monaco, 1978). It has been proposed that one consequence of reduced attentional capacity for natural language understanding is less efficient integration of new information with previously stored general world knowledge. Integration of new information with prior knowledge is fundamental to discourse comprehension. Readers and listeners generally assume that they share the same world knowledge as writers or speakers and expect to be able to interpret what they read or hear in the light of this knowledge (Brown & Yule, 1983; Clark & Marshall, 1981). Therefore, problems in the use of general world knowledge in older adults would be expected to lead to difficulties in comprehension.

A number of investigators have reported that older adults have difficulty in drawing both logical and pragmatic inferences from discourse. Thus, Cohen (1981, Experiment 1) and Light, Zelinski, and Moore (1982) have found that older adults are less likely to draw logical inferences than young adults when integration of information from several sources is required, especially when memory load is high, because the information necessary for making the inference must be retrieved from memory and/or because the order in which information is presented is not optimal for integration.

Results from studies of pragmatic implication have been mixed. The studies that have reported age-related differences in pragmatic implication have, by and large, measured retention rather than comprehension (Cohen, 1979, 1981; Till, 1985; Till & Walsh, 1980). For instance, Cohen (1981, Experiment 2) found that when tested after reading a series of short passages, older adults were less likely than young adults to infer (1c) from (1a) and (1b).

(1a) A burning cigarette was carelessly discarded.
(1b) The fire destroyed many acres of virgin forest.
(1c) A discarded cigarette started a fire.

Similarly, Cohen (1979, Experiment 2) reported that older adults were less apt to detect anomalies when brief passages contained statements that contradict general world knowledge (e.g., that a housewife who had no bread made sandwiches).

In this study, subjects heard short passages and responded after each. Hence it is possible that failure to detect anomaly resulted from failure to remember explicitly stated information (e.g., that there was no bread) rather than from accessing or using pragmatic information in long-term memory. Till and Walsh (1980) presented young and older adults with sentences such as *The chauffeur drove on the left side* and tested memory by free recall or by recall cued with nouns (here *England*) that referred to information pragmatically implied by the sentences. Young adults were better able to use the cues than older adults except when subjects were required to provide continuations for the sentences during presentation. This result suggests that older adults do not spontaneously use pragmatic information during sentence comprehension. However, Till and Walsh's choice of cued recall as a test of retention is not optimal for drawing conclusions about the use of pragmatic information during comprehension because cued recall may tap primarily retrieval processes rather than comprehension processes (McKoon & Ratcliff, 1980). The same objection may be made to Till's (1985) use of questions to tap memory for implications.

When comprehension is examined more directly, the evidence suggests that age differences in ability to use pragmatic information are negligible. Thus, Belmore (1981) found no age differences in accuracy of answers to questions requiring integration of new information with previously stored general world knowledge when prose passages had just been viewed; however, older adults were less able than young ones to answer such questions correctly after a delay. Burke and Yee (1984) observed similar priming effects for young and older adults in a lexical decision task when the target was pragmatically implied by the preceding sentence context. In a related vein, although memory rather than comprehension was studied, Hess and Arnould (1986) found that young and older adults were equally likely to falsely recognize instruments such as *broom* after reading sentences such as *She had swept the garage floor that morning,* suggesting similar encoding of implied information. Finally, Light and Anderson (1983) found no evidence of age-related differences in reliance on knowledge of routine stereotypical action sequences or *scripts* in re-membering stories about daily activities. Taken together, these results suggest that activation of pragmatic information in semantic memory proceeds in the same way regardless of age.

In what follows we present new evidence from several paradigms which converges on the conclusion that age differences in the use of pragmatic information are vir-tually nonexistent unless working memory is taxed by use of sentences that require considerable mental gymnastics if they are to be comprehended or by presentation of material irrelevant to the task at hand. These points will be clarified as we discuss each area of research.

Comparison of logical and pragmatic inferences in young and older adults

Together with Janet Capps, we investigated the question of whether young and older adults differ in their understanding of sentences carrying logical and pragmatic implications. No explicit comparison of possible age differences in these two types of implication had been undertaken previously. Harris and Monaco (1978) have suggested that comprehension of sentences carrying logical implications such as (2a) requires one to make the inference in (2b), whereas comprehension of sentences carrying pragmatic implications such as (3a) does not force one to make the inference in (3b).

(2a) Neil was forced to fly the plane.
(2b) Neil flew the plane.
(3a) Bob was able to climb the ladder.
(3b) Bob climbed the ladder.

Making pragmatic inferences that reflect shared common experience about the way in which the world works would thus seem to involve more complex semantic analyses than making logical inferences although both depend on understanding of word meanings. On this view, proponents of the processing resource hypothesis, who argue that older adults do not process the meaning of new information as effectively as young adults because of reduced processing resources or attentional capacity, might predict that older adults would be less likely to make pragmatic inferences than young adults and further that age differences in the rate of making inferences should be greater for pragmatic than for logical inferences. On the other hand, the evidence reviewed above suggests that old and young adults should be equally likely to make inferences of either type when comprehension rather than retention is measured.

The task we used was borrowed from Harris (1974), who studied comprehension of *S-complement verbs*, that is, verbs that take underlying sentences as their objects. S-complement verbs come in a variety of types. Some carry logical implications about the truth status of their sentential complements regardless of whether the verb is expressed in the affirmative or in the negative. For instance, *Harrison was sick* follows logically from either *Bill realized that Harrison was sick* or *Bill did not realize that Harrison was sick*. Other S-complement verbs carry only pragmatic implications about the truth value of their complements. For instance, *Terry believed that Robert was strong* invites the inference that *Robert was strong* (why else would Terry hold this belief?) but does not logically require it; its truth status is indeterminate. In the case of yet other classes of S-complement verbs, whether the truth or falsity of the complement is logically implied depends on whether the main verb is affirmative or negative. Contrast *Neil was forced to fly the plane*, which logically implies that *Neil flew the plane*, with *Neil was not forced to fly the plane*, which is indeterminate in truth status.

The subjects in this study were 32 young adults (mean age, 25.19; range, 20–36) and 32 older adults (mean age, 72.56; range, 58–82), all highly educated and high in verbal ability. They saw pairs of sentences such as *Neil was forced to fly the plane. Neil flew the plane.* on a computer monitor and decided whether the second sentence in the pair was true, false, or indeterminate in truth value, given the first sentence of the pair. Of the test pairs, 18 involved sentences that carried logical implications and 10 involved sentences with verbs that invited inferences. In order to follow up an informal observation made by Cohen (1979), that older adults experience particular

Table 8.1. *Proportion of correct inferences, incorrect inferences, and indeterminate responses as a function of inference type and age*

| | Logical inferences | | |
	Correct inference	Incorrect inference	Indeterminate
Young	.87	.10	.03
Old	.84	.11	.05
	Pragmatic inferences		
	Correct inference	Incorrect inference	Indeterminate
Young	.35	.12	.53
Old	.47	.21	.33

difficulty when drawing inferences from negative premises, we also varied whether the verbs in the main and complement clauses were stated in the affirmative or in the negative. Four patterns of affirmation–negation (+ +, + −, − +, and − −) were crossed with seven verb types to produce the 28 sentence pairs seen by each subject.

It is clear from Table 8.1 that there were no reliable age differences on the logical inferences either in the proportion of times that subjects made the correct inferences or in the proportion of "indeterminate" responses. On the other hand, there was a different pattern for the invited inferences. Older adults were reliably more likely to make both correct and incorrect pragmatic inferences and were less likely to respond "indeterminate." Note that age differences in the rate of indeterminate responses to sentences carrying pragmatic implications cannot be attributed to differences in response bias or cautiousness because the two age groups were nearly identical in their proportion of indeterminate responses to sentences carrying logical implications.

To obtain a more detailed picture of the results, we examined the distribution of true, false, and indeterminate responses for young and older adults for each of the 28 sentence types used in this study (seven verb types crossed with four patterns of affirmation–negation). We want to make three points about these analyses. First, overall the pattern of responses was quite similar across ages. Second, members of both age groups experienced difficulty when there were negatives in both the main and complement clauses and when the verbs involved were lexically negative. Young and older adults were alike in responding "true" to sentences with double negatives containing *Negative Implicative* verbs such as *fail, avoid, forget to, refrain from,* although the logically correct response here is "false"; the proportions of "true" responses were .60 for the young and .78 for the old. A similar situation arose for *Negative If* verbs such as *prevent, keep from, exclude, be impossible for.* In this instance, both young and older adults were likely to respond "true" for sentences having a − − pattern of affirmation–negation although Karttunen's analysis (1970) suggests that people should respond "false" to the invited inference in sentences such as *Wally was not prevented from not finishing his work.* The proportion of "true" responses for sentences of this type was .34 for the young and .69 for the old, a reliable difference. Harris (1974) who also observed this pattern of responding, suggested that the double negative is especially difficult to deal with for lexically negative verbs and that subjects may use a "two negatives make a positive" heuristic in such situations. Our results indicate that older adults may be more likely to use this strategy than young adults, when they encounter such verbs.

Third, there were only three cases out of 28, all involving pragmatic implication, in which the responses of older adults were distributed reliably differently from those of young adults. One was the just-mentioned case of Negative If verbs with double negatives. The remaining two cases involved *Nonfactive* verbs such as *say, believe, answer, claim* (Kiparsky & Kiparsky, 1970); here the older adults were more likely to make invited inferences than the young for + + and − − patterns of affirmation–negation in the main and complement clauses. For the + + sentences, pragmatic inferences were made .31 of the time by the young and .58 of the time by the old. For − − sentences, these proportions were .09 and .31 for young and old, respectively.

These results offer no support for the processing resource hypothesis which predicts that older adults, because they access general world knowledge less readily than the young, ought to make fewer pragmatic inferences. Given the distribution of responses across age, we prefer to interpret the data as evidence that older adults have difficulty in understanding sentences that rely on general world knowledge *only* when it is also necessary to engage in problem solving activity during comprehension – for instance, when sentences with double negatives and lexically negative verbs must be coped with. Such sentences are not likely to be encountered in either written or spoken discourse; thus understanding sentences that carry implications should pose few problems for older adults in their daily lives.

Use of pragmatic information in establishing coreference

Cohen (1979) found that older adults made more errors of coreference than younger adults when they recalled stories. That is, older adults attributed characteristics or actions to the wrong protagonists in the story and failed to specify adequately the antecedents of pronouns. This finding suggests that older adults may have difficulty in understanding anaphoric devices such as pronouns and noun phrases that refer to concepts that have been introduced previously in a discourse. Comprehension of anaphoric devices is important for establishing discourse coherence, that is, in determining the relation between what has been said before and what is being said now (Lesgold, 1972). Any problems that older adults may experience in determining coreference could thus contribute to comprehension failure and lack of integration of material, with subsequent forgetting a natural outcome of problems in initial understanding. We have investigated possible age differences in ability to use general world knowledge to determine coreference in a series of studies dealing with determination of the antecedents of ambiguous pronouns and noun phrases.

We first consider how young and older adults deal with pronouns. Consider the sentence fragments in (4a) and (4b):

(4a)   John apologized to Bill because he...
(4b)   John blamed Bill because he...

These fragments contain verbs which have a property that Garvey and Caramazza (1974), following Chafe (1972), call "implicit causality." Although the pronoun *he* is referentially ambiguous in these fragments because both John and Bill are masculine and singular and so agree in gender and number with *he*, we expect continuations which, in the case of *apologize,* assign the pronoun to John – that is, to the first noun – and to Bill – the second noun – in the case of *blame,* as in (4c) and (4d):

(4c)   John apologized to Bill because he stepped on his foot.
(4d)   John blamed Bill because he forgot to put the cat out.

Note that continuations that violate this expectation and assign the pronoun differently are possible in each case, as in (4e) and (4f):

(4e)   John apologized to Bill because he was so upset at the criticism.
(4f)   John blamed Bill because he was afraid he'd be accused himself.

Pragmatic considerations are very important here. Ehrlich (1980) has analyzed the sentence frame *John blamed Bill because he* . . . in the following way: "At some time, Bill does something which is probably bad. This action is a reason for John to say something to someone about Bill's action, at some later time" (p. 248).

Grober, Beardsley, and Caramazza (1978) found that when people were asked to complete sentence fragments such as these with a motive or reason appropriate to the action in the first part of the sentence, completions tended to be consistent with the implicit causality of the verb. However, when the connective *but* was used in place of *because,* the outcome was different. The completions given with *but* indicated that the pronoun had been assigned to the subject noun in the stem regardless of whether the verb biased the first noun (NP1 verbs) or the second noun (NP2 verbs). The connective *because* encourages continuations that explain the action referred to by the verb, while *but* invokes "a statement of what has happened which usually is the opposite of what might be expected on the basis of the behavior described in the main clause" (Grober et al., 1978, p. 124).

Note that assignment of the pronoun to the subject noun in the stem of the fragment is what would be expected if people simply use the strategy of assigning the pronoun to the first-mentioned individual in the stem who is likely to be the topic of the sentence. Choosing the subject is a powerful heuristic for pronoun resolution. Hobbs (1979) reports that it works about 90% of the time in written texts and about 75% of the time in dialogues he has examined. Thus, unless there is a very good reason to do otherwise – for instance, if the presuppositions involved in the use of a verb suggest that the pronoun should be assigned to the second noun phrase – people interpret a pronoun in the second clause of a complex sentence as being coreferential with the noun phrase that is signaled as topic by being in subject position. If older adults are not sensitive to the presuppositions about human interactions underlying the verbs in sentence fragments or if they are not sensitive to the meanings of various connectives such as *because* or *but,* because they do not process word meanings as deeply as young adults, we might expect to find that they are more prone to adopt a simple course of action such as that embodied in the strategy of choosing the topic in assignment of pronouns when completing sentence fragments.

Light and Capps (1983) asked groups of highly educated young and older adults, whose mean ages were 21.48 (range, 19–28) and 68.85 (range, 61–79), respectively, to perform a sentence completion task modeled after that of Grober et al. (1978). All subjects completed 60 fragments of which 24 were fillers and contained pronouns whose antecedents were made unambiguous by use of one male and one female name in the sentence fragment. The 36 test fragments involved six verbs – two which were supposed to bias pronoun assignment toward the first noun phrase (*apologize* and *accuse*) and four which were expected to bias pronoun assignment toward the second noun phrase (*blame, praise, scold,* and *forgive*) in fragments having the connective *because*. Each of the six verbs appeared three times with *because* and three times with *but*. In addition, each verb appeared alone, with a weak modal auxiliary (*can* or *may*), or with a strong modal auxiliary (*must* or *ought to*). Grober et al. found that the presence of modal auxiliaries in the stem affected the assignment of pronouns in fragments containing *because* for NP2 verbs. Strong modals increased the amount of bias, while weak modals attenuated the bias. Grober et al. suggested that strong modals express necessity while weak modals attenuate the bias of the verb and encourage choice of the first-mentioned noun as coreferential with the pronoun.

(4g) George must scold Walter because he torments the dog unmercifully.
(4h) George may scold Walter because he needs to let off steam.

In (4g) it is clear that the reasons for scolding Walter arise out of Walter's behavior, while in (4h) George may scold Walter but whether he actually decides to is more likely to depend on his own mood, physical state, or attitudes toward Walter than on anything that Walter does or does not do.

After subjects finished the sentence completion task, they were asked to read through their answers and to circle the name in each fragment that they intended as the referent of the pronoun. The results from verbs without modals are shown in Table 8.2, which gives the distribution of responses for each of the six verbs in the context of *because* and *but* connectives. Two verbs were expected to bias the first noun phrase in the context of *because*, and the results are generally in the right direction for these two verbs although the young did not split reliably on *accuse*. Of the four verbs expected to bias the second noun phrase in *because* sentences, three showed the predicted pattern while one, *forgive*, seemed to act as a NP1 verb for our subjects. For *but* fragments, both age groups showed strong preference for NP1 assignment. The important point here is that the two age groups were very similar in their responses to the connectives. In fact, when we compared the responses of the two age groups for each of the 12 verb–connective combinations, not one of the chi-squares was reliable. By contrast, when we compared the distribution of responses for *because* and *but* separately for each age group for the three verbs *blame, praise,* and *scold* which showed NP2 bias with *because,* all three showed the predicted shift from NP2 to NP1 in the presence of *but* and, more critically for our argument, both young and old showed the shift. In the case of *forgive,* which showed an unexpected majority of NP1 responses in the presence of *because,* both age groups gave an even greater number of NP1 responses in the presence of *but,* although the shift was reliable only for the young. Thus, these data give us no reason to believe that

Table 8.2. *Frequency of assignment of pronouns to NP1 and NP2 for "because" and "but" sentence fragments without modals*

Verb		Young				Old		
		NP1	NP2	Chi-square[a]		NP1	NP2	Chi-square[a]
Apologize[b]	because	23	2	3.91	because	24	3	0.59
	but	19	8		but	22	5	
Accuse[b]	because	15	11	1.58	because	18	8	0.50
	but	20	7		but	21	6	
Forgive[c]	because	19	8	2.85	because	17	8	10.21
	but	24	3		but	27	0	
Blame[c]	because	10	17	11.05	because	6	20	23.35
	but	22	5		but	24	3	
Praise[c]	because	5	21	18.17	because	7	20	13.78
	but	21	6		but	20	6	
Scold[c]	because	8	18	6.83	because	9	18	7.42
	but	18	9		but	19	8	

[a]The values of chi-square are for the comparison of NP1 and NP2 responses to *because* and *but* sentence fragments for each age group. The cell frequencies do not always sum to 27 because of unscorable responses.
[b]NP1 verbs.
[c]NP2 verbs.

there are any age differences in strategies for pronoun assignment in the absence of modals. The data obtained with modals bear out what we have just said and do not require any qualification of the claims made.

In sum, these data suggest that older adults are sensitive to the presuppositions underlying the use of verbs as well as to linguistic context during comprehension. Adults of various ages are attuned to rather subtle nuances of meanings of the words that they encounter and are able to use linguistic context to determine the coreferentiality of ambiguous pronouns whose meaning changes with the specific context in which they occur.

We have also compared the performance of young and older adults in an on-line task that taps comprehension of noun-phrase anaphors during the reading of sentences in short paragraphs such as (5).

(5) A burglar surveyed the garage set back from the street.
Several milk bottles were piled at the curb.
The banker and her husband were on vacation.
The criminal slipped away from the street lamp. (Anaphor)
A cat slipped away from the street lamp. (Unrelated)

In the Unrelated version of the paragraph [the first three lines and the last line of (5)], a new entity is introduced which does not corefer with any of the previously mentioned concepts. In the Anaphor version of the paragraph [the first four lines of (5)], the last sentence contains a referring expression, *the criminal,* which is a superordinate of the subject of the first sentence. Use of the definite article *the* signals that the concept *criminal* has been introduced earlier in the discourse and encourages the inference that the burglar mentioned in the first sentence and the criminal mentioned in the last sentence refer to the same individual. Deciding that *the criminal* and *a burglar* refer to the same individual here requires an inference inasmuch as there is no logical necessity that this be the case. It is the use of the definite article and the superordinate which, together with our assumption that discourses are coherent, leads us to make the inference because doing so results in a comprehensible paragraph (Hobbs, 1979).

When an expression such as *the criminal* is encountered during reading, previous sentences containing possible antecedents are activated or brought into working memory where connections between the information in the new sentence and prior information may be established. Dell, McKoon, and Ratcliff (1983; McKoon & Ratcliff, 1980) found that this activation process begins as soon as the anaphor is read and continues at least until the end of the sentence is reached. In their procedure, paragraphs such as (5) were presented on a computer monitor. Each sentence was printed on the screen one word at a time, with successive words presented at a 250-msec rate and remaining visible until the entire sentence was on the screen. At various points in the final sentence, a probe word was presented for recognition, with the subject's task being to respond positively if the probe appeared earlier in the paragraph and negatively if the probe did not. Subjects responded more rapidly to probes such as *burglar* when there was an anaphor in the last sentence than when the last sentence was unrelated, indicating that the initial sentence becomes available in working memory more rapidly when an anaphor is used, that is, when the last sentence can be interpreted as referring to earlier mentioned entities. The priming effect (unrelated response time minus anaphor response time) was found for probes presented immediately after the anaphor or unrelated word (250 msec later) and persisted undiminished for all probe positions to the end of the sentence.

We compared the performance of young and older adults in this paradigm to determine whether the magnitude and time course of the priming effect were similar across ages. These issues are important because failure to identify expressions as coreferring or relative slowness in doing so could seriously interfere with the ability of older adults to integrate successive parts of a discourse. Twenty-four young adults (mean age, 24.00; range, 18–34) and 24 older adults (mean age, 66.63; range, 60–75) read 135 paragraphs such as those in (5), of which 75 were fillers and 60 were experimental passages generously provided by McKoon and Ratcliff. Each paragraph was presented on a monitor using the timing parameters described by Dell et al. (1983). For the 60 experimental paragraphs, half of the probes were presented immediately after the anaphor (or unrelated word) and half were presented at the end of the sentence. Half the paragraphs ended with a sentence containing an anaphor, and half ended with an unrelated sentence. Probe position was crossed with paragraph version.

Mean response times for correct responses as well as error rates (in parentheses) are given in Table 8.3 for young and older adults as a function of paragraph version and probe position. The two age groups were similar in error rates, with young adults

Table 8.3. *Mean response times (in msec) and proportion of errors (in parentheses) in probe recognition task*

	Young			Old		
	Anaphor	Unrelated	Priming effect	Anaphor	Unrelated	Priming effect
Probe after target	726 (.09)	760 (.14)	35	1074 (.11)	1120 (.13)	46
Probe at end	747 (.08)	765 (.09)	18	1076 (.08)	1149 (.11)	73

failing to recognize the probe on .10 of the trials and older adults making errors .11 of the time. Like Dell et al., we found that probe recognition was reliably faster for the anaphor versions and that this was equally true at both probe positions. Although the older adults were overall slower to respond than the young adults, the magnitude of the priming effect did not differ for the two age groups at either probe position. Immediately after the anaphor position, the priming effect was 35 msec for the young and 46 msec for the old. At the end of the sentence, the corresponding figures were 18 msec for the young and 72 msec for the old. If anything, the presence of an anaphor was somewhat more beneficial for the older adults. These data suggest that comprehension of noun phrase anaphors during reading proceeds in the same way in young and older adults and offer additional evidence that pragmatic inferences are readily made by older adults.

The starting point for our inquiry into language comprehension in old age was the claim that problems in understanding are the underlying cause of memory deficits. In the study just described, we found no reliable age differences in the magnitude or time course of the priming effect, indicating similar comprehension across ages and similar availability of information shortly after reading a sentence. We might, therefore, predict that there should be no age differences in subsequent retention of the paragraphs. To test this prediction, we gave our subjects a recognition test consisting of 24 first sentences from the experimental paragraphs, intermixed with 24 new sentences that had not been seen previously. Discrimination between old and new test sentences for both age groups was very good, with d''s of 2.88 and 2.23, for young and older adults respectively. Nevertheless, the young adults' scores were reliably higher. Despite the absence of age differences in comprehension, we observed an age-related decrement in retention of the materials used in the comprehension task. Similar dissociations between comprehension and memory have been reported by Burke (Burke & Harrold, this volume; Burke, White, & Diaz, 1987; Burke & Yee, 1984); Howard (this volume), and Mitchell and Perlmutter (1986) and pose a theoretical puzzle to which we return in the Conclusions at the end of the chapter.

Working-memory constraints on pragmatic implication

Thus far, we have seen no evidence for age-related differences in determining co-reference even when inferences based on general world knowledge are required.

These studies, however, have dealt with tasks that do not make heavy demands on working-memory capacity. They have involved only small amounts of material, sentence fragments, pairs of sentences, or short paragraphs. Even in the case in which a paragraph-length narrative was used, demands on attentional capacity in working memory were relatively low because the materials were presented in written form. We have carried out several experiments which systematically manipulate demands on working memory, and these do, in general, suggest that the referential processes needed to establish coherence are adversely affected in old age by increases in working-memory load.

One source of evidence that increasing working-memory load has a relatively greater impact on determining coreferentiality by older adults comes from a set of experiments conducted by Light and Capps (1986), using materials such as those in (6), which were adapted from Hirst and Brill (1980).

(6a) Henry spoke at a meeting while John drove to the beach.
He brought along a surfboard.
(6b) Henry spoke at a meeting while John drove to the beach.
He lectured on the administration.

A decision as to the antecedent of the pronoun *he* in these examples cannot be made on the basis of number or gender because both possibilities are male and singular. Rather an inference based on general world knowledge must be made. Surfboards are generally found at the beach, but lectures rarely occur on the beach. We asked 24 young (mean age, 26.32; range, 21–37) and 24 older (mean age, 69.91; range, 62–82) subjects to listen to sentence pairs such as those in (6) and to decide for each one whether it was John or Henry who was being referred to in the second sentence.

To assess the effects of memory load, we varied the number of sentences intervening between the context setting sentence and the sentence containing the pronoun. Each subject heard one block of items with no intervening sentences and one block of items with two intervening sentences as in (7).

(7) John stood watching while Henry jumped across a ravine.
The ground was so rocky and uneven that only goats used this path.
There were no flowers but a few weeds grew here and there.
He fell in the river.

The intervening sentences were designed to avoid biasing pronoun assignment to either John or Henry, and in general could be said to "background" the information in the first sentence of a set so that it might no longer be available in consciousness or working memory (Chafe, 1972). If older adults have less working-memory capacity, they may experience difficulty in choosing the appropriate referent when irrelevant material intervenes between an anaphor and its antecedent. This could happen either because older adults are less able to remember the information required for specification of pronoun antecedents when the pronoun and its referent are separated by intervening material or because they are less able to integrate the old and new information when greater amounts of material are presented.

We have already seen that older adults are able to use general world knowledge in resolving pronoun anaphors under the conditions of low memory load which ob-

Table 8.4. *Proportion of consistent pronoun choices as a function of age and number of intervening sentences*

	Number of intervening sentences		
	0	2	Mean
Young	.97	.93	.95
Old	.95	.83	.89
Mean	.96	.88	

Source: L. L. Light & J. L. Capps (1986). Comprehension of pronouns in young and older adults. *Developmental Psychology, 22,* 583. Copyright 1986 by the American Psychological Association, Inc. Adapted by permission.

tained in the sentence completion task described earlier in the chapter, and we did not anticipate age differences in the present task when there were no intervening sentences. Thus, we predicted an interaction between age and number of intervening sentences, and this was precisely what we found. Table 8.4 gives the mean proportion of referent choices consistent with contextual bias as a function of age and number of intervening sentences. The performance of young and old did not differ reliably when there were no intervening sentences (see also LeDoux, Blum, & Hirst, 1983), but the age difference was reliable when there were two intervening sentences.

We conducted a follow-up study (Light & Capps, 1986) to tease apart whether older adults rely less on pragmatic constraints to make pronoun assignments when memory load is high because they are unable to retrieve the relevant information from the context-setting sentences or because they are unable to integrate this information with the information in the sentence containing the pronoun. To discriminate between these two possibilities, we replicated the condition with two intervening sentences with new groups of 16 young (mean age, 23.50; range, 19–28) and 16 older (mean age, 65.50; range, 58–69) adults with one added twist to the procedure: Subjects were asked to recall in writing the first sentence in each set after making a pronoun assignment. Given that there were only two possible antecedents, John and Henry, subjects should be able to make pronoun assignments based on pragmatic constraints even if they remember only one clause of the context-setting sentence. It should not matter whether the remembered clause is consistent with the pragmatic information in the pronoun sentence or not; if the remembered clause contains a name that is an unlikely candidate for being the antecedent, the other name can be chosen. Thus, if failure to use pragmatic constraints in pronoun assignment is due to inability to retrieve relevant information, we should find that assignments inconsistent with the bias established by the context are made primarily when subjects remember neither clause of the context-setting sentence. Problems in integration of information would be manifested in inconsistent assignments even when relevant information can be recalled.

As expected, the two age groups differed in their use of pragmatic constraints. The young made pronoun assignments consistent with the bias induced by the context-setting sentences .94 of the time, while the old did so on .86 of the trials. When we scored recall of the context-setting sentences, we found that young adults had more instances of recalling both clauses correctly than did the old, with proportions correct of .94 and .65, respectively. The young also had fewer instances of recalling neither clause correctly (.03 versus .13). More to the point, however, when we conditionalized consistent pronoun assignment on correct recall of both clauses, we found that the probability of choosing the biased referent was .97 for the young and .98 for the old. The conclusion we draw from these findings, together with those of the first study we have described from this series, is that older adults' failure to use pragmatic constraints in pronoun assignment is due primarily to problems in remembering the appropriate contextual information. When contextual information can be retrieved, age differences disappear.

In the studies just described, availability of information needed to draw pragmatic inferences was manipulated by varying the amount of material that intervened between the two sentences to be integrated. This is by no means the only way to manipulate availability of information in working memory. Consider the differences between (8a) and (8b):

(8a)   Next door to us there's an old man who's completely blind. He lives quite alone and nobody ever goes to visit him, but he seems to manage quite well. He has a guide dog and goes out with the dog every day to do his shopping. We often see him sitting on his porch reading his newspaper.

(8b)   Next door to us there's an old man who's completely blind. He lives with his unmarried sister who works as housekeeper for a banker. She works long hours and rarely seems to get any time off to be with her brother. We often see him sitting on his porch reading his newspaper.

In both versions, the blindness of the neighbor is introduced in the first sentence and the anomalous fact that he reads the newspaper is reported in the last sentence. To detect the anomaly here requires us to note that the old man is blind and to relate this information not only to the fact in the last sentence but to our general world knowledge that reading requires vision (ignoring the possibility of Braille newspapers). In neither version is the blindness explicitly mentioned after the first sentence, and in both versions two sentences, with approximately the same number of words, intervene between the two crucial pieces of stated information. Yet the anomaly seems to be more obvious in (8a) than in (8b), because although blindness is not mentioned again in (8a), the salience of the old man and his blindness to the discourse is maintained. We learn that he manages quite well and that he has a guide dog. These facts (which also require inferences for their salience to be appreciated) help to keep the old man and his physical disability active in working memory, or foregrounded, so that relevant new information can be assessed and integrated with what we already know about him. In (8b), on the other hand, a new character is introduced and facts about her are then related. Here the old man and his physical disability are no longer the focus of the discourse; they are in the background.

Lesgold, Roth, and Curtis (1979) have found that people take longer to read sentences related to prior information that has been backgrounded than to read sen-

Table 8.5. *Proportion of correct responses as a function of age, foregrounding, and question type*

	Young	Old
Foreground		
Inference	.84	.84
Fact	.93	.94
Background		
Inference	.80	.74
Fact	.91	.83

tences related to foregrounded information. Together with Asha Singh, we were interested in determining whether with amount of information held constant, varying the nature of the intervening material would affect the ease with which anomaly can be detected and whether the effects of backgrounding would be the same across age. If relevant information is no longer in working memory because it has been backgrounded by a momentary shift in topic, older adults may experience relatively greater difficulty in detecting anomaly than they do when the topic is maintained in the foreground. The reason for expecting this is that backgrounded information may need to be retrieved from long-term memory and older adults are less effective in memory search than young adults. In addition, older adults may be more prone to forgetting backgrounded information altogether. Cohen (1979) has found that older adults are not as good at detecting anomaly as young adults and has called attention to the importance of knowing when new information should *not* be integrated with prior information if discourses are to be properly understood. We were concerned with exploring the generality of Cohen's finding and specifying the conditions under which it holds.

To this end, we presented 33 young adults (mean age, 23.42; range, 19–32) and 32 older adults (mean age, 67.56; range, 60–76) with 16 short passages similar to those in (8a) and (8b). Some of these passages were adapted from Cohen's materials whereas others were new passages written for this study. Half of the passages contained an anomaly and half did not [in the normal versions of (8), the old man was seen smoking his pipe]. In addition, for each subject, half of the passages were in the foregrounded condition and half were in the backgrounded condition. After hearing each passage, subjects were asked whether it contained an anomaly and, if so, to indicate the nature of the problem (inference question). They were then asked a question about one of the pieces of information needed to detect the anomaly (fact question). For instance, in the case of (8), the fact question was "What handicap does the man next door have?"

Positive responses to the anomaly question were counted as correct for anomalous items only when an adequate reason for viewing the passage as peculiar was stated. Table 8.5 shows the proportion of correct responses for each age group as a function of foregrounding and response type (inference vs. fact questions), collapsing across the anomaly factor which did not interact with age. Two aspects of these data are particularly worthy of mention. First, subjects were more accurate in detection of anomaly in the foregrounded versions of these passages, and as anticipated, the negative impact of backgrounding was greater for older adults. The mean proportions of correct anomaly detections in the foregrounded versions were .84 and .84, for young and old, respectively, with the corresponding figures for the backgrounded versions being .80 and .74. Second, although subjects were more likely to be correct on facts than on inferences, this variable did not interact with either foregrounding or age. That is, backgrounding did not simply reduce people's ability to draw inferences when they could remember relevant factual information; rather, that factual information itself was less available in the backgrounded condition. In addition, when we conditionalized anomaly detection on correct fact recall, the age difference disappeared, with the conditional proportions being .85 for the young and .84 for the old. We interpret these results as further support for the view that under optimal conditions young and older adults are equally good at utilizing general world knowledge to determine when an inference is appropriate, but that when relevant information is less available in working memory, older adults will experience more trouble than young ones. The present results also suggest that older adults have difficulty in retrieving information following a topic shift.

Thus far our story has been a consistent one. We have found no age differences in ability to deal with pragmatic information except when working memory is somehow burdened. We do, however, have some data that seem to contradict this position. These data come from a pair of studies carried out by Light and Anderson (1985) which compared young and older adults' ability to determine the antecedent of an ambiguous pronoun in the last sentence of a fairly long (12-sentence) paragraph containing several possible referents. Young adults performed better than older adults on this task both when asked to recall the antecedent and when asked to pick out the antecedent from three possibilities offered by the experimenter on a recognition test. They were also more likely to recall or recognize specific facts that did not require inferences. These findings reinforce our belief that forgetting of relevant information is a major source of older adults' problems in establishing discourse coherence through inferences based on general world knowledge.

Two aspects of Light and Anderson's (1985) results are less readily dealt with in this framework. To understand why, one detail of the experimental design must be considered. The distance of the sentence containing the pronoun referent from the end of the paragraph was varied. Daneman and Carpenter (1980) found that accuracy in recalling the antecedent of the pronoun in the last sentence was a function of how far back in the paragraph the antecedent had been mentioned. This result suggests that antecedents of pronouns are readily identifiable if the relevant information is available in working memory, as would be the case when the pronoun-referent distance is small. When the pronoun-referent distance is greater, locating the relevant information requires a search of long-term memory. Because older adults have less working-memory capacity, we expected that they would need to begin searching long-term memory at smaller pronoun-referent distances. Because search is fallible and the relevant information may not be accessed, we predicted an interaction between age and pronoun distance. We found pronoun-referent distance effects for both age groups, but no interaction. We suspect that the sheer length of our paragraphs (12 sentences) and the presence of from three to ten possible antecedents in addition to the target create sufficient memory load to swamp any interaction. This is, however, clearly an ad hoc analysis.

Further, Light and Anderson (1985) collected several estimates of working-memory capacity including traditional span measures and a sentence span measure that Daneman and Carpenter (1980) found to be highly predictive of both pronoun identification and fact memory. Although Light and Anderson found moderately strong correlations among span measures, none of the span measures were very successful in predicting either recall or recognition, and partialing out span measures did not affect the size of the large negative correlation between age and memory test scores. If working-memory capacity is a factor in limiting successful discourse integration involving pragmatic inference, it should be possible to use an individual-differences approach to predict performance on criterion tasks (see Hartley, this volume, and Kemper, this volume, for related arguments). However, our foray into this enterprise was not very successful. This is clearly an area in which further investigation is needed.

Conclusions

The research discussed in this chapter has shown that young and older adults are equally sensitive to pragmatic constraints in discourse except when memory load is high. Young and older adults were equally able to understand S-complement sentences containing verbs that invited inference except when double negatives were used; in such cases, we believe that normal language comprehension processes are replaced by problem solving activity which is impeded by reduced working-memory capacity in old age. Determination of the coreferentiality of pronouns in sentence fragments was affected by the complex presuppositions about the nature of interpersonal relationships that underlie the use of verbs of implicit causality, as well as by the presence of particular conjunctions and modal auxiliaries, in the same way in young and older adults. In addition, the magnitude and time course of priming effects during comprehension of sentences containing noun phrase anaphors appear to be constant across the adult years. Thus, we have found no evidence for age differences in the extent to which young and older adults are likely to make inferences based on general world knowledge or in the degree to which fairly subtle changes in linguistic context affect comprehension.

When language comprehension takes place under conditions of high memory load, age-related differences appear which suggest that older adults have comprehension deficits. Our claim, however, is that these comprehension deficits are not the result of deficient semantic processing of individual words or sentences but rather arise when relevant prior information is not available. That is, we believe that many comprehension failures are really memory failures in disguise. Thus, young and older adults were equally able to use pragmatic information to determine the antecedent of a pronoun in one sentence *if* they were able to remember relevant contextual information from a previous sentence. Because older adults were less apt to remember this contextual information when it was followed by two irrelevant sentences, however, their ability to determine coreferentiality was more impaired under such circumstances than that of young adults. Real-life parallels to our experiments such as interruptions of a conversation are for this reason more likely to have a negative impact on integration of information in a discourse by older adults. Change of topic may also be particularly detrimental to older adults' comprehension of natural language; anomaly detection was problematic for older adults only when relevant information was backgrounded and this information was forgotten. Finally, long narratives containing many potential antecedents may be a source of comprehension difficulty for older adults because relevant information may be difficult to remember or to manipulate in working memory.

Cohen (1979, 1981) has suggested that older adults are impaired in drawing inferences even when they are as able as young adults to remember facts. The results we have presented in this chapter indicate, somewhat to the contrary, that older adults are just as likely to draw inferences as younger adults *except* when they cannot remember relevant facts, a problem that occurs when memory load is high. Prior inputs that cannot be remembered cannot be integrated with current information. Interestingly enough, there is also evidence that older adults are *more* likely than young adults to make pragmatic inferences under some circumstances. Reder, Wible, and Martin (1986) found that immediately after reading a story, older adults were less likely than young adults to correctly identify highly plausible inferences as new statements on a recognition test but were just as accurate in judging whether statements were plausible, given what they had read. This result, coupled with the fact that older adults were slower on recognition than on plausibility judgment in this condition while the reverse was true for young adults, led Reder et al. to conclude that older adults are apt to make recognition judgments by evaluating the plausibility of statements rather than by searching memory; they argue that older adults prefer the plausibility strategy either because their memory is impaired so that specific information is less available or because memory search is deemed effortful. Their results, like ours, are inconsistent with the view that older adults are less likely than young adults to make inferences.

Although the focus of this chapter has been on natural language understanding rather than memory, we believe that our results offer a challenge for hypotheses about memory and aging that posit that the decline of memory in old age is due to impoverished semantic analysis of words and sentences. We have found no evidence for impoverished semantic analysis of words or sentences during language comprehension. When we examined both on-line comprehension of noun phrase anaphors and subsequent memory for the sentences containing their antecedents, we found no age differences in the amount or duration of priming, but age differences in memory were nevertheless observed. This dissociation between comprehension and memory, also observed in studies by Howard (this volume) and by Burke (Burke, White, & Diaz, 1987), is not consistent with the resource deficit hypothesis proposed by Craik and his associates (e.g., Craik & Byrd, 1982; Craik & Rabinowitz, 1984).

Of course, it could be argued that it is *encoding* rather than *comprehension* which is the problem. Perhaps older adults have no problem in understanding language but simply lay down less semantically elaborated memory traces of whatever they have understood (Craik & Rabinowitz, 1984). The problem with this approach is that there does not seem to be any clear theoretical analysis of why this should occur. If comprehension is unimpaired, what does it mean to say that encoding is impoverished? What mechanisms are involved in moving from a representation that is adequate during "comprehension" to a representation that is less satisfactory during "encoding"? Why, after achieving comprehension, would older adults engage in encoding strategies that produce less good memory representations?

To say that limitations in attentional capacity lead to use of less efficient encoding processes does not seem to be a satisfactory answer. It is precisely those semantic processes involved in comprehension that we might expect to suffer from reduced capacity. The point at which "comprehension" leaves off and "encoding" begins has never been defined. Certainly in laboratory tasks involving intentional learning, people may engage in postcomprehension mnemonic activities, such as rehearsal or elaboration. In such situations, comprehension and encoding operations may compete for the same limited pool of attentional resources, with encoding operations given lower priority if attentional capacity is reduced, as it appears to be in old age (Light & Anderson, 1983). However, these situations are probably the exception rather than the rule. Real life more closely approximates conditions of incidental learning in which intentional postcomprehension processing is likely to be minimal; yet age differences in memory are observed under incidental as well as intentional learning conditions (Burke & Light, 1981). We are thus left with a set of questions that will need to be answered before we can arrive at an understanding of the relation between language comprehension and memory in old age.

References

Belmore, S. M. (1981). Age-related changes in processing explicit and implicit language. *Journal of Gerontology*, *36*, 316–322.

Brown, G., & Yule, G. (1983). *Discourse analysis*. Cambridge: Cambridge University Press.

Burke, D. M., & Light, L. L. (1981). Memory and aging: The role of retrieval processes. *Psychological Bulletin*, *90*, 513–546.

Burke, D. M., & Peters, L. J. (1986). Word associations in old age: Evidence for consistency in semantic encoding during adulthood. *Psychology and Aging*, *1*, 283–292.

Burke, D. M., White, H., & Diaz, D. L. (1987). Semantic priming in young and older adults: Evidence for age-constancy in automatic and attentional processes. *Journal of Experimental Psychology: Human Perception and Performance*, *13*, 79–88.

Burke, D. M., & Yee, P. L. (1984). Semantic priming during sentence processing by young and older adults. *Developmental Psychology*, *20*, 903–910.

Chafe, W. L. (1972). Discourse structure and human knowledge. In J. Carroll & R. Freedle (Eds.), *Language comprehension and the acquisition of knowledge* (pp. 41–69). Washington, DC: Winston.

Clark, H. H., & Marshall, C. R. (1981). Definite reference and mutual knowledge. In A. K. Joshi, B. L. Webber, & I. A. Sag (Eds.), *Elements of discourse understanding* (pp. 10–63). Cambridge: Cambridge University Press.

Cohen, G. (1979). Language comprehension in old age. *Cognitive Psychology*, *11*, 412–429.

Cohen, G. (1981). Inferential reasoning in old age. *Cognition*, *9*, 59–72.

Craik, F. I. M., & Byrd, M. (1982). Aging and cognitive deficits: The role of attentional resources. In F. I. M. Craik & S. Trehub (Eds.), *Aging and cognitive processes* (pp. 191–211). New York: Plenum.

Craik, F. I. M., & Rabinowitz, J. C. (1984). Age differences in the acquisition and use of verbal information: A tutorial review. In H. Bouma & D. G. Bouwhuis (Eds.), *Attention and performance X: Control of language processes* (pp. 471–499). Hillsdale, NJ: Erlbaum.

Daneman, M., & Carpenter, P. A. (1980). Individual differences in working memory and reading. *Journal of Verbal Learning and Verbal Behavior*, *19*, 450–466.

Dell, G. S., McKoon, G., & Ratcliff, R. (1983). The activation of antecedent information during the processing of anaphoric reference in reading. *Journal of Verbal Learning and Verbal Behavior*, *22*, 121–132.

Ehrlich, K. (1980). Comprehension of pronouns. *Quarterly Journal of Experimental Psychology*, *32*, 247–255.

Eysenck, M. W. (1974). Age differences in incidental learning. *Developmental Psychology*, *10*, 936–941.

Garvey, C., & Caramazza, A. (1974). Implicit causality in verbs. *Linguistic Inquiry*, *5*, 459–464.

Geis, M. L., & Zwicky, A. M. (1971). On invited inferences. *Linguistic Inquiry*, *2*, 561–566.

Grober, E. H., Beardsley, W., & Caramazza, A. (1978). Parallel function strategy in pronoun assignment. *Cognition*, *6*, 117–133.

Harris, R. J. (1974). Memory and comprehension of implications and inferences of complex sentences. *Journal of Verbal Learning and Verbal Behavior*, *13*, 626–637.

Harris, R. J., & Monaco, G. E. (1978). Psychology of pragmatic implication: Information processing between the lines. *Journal of Experimental Psychology: General*, *107*, 1–22.

Hartley, J. T., Harker, J. O., & Walsh, D. A. (1980). Contemporary issues and new directions in adult development of learning and memory. In L. W. Poon (Ed.), *Aging in the 1980s: Psychological issues* (pp. 239–252). Washington, DC: American Psychological Association.

Hasher, L., & Zacks, R. T. (1979). Automatic and effortful processes in memory. *Journal of Experimental Psychology: General*, *108*, 356–388.

Hess, T. M., & Arnould, D. (1986). Adult age differences in memory for explicit and implicit sentence information. *Journal of Gerontology*, *41*, 191–194.

Hirst, W., & Brill, G. A. (1980). Contextual aspects of pronoun assignment. *Journal of Verbal Learning and Verbal Behavior*, *19*, 168–175.

Hobbs, J. R. (1979). Coherence and coreference. *Cognitive Science*, *3*, 67–90.

Howard, D. V. (1980). Category norms: A comparison of the Battig and Montague (1968) norms with the responses of adults between the ages of 20 and 80. *Journal of Gerontology*, *35*, 225–231.

Hultsch, D. F., & Dixon, R. A. (1984). Memory for text materials in adulthood. In P. B. Baltes & O. G. Brim, Jr. (Eds.), *Life-span development and behavior* (Vol. 6, pp. 77–108). New York: Academic Press.

Karttunen, L. (1970). On the semantics of complement sentences. *Papers from the Sixth Regional Meeting Chicago Linguistic Society*, 328–339.

Kiparsky, P., & Kiparsky, C. (1970). Fact. In M. Bierwisch & K. E. Heidolph (Eds.), *Progress in linguistics* (pp. 143–173). The Hague: Mouton.

LeDoux, J. F., Blum, C., & Hirst, W. (1983). Inferential processing of context: Studies of cognitively impaired subjects. *Brain and Language*, *19*, 216–224.

Lesgold, A. M. (1972). Pronominalization: A device for unifying sentences in memory. *Journal of Verbal Learning and Verbal Behavior*, *11*, 316–323.

Lesgold, A. M., Roth, S. F., & Curtis, M. E. (1979). Foregrounding effects in discourse comprehension. *Journal of Verbal Learning and Verbal Behavior*, *18*, 291–308.

Light, L. L. (1988). Language and aging: Competence versus performance. In J. E. Birren & V. L. Bengtson (Eds.), *Emergent theories of aging* (pp. 177–213). New York: Springer.

Light, L. L., & Anderson, P. A. (1983). Memory for scripts in young and older adults. *Memory & Cognition*, *11*, 435–444.

Light, L. L., & Anderson, P. A. (1985). Working-memory capacity, age, and memory for discourse. *Journal of Gerontology*, *40*, 737–747.

Light, L. L., & Capps, J. L. (1983). *Comprehension of implicit causality in young and older adults*. Unpublished manuscript, Pitzer College, Claremont, CA.

Light, L. L., & Capps, J. L. (1986). Comprehension of pronouns in young and older adults. *Developmental Psychology, 22*, 580–585.

Light, L. L., Zelinski, E. M., & Moore, M. (1982). Adult age differences in reasoning from new information. *Journal of Experimental Psychology: Learning, Memory, and Cognition, 8*, 435–447.

McKoon, G., & Ratcliff, R. (1980). The comprehension processes and memory structures involved in anaphoric reference. *Journal of Verbal Learning and Verbal Behavior, 19*, 668–682.

Mitchell, D. B., & Perlmutter, M. (1986). Semantic activation and episodic memory: Age similarities and differences. *Developmental Psychology, 22*, 86–94.

Perlmutter, M. (1978). What is memory aging the aging of? *Developmental Psychology, 14*, 330–345.

Reder, L. M., Wible, C., & Martin, J. (1986). Differential memory changes with age: Exact retrieval versus plausible inference. *Journal of Experimental Psychology: Learning, Memory, and Cognition, 12*, 72–81.

Salthouse, T. A. (1982). *Adult cognition: An experimental psychology of human aging.* New York: Springer-Verlag.

Schaie, K. W. (1980). Cognitive development in aging. In L. K. Obler & M. L. Albert (Eds.), *Language and communication in the elderly* (pp. 7–25). Lexington, MA: Lexington Books.

Simon, E. (1979). Depth and elaboration of processing in relation to age. *Journal of Experimental Psychology: Human Learning and Memory, 5*, 115–124.

Till, R. E. (1985). Verbatim and inferential memory in young and elderly adults. *Journal of Gerontology, 40*, 316–323.

Till, R. E., & Walsh, D. A. (1980). Encoding and retrieval factors in adult memory for implicational sentences. *Journal of Verbal Learning and Verbal Behavior, 19*, 1–16.

9 Capacity theory and the processing of inferences

Rose T. Zacks and Lynn Hasher

The study of adult age differences in comprehension of and memory for text is a now burgeoning enterprise in cognitive gerontology, in part because of the potential for direct application of the findings to everyday life. To date, the work on discourse processing suggests the existence of age deficits of varying magnitudes, deficits that are largely quantitative rather than qualitative in nature. The work thus suggests that older adults use the same processing mechanisms as younger adults but with poorer results (e.g., Mandel & Johnson, 1984; Zelinski, Light, & Gilewski, 1984).

Beyond this summary the literature yields few simple generalizations; indeed, the findings on any given variable (e.g., educational level) tend to be complex and inconsistent. Consider the literature on the recall of ideas that differ in their importance to the meaning structure of the text. The usual finding with young adults (called the "levels effect") is that the probability of recalling information from text is directly related to the information's importance level in the text as defined by a model (e.g., Kintsch's, 1974) of the hierarchical structure of that text. When young and elderly adults have been compared, different experiments have produced contradictory results (for a recent review, see Zelinski et al., 1984; see also Cohen, this volume). The most frequent findings are (1) parallel levels effects for younger and older adults (e.g., Zelinski et al., 1984); or (2) an exaggerated levels effect for the older adults, with the greatest age deficit seen at low importance levels (e.g., Dixon, Hultsch, Simon, & von Eye, 1984, for high verbal ability subjects; Spilich, 1983). However, there is also an occasional finding of a diminished levels effect for older adults with the greatest age deficit at high importance levels (e.g., Dixon et al., 1984, for low verbal ability subjects).

Conflicting results of this sort suggest the likelihood that additional variables are operating. In the case of the levels effect, such variables as education, verbal ability, and characteristics of the experimental texts (e.g., the familiarity of the text structure and/or its content) might mediate the variable aging trends (Dixon et al.,

The research reported here and the preparation of this chapter were supported by National Institute of Mental Health Grant MH33140, Army Research Institute Grant MDA903-82-C-0317, and National Institute of Aging Grant AG04306, as well as by Biomedical Research Grants from Temple and Michigan State Universities. The authors acknowledge the invaluable assistance of the following individuals: Bonnie Doren, Verneda Hamm, Mary Attig, Betty Goldstein, and Natalie Davidson.

154

1984; Meyer & Rice, 1981). The suggestion that such variables interact with age differences is consistent with Jenkins's (1979) tetrahedral model of memory which argues that memory performance in a particular situation is a joint function of the characteristics of the subjects, of the materials they are required to remember, of the acquisition conditions, and of the criterial tasks. Indeed, Jenkins's model has been used in attempts to organize the findings on age differences in memory for both nonstructured and prose materials (Craik & Byrd, 1982; Hultsch & Dixon, 1984).

We are sympathetic with the general goals of identifying and classifying the multiple factors that control age differences in memory for text. However, we believe that pursuit of these goals will benefit from theoretical analyses which indicate the specific characteristics of subjects, materials, and tasks that might be functional in a particular situation. Thus, we chose a different approach to the general problem of age differences in discourse comprehension and memory.

The theoretical orientation guiding our research on discourse processing derives from limited-capacity attention theory (Kahneman, 1973). We began our research program with a general limited-capacity framework which made few specific claims about either the nature of capacity constraints on text processing or age differences. The initial framework and its associated research led us to elaborate on our capacity model in such a way as to increase the precision of our analysis of age differences in discourse processing. In this paper we trace the development of our thinking by reporting on a line of research that at first seemed to support and then to constrain the value of our initial general-capacity model. We also outline our elaborated view on which future research will be based.

The general-capacity theory and age differences in discourse processing

Two central assumptions of any limited-capacity model based on Kahneman's (1973) ideas are that (1) information processing is constrained by the amount of cognitive capacity (or mental resources) available at a given moment; and (2) that cognitive activities vary in the mental resources they require for maximal performance. In particular, automatic processes require very minimal amounts of capacity whereas effortful processes require significant resources (Hasher & Zacks, 1979, 1984). The fundamental aging assumption of a capacity-based theory of adult age differences in cognition is that available capacity declines with advancing age (e.g., Craik, 1983; Craik & Rabinowitz, 1983, 1984; Hasher & Zacks, 1979, 1984). The negative impact of this decline in mental resources should be minimal for automatic processes and should be increasingly severe the more demanding of capacity a particular effortful cognitive activity is.

Probably the most well known capacity-decline model of aging deficits in cognition is that of Craik and his colleagues (e.g., Craik, 1983; Craik & Byrd, 1982; Craik & Rabinowitz, 1983, 1984). This view assumes that aging deficits are due to a reduction in the "processing resources" needed to energize mental operations. For memory encoding, the major consequence of this reduction of resources is impaired semantic processing of to-be-remembered stimuli. Craik and his colleagues do not assume an absolute deficiency of semantic processing in older adults. The encoding of general, stereotypical aspects of meaning is preserved because the activation of these semantic attributes is largely automatic. However, the reduced processing resources do result in a diminished degree of elaboration and precision of semantic processing: Processing yielding rich, distinctive, and precise memories "is effortful and requires greater amounts of processing resources than [older adults] have available" (Craik, 1983, p. 112). A similar analysis applies to retrieval operations. The reduced processing resources of older adults result in a decrease in the occurrence of self-initiated and effortful retrieval operations. Where such operations are essential for good performance (e.g., free-recall tests), age differences will be seen, but where effortful retrieval operations are largely bypassed by strong environmental support for retrieval (e.g., perceptual learning tasks), age differences will be small or nonexistent.

Various findings, mainly from list memory experiments, support Craik's aging model. These include results indicating that young adults whose capacity for a target task is reduced by having them operate under divided attention constraints perform similarly to older adults (Rabinowitz, Craik, & Ackerman, 1982), and findings of relatively small age differences when the learning materials, the orienting task, and the memory test "drive" or "force" effective processing at encoding and retrieval (for a summary, see Craik, 1983). Findings from our laboratories are also consistent, at least in broad outline, with a reduced-capacity view of adult age differences in cognition: On the one hand, we have found no age differences in a memory task dependent on automatic encoding mechanisms (Attig & Hasher, 1980); on the other hand, we have obtained a significant age deficit in a memory task dependent on effortful processing (Zacks, 1982). Such findings, together with our own theoretical framework for cognitive processes (Hasher & Zacks, 1979, 1984), encouraged us to use a capacity model in our studies of discourse comprehension in older adults. (Cohen, this volume, also discusses capacity-based models of age differences in cognition.)

Application of a general-capacity framework to discourse processing

The value of capacity accounts of aging effects depends on the identification of mental activities that vary in their demands on cognitive capacity. Such identification is the basis of specific predictions of age-sensitive and age-insensitive cognitive operations. Because discourse processing clearly involves the coordinated occurrence of multiple-component processes which vary widely in their demands on cognitive capacity (cf. LaBerge & Samuels, 1974; Stanovich & West, 1983), this area seems to us to provide an ideal arena in which to test capacity models of adult age differences. Comparisons can be made between processes such as that of lexical access which tend to place minimal demands on capacity (Stanovich & West, 1983) and processes such as that of generating an anaphoric inference which can be highly demanding of capacity, particularly when there is little contextual support for the inference (LeDoux, Blum, & Hirst, 1983).

A review of the relevant literature provides some findings suggestive of the validity of a capacity-decline analysis of age differences. As this analysis predicts, there seems to be little or no age deficit in aspects of word meaning activation which have been identified as automatic in research with young adults. For example, word naming and lexical decision tasks have revealed minimal age differences either in lexical access time (Bowles & Poon, 1985; Cerella & Fozard, 1984; Mueller, Kausler, & Faherty, 1980; Waugh & Barr, 1982) or in semantic priming effects (Cerella & Fozard, 1984; Howard, 1983; Howard, McAndrews, & Lasaga, 1981; but see Madden, 1985).

Not all aspects of the lexical–semantic processing of words show age invariance, however. For example, in addition to investigating age differences on a lexical decision task (and finding none), Bowles and Poon (1985) compared younger and older adults on a task that required them to name the target words corresponding to definitions provided by the experimenter. Bowles and Poon argue that the definition of a word provides only indirect access to the lexical (i.e., phonetic) information needed to name the word, and that age-sensitive retrieval processes are involved in finding that information. If these age-sensitive retrieval processes are capacity demanding (as implied by Bowles and Poon), then the finding in this study of an age deficit on the word retrieval task is consistent with the reduced-capacity view.

A considerable body of research on memory for the content of text is also consistent with the general-capacity view. The age deficits are widespread; they occur whether the text is read or heard, whether the retention test is immediate or delayed, and whether recall or recognition tests are used (Hultsch & Dixon, 1984; Kausler, 1982; Salthouse, 1982). Adults with superior verbal–intellectual ability do seem to demonstrate some protection from aging declines in discourse processing (e.g., Hultsch & Dixon, 1984; Hultsch, Hertzog, & Dixon, 1984). However, given the possibility that high verbal ability subjects have greater capacity or that they use more efficient processing strategies than do those with lower verbal ability (cf. Cohen, this volume), even this last trend may fit a capacity model. Thus, the bulk of the literature on prose processing, from semantic activation to recall, is consistent with a general-capacity view of age deficits.

Our own research began as an attempt to apply the general-capacity framework to the ability to form and remember inferences. The first of two major reasons to focus on inferences is that they are widely believed to be critical to the process of understanding discourse (e.g., Bransford, 1979; Harris, 1981). Indeed, the formation of a coherent and integrated representation of a text typically requires the generation of anaphoric, causal, and other types of inferences to connect the various pieces of explicit information to one another (e.g., Clark, 1977; Garrod & Sanford, 1981). Second, unlike the task of memorizing lists of unrelated items, all adults have had considerable practice at understanding and remembering discourse, possibly making text processing tasks more familiar than others to elderly adults.

Because the encoding of implicit information is considered to involve processing beyond that required for encoding of explicit text information (e.g., Clark, 1977), the general-capacity view predicts a greater age deficit in processing implicit as compared to explicit text information. A number of studies have obtained results consistent with this prediction (Cohen, 1979, 1981; Light & Capps, 1986; Light, Zelinski, & Moore, 1982). However, there are some studies, including those of

Belmore (1981) and Till (1985), that did not find a greater age deficit for implicit than for explicit information.

As noted by Reder, Wible, and Martin (1986), analysis of the inferences used in the various studies suggests a possible resolution of these conflicting results. Specifically, it is likely that across studies, the inferences used varied in their demands on cognitive capacity. In cases where the inferences require only a minimal increment of capacity beyond that required for processing of explicit information, it would not be surprising if the usual finding of a greater age deficit for inferential than for explicit information does not hold. More effortful inferences should, of course, show the expected pattern of age differences.

Consider now the contrast between the materials used by Belmore (1981) and those used by Cohen (1979). To judge from the samples provided, Belmore's inferences were based on obvious connections between text information and basic knowledge about how the world works. For example, one passage required the subjects to infer that a vase located on the dinner table contained the roses that some dinner guests were admiring. For such inferences, limited processing of the texts would have sufficed. By contrast, Cohen's inferences appear to have required the integration of specific, detailed information from within the texts and so to have been more demanding of capacity than were the well-learned, preexisting connections used by Belmore. The conflict between Belmore's and Cohen's results on age differences in inferential processing can then be attributed to the use by Belmore of relatively nondemanding inferences and by Cohen of relatively demanding inferences. The research described next provides some data relevant to this line of argument.

Experiments

A major goal of our experiments on age differences in inference generation is the testing of two predictions of the capacity-decline view: (1) that there is an age deficit in inference generation, and (2) that the age deficit is greater for difficult, capacity-demanding inferences than for easy, relatively noncapacity-demanding inferences. To vary ease of inference generation, we used the following scheme, borrowed from Alba (1981). For each paragraph-length passage, a piece of information, *central* to an understanding of the passage, was designated the *target* fact. For example, in the passage entitled *The Artist*, the central event is a phone call that the artist receives while *busily painting one day*. Essential to a correct understanding of this passage is the encoding of the target fact that the artist was told in the phone call that he had 3 more months to live (rather than to finish the painting he was working on). Three versions of each passage were written in such a way as to vary the difficulty of arriving at the proper interpretation of the target fact.

In the *explicit* version, the target fact is actually presented. In the other two, the target information is implicit and so its encoding requires an inference. In the *expected inference* condition, there is strong contextual support for the target inference from the beginning of the paragraph (e.g., in the first sentence it is stated that the artist was expecting a phone call from his doctor's office). Drawing an inference in this condition should be relatively easy, requiring only the most obvious elaborations of the explicitly presented information. Furthermore, although in a number of cases the correct inference requires the activation of the typically less probable interpretation of a homophone (e.g., *camera* shot rather than *rifle* shot in a passage about a safari), Hess and Higgins (1983; Hess, 1984) have recently demonstrated that older adults, like younger ones, are sensitive to the semantic context in their interpretation of such words.

By contrast to the expected condition, drawing the correct inference in the *unexpected* condition should be considerably more effortful. The potential for increased effort demands derives from the lack of initial contextual support for the target inference (no mention is made about expecting a doctor's call), and from the fact that the initial context misleads the listener into drawing an incorrect inference (the artist is said to be concerned about an exhibit deadline). It is only later in the passage when a piece of information inconsistent with the initial interpretation is presented (the artist's shock at hearing bad news from his doctor is mentioned) that the subjects are led to question their first interpretation of the passage. At this point, the incorrect inference must be suppressed, and memory of the preceding text has to be searched to find the basis for the correct inference and thus for a coherent representation of the passage. Our expectations were that the unexpected condition would be particularly difficult for older adults, and that the age deficits would be greater for the unexpected than for the expected condition.

Across experiments, we have used both oral and self-paced visual presentation procedures. The differences between these procedures enable a test of the capacity decline view. Specifically, a self-paced procedure allows subjects to vary their reading rate in response to high processing demands. If older subjects do slow down when demands increase (e.g., when an inference is required), the result (in comparison with oral presentation) could be a smaller age deficit in inference generation, especially for easy inferences. (For a similar line of reasoning and for confirming data, see Cohen, 1981.) Furthermore, the self-paced condition allows for the collection of reading times. Our assumption, shared with many in this research domain (e.g., O'Brien & Myers, 1985), is that reading time measures offer a window into underlying cognitive processes, and so should add to our understanding of the impact of reduced capacity on inference generation.

Methods

What follows is a detailed description of an experiment that used a self-paced presentation procedure in which subjects read experimental passages displayed one sentence at a time on a video monitor. Reference will also be made to the results of an experiment (Zacks, Hasher, Doren, Hamm, & Attig, 1987) in which the same materials were read to the subjects at a normal reading rate. The materials used in these experiments consisted of explicit, expected, and unexpected versions of each of 12 passages. Each passage described a concrete scene or event (e.g., a father and son preparing dinner, an individual waiting for a ride home from work). In developing the materials, we tried to use content that would be equally familiar to the

Table 9.1. *Example of the materials used in the research*

The artist

Explicit and expected versions (in the latter, the phrase in parentheses is omitted)
    The artist was busily painting one day when he received the phone call he had been expecting from his doctor's office.
    He was concerned about the results of a series of lab tests he had taken.
    The artist was told he had three more months (to live).[a]
    He was shocked to hear this kind of news from his doctor.[b]
    Although he had not been feeling well, he still had not expected to hear such bad news.[c]
    His doctor expressed sympathy and hung up.
    Suddenly, the painting was no longer important.
    The artist mixed himself a stiff drink.

Unexpected version
    The artist was concerned about having his painting ready for the exhibit deadline.
    While he was busily painting one day, he received a phone call.
    The artist was told he had three more months.[a]
    He was shocked to hear this kind of news from his doctor.[b]
    Although he had not been feeling well, he still had not expected to hear such bad news.[c]
    His doctor expressed sympathy and hung up.
    Suddenly, the painting was no longer important.
    The artist mixed himself a stiff drink.

Control questions
    What was the artist doing when the phone call came?
    What did the artist do after he got off the phone?

Question on the target fact
    The artist was told he had three more months to do what?

[a]The sentence in which the target inference should occur in the expected condition.
[b]The critical sentence in the unexpected condition and the comparison sentence in the other two conditions.
[c]The postcritical sentence.

older and younger subjects. Data from a pilot study suggest that we were successful in achieving this goal. When allowed to consult a printed version of the passages, neither age group displayed significant problems with answering comprehension questions about the passages. In addition to the passages, the experimental materials included direct questions (e.g., *The artist was told he had three more months to do what?*) which were used to test retention for both target and control information. The latter was relatively unimportant information which was explicitly stated in all three versions of the passage. A complete example of one set of the materials is presented in Table 9.1.

It should probably be acknowledged that we designated the target facts as central information and the control facts as peripheral information, not on the basis of a formal analysis of passage structure such as that of Kintsch (1974), but on more intuitive grounds. Nonetheless, our intuitions are supported by data from a pilot study in which (young adult) subjects read and produced written recalls of the passages. According to the importance level research, if we were correct in assuming that the target information was more important than the control information for each passage, then the probability of recalling the target information should correspondingly be greater than the probability of recalling the control information. This indeed is what we found. For example, for the explicit versions, the mean percentages recalled were 82% and 45%, respectively. Additionally, it can be noted that although age differences in importance level effects were not a central concern of our research, the fact that the target and control information for each paragraph differed in importance level allows our data to address this issue.

Every subject read a single version of each of the 12 passages, with four each from the expected, unexpected, and explicit conditions. Across subjects, an equal number processed each of the passages in each of the three versions. This meant that the *same* target information was tested in the explicit condition and in the two implicit conditions, and that comparisons between explicit and inferential information and between easy and hard inferential information were not complicated by differences in other variables such as importance level.

Each passage was presented one sentence at a time at a rate controlled by the subject who pressed a button whenever he or she was ready for the next sentence. Each button press resulted in the erasure of the current sentence and the presentation of the next one. The subjects read the first six passages and then were tested with the target and control questions on those; then the same procedure was followed for the remaining six passages. On the retention test, the questions appeared on the video screen but were answered orally by the subjects.

Thirty subjects from each of two age groups (means = 19.7 and 72.3 years) participated in the study. The young subjects were university undergraduates who participated for course credit. The older adults were community residents, who were in reasonably good health for their age and who were paid for their participation. The younger subjects were mostly freshmen and sophomores; the older subjects had a mean of 14.2 years of education. In addition, all subjects were administered the vocabulary subtest of the Wechsler Adult Intelligence Scale – Revised (WAIS-R). The mean standardized scores on this instrument were 11.23 for the younger adults and 12.27 for the older ones.

Results and discussion

We first describe the results for the recall data and then the reading time results. Table 9.2 presents the percentage correct recall of the control and target information as a function of passage version and age. From the table it is clear that an importance level effect was obtained for both age groups and that it was approximately equal in magnitude across ages: The average target–control difference was 16.2% for the younger subjects and 19.3% for the older ones.

Because the target and control questions tested different information, we examined age and version differences for each type of question separately. In the separate analysis of the control information recall, the only significant effect was that for age, with the age deficit being 12.8%. By contrast, the analysis of the data on target information recall revealed significant main effects of both age and passage version and a

Table 9.2. *Percentage recall of control and target information*

Passage	Control information		Target inferences	
	Younger	Older	Younger	Older
Explicit	74.6%	63.8%	98.3%	90.0%
Expected	78.8%	65.8%	92.5%	92.5%
Unexpected	78.8%	64.2%	90.0%	69.2%
Mean	77.4%	64.6%	93.6%	83.9%

significant Age × Version interaction. For both age groups, the lowest level of recall of the target information occurred in the unexpected condition. (For the younger subjects, only the explicit–unexpected difference was significant; for the older ones, the unexpected condition differed significantly from the other two.) However, the striking aspect of the target recall data is the poor performance of the older subjects on the unexpected inferences relative to their performance in the other two inference conditions. The age deficit in the unexpected condition was 20.8% as contrasted to 8.3% in the explicit and 0% in the expected condition. (Although relatively small, the age difference for the explicit condition was nonetheless significant.)

The target recall results can be related to the existing literature on age difference in inference generation and to the reduced-capacity views of aging. With regard to the former, the results replicate in a single experiment both the finding of no age difference in inference generation (the expected condition; cf. Belmore, 1981) and the finding of a significant age deficit (the unexpected condition; cf. Cohen, 1979). Our earlier suggestion that inference difficulty was a likely source of the conflicts in the literature is therefore supported.

As to the relevance of these findings to reduced-capacity models, one prediction of such views was clearly confirmed. Specifically, the age deficit was largest in the most demanding condition – the unexpected inference condition. However, another fairly direct prediction of the reduced-capacity view, that the age deficit in the expected condition should be intermediate between the other two conditions, was not supported.

This apparent disconfirmation of the capacity view should probably be evaluated in the light of other data from our research program which suggests that the disconfirming outcome is tied to the self-paced presentation mode of the current experiment. That is, because they could slow down their reading rate, the older adults were apparently able to compensate somewhat for their reduced capacity. At the least, they could compensate sufficiently to handle, without deficit, the relatively small increases in capacity needed for the generation of Expected inferences.

A different pattern of target recall was obtained in another experiment that utilized the same materials and same general design but an oral presentation procedure (Zacks et al., 1987). These data, along with the target recall data of the self-paced reading study, are shown in Figure 9.1. It can be seen in the figure that the overall

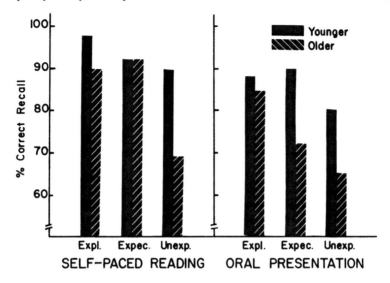

Figure 9.1. Percentage correct recalls of the target information in the self-paced reading and oral presentation studies. (Adapted in part from Zacks et al., 1987, by permission of *The Journal of Gerontology*, vol. 42, no. 4, 1987.)

performance level was lower in the oral presentation experiment than in the self-paced reading experiment. However, more important is the fact that in contrast to the reading situation, the oral presentation mode resulted in a significant age deficit for both the expected and the unexpected inferences. Apparently, when they are not allowed to control the rate of information input, the older subjects are not able to handle as efficiently as younger subjects the processing demands of either easy or difficult inferences (cf. Cohen, 1981). Another important point highlighted by this comparison of the target recall results of the two experiments is that the processing demands of a particular text variable cannot be established in isolation from a consideration of the presentation mode and its influence on momentary demands on processing capacity.

We turn now to the reading time data of the self-paced study. We will focus in particular on aspects of these data that might provide further insight into the large age deficit in encoding of unexpected inferences. Because sentences varied in length, reading times were computed per word. Consistent with the widely observed slowing of mental processing in older adults (e.g., Salthouse, 1982), the older adults paced themselves more slowly (mean reading time per word = 502 msec) through the passages than did the younger adults (mean = 340 msec).

Three sentences were singled out for specific analysis of their reading times. (These sentences are marked in the example in Table 9.1.) The first of these was the sentence that explicitly stated the target information in the explicit condition and that invited the target inference in the expected condition. The analysis of this sentence was relatively uninformative, with no effects of passage version being

Table 9.3. *Reading speed (in msec/word) for
inference, critical, and postcritical sentences*

	Explicit	Expected	Unexpected
Younger subjects			
Inference	318	350	323
Critical	347	347	396
Postcritical	284	299	325
Older subjects			
Inference	469	495	506
Critical	514	496	577
Postcritical	423	437	476

found for either age group. This was probably due to the relative insensitivity of whole-sentence reading times to small increments in processing demands such as would be produced by the easy, expected inferences.

Much more intriguing was the pattern of data for the sentence in which the target inference is first clued in the unexpected passage versions. It is here that subjects reading an unexpected passage first receive information that is incongruent with their initial interpretation of the passage. For example, in the unexpected version of the artist passage, subjects assume that the artist is concerned about the exhibit deadline until they read "He was shocked to hear this kind of news from his doctor." Subjects in the explicit and expected versions read the identical sentence, but these subjects already know that the artist was worried about his doctor's report. No differences are expected between these two conditions. However, in the unexpected condition, reading speed for this sentence, called "critical" in Tables 9.1 and 9.3, should be considerably slower. And indeed, this pattern prevails (see Table 9.3) with a reliable difference among versions that is entirely due to the slower reading of the critical sentence in the unexpected version. Reading times for this sentence in the explicit and expected versions did not differ from each other, and as with all the reading time results, the older subjects read this sentence more slowly than the younger subjects.

We also expected, but did not find, a significant Age × Version interaction, with the older subjects showing less of an effect of passage version than the younger ones. Our reasoning here was as follows: The slowdown in reading time for the critical sentence in the unexpected condition reflects the extra processing needed to generate the target inferences in this condition. Because older subjects are less likely than younger ones to generate these inferences (and the recall data support this supposition), they should show less of a slowdown than the younger subjects. But they do not: There was not even the slightest hint of the predicted interaction.

In order to explore this issue further, we looked at the reading times for the sentence immediately following the critical sentence. We were led to this analysis by a suggestion of Mary Attig's as well as by some recent work of O'Brien and Myers (1985). In research with young adults, O'Brien and Myers obtained data suggesting that an unanticipated word in the midst of a passage leads to reprocessing of the text preceding the surprise. This covert reprocessing occurs during the reading of the remainder of the passage, reducing reading speed and resulting in superior memory for early portions of passages containing unpredicted words. Although we have no appropriate measure of passage recall to compare to O'Brien and Myers's, the reading times for the postcritical sentence are relevant to this type of theoretical argument.

In analyzing the reading times for the postcritical sentence (also shown in Table 9.3), we expected to see a "spillover" slowdown from the preceding sentence in the unexpected condition. The slowdown would reflect a continuation of the reprocessing of the text that was initiated by the critical sentence. Because our original concept was that the older subjects would be limited in the amount of reprocessing they could carry out, we expected them to show a smaller spillover effect than the younger adults. The analysis of the postcritical sentence reading times revealed (unsurprisingly) that the older adults read this sentence more slowly than the younger adults; additionally, the effect of passage version was as predicted, with the slowest times in the unexpected condition. However, once more our expectations about age differences were disconfirmed: The spillover effect in the unexpected condition was of approximately the *same* magnitude for younger and older adults (interaction $F < 1$).

The data from this experiment make it clear that both younger and older adults realize that the critical sentence in the unexpected version requires special processing, resulting in slower reading rates. This slowdown also spills over to the succeeding sentence. Because these effects on reading time are similar for both age groups, the reading time data do not clearly point to a specific locus of deficit that would account for the older adults' depressed recall of the target inferences in the Unexpected condition. However, a number of possibilities can be suggested. One is that despite the slowdown in reading time, the older subjects are still less likely than the young to draw the appropriate inference, perhaps because they are unable to retrieve enough of the preceding text to do so (cf. Glanzer, Fischer, & Dorfman, 1984; Glanzer & Nolan, 1986). Another possibility is that having drawn the correct inference, the older subjects fail to completely reinterpret the passage as a whole and therefore they fail to integrate the inference into a coherent text representation.

In general, our working assumption is that the difficulty of the unexpected passages stems from the need to juggle making of the inference with the task of reinterpretion and integration of the text as a whole. We assume that the young are more successful at handling these two tasks than the elderly, leaving the former with access to a variety of cues that can help them to answer the inference probe question. The older adults' reduced probability of answering the target question may stem in part from a lowered probability of generating the critical inference during comprehension. However, they may also have problems even when they succeed in generating the critical inference. In this case, the failure to encode a well-integrated representation of the text may have left them with fewer cues with which to access the target information on the recall test.

Such an explanation of the inference recall results is broadly consistent with the general capacity view with which we began. Certainly, it is compatible with this view to argue that the reduced capacity of the elderly decreases their ability to retain new information while reconsidering earlier information. However, although this argument is compatible with the general-capacity model, it is not specifically derived from it. Our current view is that an unelaborated capacity view lacks the analytic power to provide a detailed specification of the nature of age differences in processes such as inference generation and text reinterpretation. Because of this, we were motivated to develop a more analytic model, one that can be readily tied to specific models of text processing. In the final portion of this chapter, we outline this model.

Capacity theory revisited: The elaborated model

Our revised capacity model represents an attempt to mesh general-capacity theory with current conceptualizations of discourse processing mechanisms, especially those involved in inference generation. The model ties the notion of capacity to that of working memory (e.g., Anderson, 1983; Baddeley, 1981; Baddeley & Hitch, 1974; Daneman & Carpenter, 1980, 1983; Klapp, Marshburn, & Lester, 1983).[1] Working memory (as distinguished from short-term memory; see Klapp et al., 1983) is assumed to have *both* storage and processing functions which trade off for capacity (e.g., Baddeley & Hitch, 1974; Daneman & Carpenter, 1980, 1983). Beyond this basic idea, the functions and operating mechanisms of working memory have as yet to be clearly defined. In fact, it is likely that the way that this system functions is highly task specific (Richardson, 1984). If so, hypotheses about age changes in working memory must be tied to a model of the experimental tasks.

We assume that in the case of text processing, two types of information are served by the storage function of working memory: (1) information derived from preceding text; and (2) prior knowledge activated from long-term memory. The more of both types of information that can be stored in working memory, the deeper will be the understanding of subsequent text (e.g., Daneman & Carpenter, 1980). The recent research of Glanzer et al. (1984; see also Glanzer & Nolan, 1986) provides striking evidence that the efficient operation of comprehension mechanisms is dependent on having prior text information (especially the last sentence or two) available in working memory.

The processing function of working memory encompasses a variety of processes that occur during text encoding. Some operate at the level of individual words and phrases and are closely tied to the words that are currently being processed. Included here are lexical access, sentence parsing, and derivation of propositions. These "within-proposition" processes are not heavily dependent on the storage functions of working memory. Contrasted with these are "between-proposition"[2] or higher-level activities such as the integration of new with prior information, the formation of inferences, and the derivation of summary propositions. These latter functions all require that the relevant information be available in the storage component of working memory. (This particular view of text processing builds upon such hierarchical models as those of LaBerge & Samuels, 1974, and of Graesser, Hoffman, & Clark, 1980).

The aging assumptions of our revised capacity model are (1) that aging is associated with an overall decline in working-memory capacity, and (2) that this capacity decline is unevenly distributed among the various storage and processing components of working memory. In particular, the major direct impact of aging will be found in a reduced storage capacity in working memory. In turn, the reduced storage capacity will impact most heavily on between-proposition processing, because between-proposition processes such as inference generation require that critical information be available in working memory (cf. Glanzer et al., 1984). By contrast to the direct effects of aging on buffer storage and to the indirect effects on between-proposition processing, we assume that the capacity allocated to within-proposition or ongoing processing is maintained at a level similar to that in young people. (See Light and Anderson, 1983, for another argument that older individuals give high priority to on-line discourse processing at the expense of other encoding processes.) The rationale for assuming this particular allocation of capacity decline is three fold: (1) The initial stages of within-proposition processing (e.g., lexical access) tend to be stimulus driven and automatic. (2) Social convention and other pragmatic considerations demand of a person supposedly conversing, reading, or listening that he or she will at least decode individual words and phrases. This means that even when within-proposition encoding puts relatively high demands on processing capacity, older adults will put a high priority on this type of encoding. (3) Finally, a number of recent empirical findings suggest that variables influencing demand on the buffer have a special impact on the elderly. For example, Light and Capps (1986) have shown that the age deficit in the ability to determine the referent of a pronoun increases with an increase in the time span over which the antecedent information must be held in working memory (see also Cohen & Faulkner, 1984; Wright, 1981).

Although the research described in this chapter does not provide a definitive test of the elaborated model, its results are readily interpreted in terms of the model. For example, the presumed reduction in older adults' buffer storage capacity provides an explanation of their depressed recall of the unexpected target inferences in the self-paced reading study: In comparison to younger subjects, older adults have available in working memory less of the information that is needed for generating the correct inference and for integrating it into a revised text representation. Furthermore, because the constraints on buffer capacity determine both the "window" of preceding text that can be maintained in working memory and the amount of text information that at any one time can be reactivated from the long-term store, older subjects may be at a disadvantage even when (as in this study) they can control the rate of information flow: The slowed reading is unable to compensate completely for their inability to hold enough relevant information in working memory simultaneously.

Obviously, considerable research will need to be done to establish the value of the elaborated capacity model and the validity of speculations such as those of the preceding paragraph (but see also Light and Albertson, this volume). However, we believe that our adoption of a working-memory analysis and our assumptions regarding the allocation of capacity declines associated with aging add considerable power to the general-capacity view, a view that has had at least moderate success in accounting for standard memory findings in cognitive gerontology (cf. the earlier discussion of Craik's capacity theory). It is our working hypothesis that such an analysis will enable us to specify exactly where inference generation in older adults breaks down and so ultimately help us to determine how it might be repaired.

Notes

1 We acknowledge that most discussions of working memory distinguish between a phonemic response buffer (or articulatory loop) and a central executive processor (e.g., Baddeley, 1981; Baddeley & Hitch, 1974; Richardson, 1984). The phonemic response buffer seems to have limited functions; it serves as a source of supplementary storage capacity in tasks (e.g., memory span) that formally require the maintenance of accurate serial-order information (Richardson, 1984). Because we are not interested in such tasks, we ignore the phonemic response buffer in what follows and treat the term "working memory" as a synonym for the central executive processor.
2 It is of course only roughly true that within-proposition processing places less demand on storage capacity than does between-proposition processing. For example, the encoding of certain multi-argument propositions can place relatively high demands on storage capacity in working memory. Nonetheless, we think it useful to distinguish between aspects of encoding that typically place a relatively high load on storage capacity and those that do not. Furthermore, it should be noted that we believe that the factors that influence storage demands are somewhat independent of those that influence ongoing processing demands. Because of our assumptions about the preservation of ongoing processing activities in the face of reduced capacity, age differences should be more sensitive to the former than to the latter.

References

Alba, J. (1984). Nature of inference representation. *American Journal of Psychology, 97,* 215–233.

Anderson, J. R. (1983). *The architecture of cognition.* Cambridge, MA: Harvard University Press.

Attig, M., & Hasher, L. (1980). The processing of frequency of occurrence information by adults. *Journal of Gerontology, 35,* 66–69.

Baddeley, A. D. (1981). The concept of working memory: A view of its current state and probable future development. *Cognition, 10,* 17–23.

Baddeley, A. D., & Hitch, G. (1974). Working memory. In G. Bower (Ed.) *The psychology of learning and motivation* (Vol. 8, pp. 47–89). New York: Academic Press.

Belmore, S. M. (1981). Age-related changes in processing explicit and implicit language. *Journal of Gerontology, 36,* 316–322.

Bowles, N. L., & Poon, L. W. (1985). Aging and the retrieval of words in semantic memory. *Journal of Gerontology, 40,* 71–77.

Bransford, J. D. (1979). *Human cognition: Learning, understanding, and remembering.* Belmont, CA: Wadsworth.

Cerella, J., & Fozard, J. L. (1984). Lexical access and age. *Developmental Psychology, 20,* 235–243.

Clark, H. H. (1977). Inferences in comprehension. In D. LaBerge & S. J. Samuels (Eds.), *Perception and comprehension* (pp. 243–263). Hillsdale, NJ: Erlbaum.

Cohen, G. (1979). Language comprehension in old age. *Cognitive Psychology, 11,* 412–429.

Cohen, G. (1981). Inferential reasoning in old age. *Cognition, 9,* 59–72.

Cohen, G., & Faulkner, D. (1984). Memory for text: Some age differences in the nature of information that is retained after listening to texts. In H. Bouma & D. G. Bouwhuis (Eds.), *Attention and performance X: Control of language processes* (pp. 501–514). Hillsdale, NJ: Erlbaum.

Craik, F. I. M. (1983). On the transfer of information from temporary to permanent memory. *Philosophical Transactions of the Royal Society of London, B302,* 341–359.

Craik, F. I. M., & Byrd, M. (1982). Aging and cognitive deficits: The role of attentional resources. In F. I. M. Craik & S. E. Trehub (Eds.), *Aging and cognitive processes* (pp. 191–211). New York: Plenum.

Craik, F. I. M., & Rabinowitz, J. C. (1983, August). *Processing resources in relation to memory encoding and retrieval.* Paper presented at the American Psychological Association Annual Meeting, Anaheim, CA.

Craik, F. I. M., & Rabinowitz, J. C. (1984). Age differences in the acquisition and use of verbal information: A tutorial review. In H. Bouma & D. G. Bouwhuis (Eds.), *Attention and performance X: Control of language processes* (pp. 471–499). Hillsdale, NJ: Erlbaum.

Daneman, M., & Carpenter, P. A. (1980). Individual differences in working memory and reading. *Journal of Verbal Learning and Verbal Behavior, 19,* 450–466.

Daneman, M., & Carpenter, P. A. (1983). Individual differences in integrating information between and within sentences. *Journal of Experimental Psychology: Learning, Memory, and Cognition, 9,* 561–584.

Dixon, R. A., Hultsch, D. F., Simon, E. W., & von Eye, A. (1984). Verbal ability and text structure effects on adult age differences in text recall. *Journal of Verbal Learning and Verbal Behavior, 23,* 569–578.

Garrod, S., & Sanford, A. (1981). Bridging inferences and the extended domain of reference. In J. Long & A. Baddeley (Eds.), *Attention and performance IX* (pp. 331–346). Hillsdale, NJ: Erlbaum.

Glanzer, M., Fischer, B., & Dorfman, D. (1984). Short-term storage in reading. *Journal of Verbal Learning and Verbal Behavior, 23,* 569–578.

Glanzer, M., & Nolan, S. D. (1986). Memory mechanisms in text comprehension. In G. Bower (Ed.), *The psychology of learning and motivation* (Vol. 20, pp. 275–317). New York: Academic Press.

Graesser, A. C., Hoffman, N. L., & Clark, L. F. (1980). Structural components of reading time. *Journal of Verbal Learning and Verbal Behavior, 19,* 135–151.

Harris, R. J. (1981). Inferences in information processing. In G. Bower (Ed.), *The psychology of learning and motivation* (Vol. 15, pp. 81–128). New York: Academic Press.

Hasher, L., & Zacks, R. T. (1979). Automatic and effortful processes in memory. *Journal of Experimental Psychology: General, 108,* 356–388.

Hasher, L., & Zacks, R. T. (1984). Automatic processing of fundamental information: The case of frequency of occurrence. *American Psychologist, 39,* 1372–1388.

Hess, T. M. (1984). Effects of semantically related and unrelated contexts on recognition memory of different-aged adults. *Journal of Gerontology, 39,* 444–451.

Hess, T. M., & Higgins, J. N. (1983). Context utilization in young and old adults. *Journal of Gerontology, 38,* 65–71.

Howard, D. V. (1983). The effects of aging and degree of association on the semantic priming of lexical decisions. *Experimental Aging Research, 9,* 145–151.

Howard, D. V., McAndrews, M. P., & Lasaga, M. I. (1981). Semantic priming of lexical decisions in young and old adults. *Journal of Gerontology, 36,* 707–714.

Hultsch, D. F., & Dixon, R. A. (1984). Memory for text materials in adulthood. In P. B. Baltes & O. G. Brim, Jr. (Eds.), *Life-span development and behavior* (Vol. 6, pp. 78–108). New York: Academic Press.

Hultsch, D. F., Hertzog, C., & Dixon, R. A. (1984). Text recall in adulthood: The role of intellectual abilities. *Developmental Psychology, 20,* 1193–1209.

Jenkins, J. J. (1979). Four points to remember: A tetrahedral model of memory experiments. In L. Cermak & F. I. M. Craik (Eds.), *Levels of processing in human memory* (pp. 429–461). Hillsdale, NJ: Erlbaum.

Kahneman, D. (1973). *Attention and effort.* Englewood Cliffs, NJ: Prentice-Hall.

Kausler, D. H. (1982). *Experimental psychology and human aging.* New York: Wiley.

Kintsch, W. (1974). *The representation of meaning in memory.* Hillsdale, NJ: Erlbaum.

Klapp, S. T., Marshburn, E. A., & Lester, P. T. (1983). Short-term memory does not involve the "working memory" of information processing: The demise of a common assumption. *Journal of Experimental Psychology: General, 112,* 240–264.

LaBerge, D., & Samuels, S. J. (1974). Toward a theory of automatic information processing in reading. *Cognitive Psychology, 6,* 293–323.

LeDoux, J. F., Blum, C., & Hirst, W. (1983). Inferential processing of context: Studies of cognitively impaired subjects. *Brain and Language, 19,* 216–224.

Light, L. L., & Anderson, P. A. (1983). Memory for scripts in young and older adults. *Memory & Cognition, 11,* 435–444.

Light, L. L., & Capps, J. L. (1986). Comprehension of pronouns in young and older adults. *Developmental Psychology, 22,* 580–585.

Light, L. L., Zelinski, E. M., & Moore, M. (1982). Adult age differences in reasoning from new information. *Journal of Experimental Psychology: Learning, Memory, and Cognition, 8,* 435–447.

Madden, D. J. (1985). Age-related slowing in the retrieval of information from long-term memory. *Journal of Gerontology, 40,* 208–210.

Mandel, R. G., & Johnson, N. S. (1984). A developmental analysis of story recall and comprehension in adulthood. *Journal of Verbal Learning and Verbal Behavior, 23,* 643–659.

Meyer, B. J. F., & Rice, G. E. (1981). Information recalled from prose by young, middle, and old adult readers. *Experimental Aging Research, 7,* 253–268.

Mueller, J. H., Kausler, D. H., & Faherty, A. (1980). Age and access time for different memory codes. *Experimental Aging Research, 6,* 445–449.

O'Brien, E. J., & Myers, J. L. (1985). When comprehension difficulty improves memory for text. *Journal of Experimental Psychology: Learning, Memory, and Cognition, 11,* 12–21.

Rabinowitz, J. C., Craik, F. I. M., & Ackerman, B. P. (1982). A processing resource account of age differences in recall. *Canadian Journal of Psychology, 36,* 325–344.

Reder, L. M., Wible, C., & Martin, J. (1986). Differential memory changes with age: Exact retrieval versus plausible inference. *Journal of Experimental Psychology: Learning, Memory, and Cognition, 12,* 72–81.

Richardson, J. T. E. (1984). Developing the theory of working memory. *Memory & Cognition, 12,* 71–83.

Salthouse, T. A. (1982). *Adult cognition: An experimental psychology of human aging.* New York: Springer-Verlag.

Spilich, G. J. (1983). Life-span components of text processing: Structural and procedural differences. *Journal of Verbal Learning and Verbal Behavior, 22,* 231–244.

Stanovich, K. E., & West, R. F. (1983). On priming by a sentence context. *Journal of Experimental Psychology: General, 112,* 1–36.

Till, R. E. (1985). Verbatim and inferential memory in young and elderly adults. *Journal of Gerontology, 40,* 316–332.

Waugh, N. C., & Barr, R. A. (1982). Encoding deficits in aging. In F. I. M. Craik & S. Trehub (Eds.), *Aging and cognitive processes* (pp. 183–190). New York: Plenum.

Wright, R. E. (1981). Aging, divided attention, and processing capacity. *Journal of Gerontology, 36,* 605–614.

Zacks, R. T. (1982). Encoding strategies used by young and elderly adults in a keeping track task. *Journal of Gerontology, 37,* 203–211.

Zacks, R. T., Hasher, L., Doren, B., Hamm, V., & Attig, M. S. (1987). Encoding and memory of explicit and implicit information. *Journal of Gerontology, 42,* 418–422.

Zelinski, E. M., Light, L. L., & Gilewski, M. J. (1984). Adult age differences in memory for prose: The question of sensitivity to passage structure. *Developmental Psychology, 20,* 1181–1192.

10   Age differences in memory for texts: Production deficiency or processing limitations?

Gillian Cohen

Studies of the effects of aging on memory for written and spoken texts have now accumulated to the point where a complex pattern of convergent and divergent results is apparent. Recent reviews have sought to make sense of this pattern and to identify the sources of the many discrepancies between different studies by analyzing the interactive relationships between attributes of the text, the learner, and the task (Hultsch & Dixon, 1984; Meyer & Rice, in press). The outcome of these reviews is that we are much better able to identify the circumstances in which old people are likely to remember texts less well than young people. We can identify the type of texts, the kind of people, and the kind of memory tasks that will, in combination, be most likely to exhibit an age-related deficit.

But why does ability to remember information from texts decline in old age? Researchers are currently focused on finding a theoretical explanation that can illuminate the underlying causes of age-related changes. The explanations that are commonly put forward can be divided into two classes, those that attribute the deficits to faulty strategies (the production deficiency explanation) and those that attribute them to processing limitations (the processing capacity explanation). This chapter attempts to assess the power and scope of these explanations using two criteria: how far the theory generates predictions that are precise and unambiguous, and how far the empirical evidence conforms to the predictions. The importance of these issues is underlined by the fact that other authors in this volume (Zacks and Hasher; Zelinski) have also homed in on the same questions.

The production deficiency explanation

The production deficiency explanation claims that elderly people do not spontaneously adopt the optimal strategies for processing texts. According to this explanation, young people are very familiar with the task of reading or listening to texts and memorizing the content. They have received intensive training and practice and have developed those strategies of encoding and organization that are best fitted for the task. Older people, on the other hand, are disadvantaged because text processing is a relatively unfamiliar task for them and they may never have received appropriate

This work was supported by a grant from the Economic and Social Research Council (ESRC), U.K.

training. In addition, their interests and intentions may differ from those of young people so that they attach importance to different aspects of the text. The production deficiency explanation has been invoked by several researchers (e.g., Schaie & Labouvie-Vief, 1974) to account for some, at least, of the observed age difference.

Two different versions of the production deficiency hypothesis can be distinguished, a "strong" version and a "weak" one.

The strong production deficiency explanation

The strong version claims that the elderly, whether from schooling, custom, inexperience, or inclination, employ nonoptimal strategies for processing texts although they *could* employ more appropriate ones if they were trained, guided, or persuaded to do so. This explanation has always suffered from an inherent implausibility. The kind of deficits typically observed in old people's memory for texts are such that it strains credulity to suppose that they deliberately choose to adopt the strategies that produce such defective performance. Although it is just conceivable that the elderly might choose to process the details of a text and neglect the gist, or might attend to what is explicit and ignore the implications, it is hardly likely that they would deliberately fail to understand logical relationships, or to link agents and actions or pronouns and referents. Moreover, it is even more unlikely that they would persist in such strategies when they found that these did not enable them to meet the task requirements.

In spite of its implausibility, several researchers have expressed views consistent with a strong production deficiency hypothesis. Meyer and Rice (1981), for example, claim that changes in educational methods and in life experience account for different styles of text processing that characterize the age groups. They suggest that the young are trained to extract the gist, whereas the older generation were drilled in rote learning. Craik and Rabinowitz (1984) believe that "older people are less able or less willing to initiate and carry out higher level cognitive operations. The older person still has the potential to carry out such operations, however, as shown by the fact that inefficient processing can be 'repaired' by structuring the task appropriately" (p. 490). Dixon, Hultsch, Simon, and von Eye (1984, p. 577) and Hultsch and Dixon (1984, p. 95) also entertain the idea that "the tendency of older adults to recall fewer details of the story may reflect the use of qualitatively different retrieval strategies and criteria for remembering."

The strong production deficiency hypothesis generates several predictions. These are:

(1) Age differences will be qualitative rather than purely quantitative.
(2) Training and practice will induce better strategies and so reduce or eliminate age differences.
(3) Individuals with high verbal ability will have good strategies and so will show little or no age deficit in memory for text.

It should be noted, though, that testing these predictions is severely hampered by vagueness in the definition of what is meant by "strategy" and by the difficulty of identifying subjects' strategies.

According to the first prediction, the production deficiency explanation is more compatible with qualitative differences in memory for texts, whereas a processing capacity explanation is required when purely quantitative differences are observed. If age groups differ in *what* they remember, it is taken as an indication that they are using different strategies; if they differ only in *how much* they remember, it is taken to indicate that old and young are doing much the same thing, but the old are doing it less efficiently. Not surprisingly, most experiments yield age effects that are both quantitative and qualitative. Although in some studies (e.g., Zelinski, this volume) the response pattern does not vary with age, and differences are purely quantitative, it is rare to find the purely qualitative differences predicted to result from production deficiencies.

In accordance with the second prediction, if age differences can be eliminated or significantly reduced by practice or instruction, the initial deficit must, it is argued, have been due to the use of faulty strategies by the elderly and the improvement occurs because, after training, these strategies are replaced by more appropriate ones. In fact, the logic of this prediction is flawed. The finding that age deficits can sometimes be eliminated by practice and training does not entitle us to conclude that the improvement in performance is wholly due to a change of strategy. Processing operations such as recoding are known to benefit from practice (Grant, Storandt, & Botwinick, 1978); thus people may be continuing to use the same strategies but may be executing them less effortfully and more efficiently. In any case, there is very little evidence that age differences are diminished by practice (Kausler, 1982).

In most of the Cohen and Faulkner studies cited in this chapter, subjects were presented with practice texts followed by 12–18 experimental texts, so there was ample opportunity for the elderly to discover that their strategies did not serve them well and to change or modify them accordingly. However, age differences were not reduced by practice and there was no sign of older subjects shifting spontaneously to better strategies. One exception to this pattern is a study by Meyer and Rice (1981) in which there was a weak interaction of Age × Practice such that an age deficit on the first text was reduced on the second text. However, because this effect was predominantly due to occasions when the text with the most difficult structure was presented first, the trend toward reduced age differences can be attributed to the relaxation of the processing demands rather than a strategy shift.

Evidence relevant to the third prediction – that text memory will be preserved in highly verbal individuals – is less clear-cut. Many researchers, including Meyer and Rice (1983) and Dixon et al. (1984), have noted that age deficits in text memory are much less evident in old people with high levels of verbal ability or education. Verbal ability is usually measured by some form of vocabulary test. It is far from clear, though, why having a good vocabulary should, in itself, ensure the use of optimal text-processing strategies. Perhaps good vocabulary and good strategies are not so much cause and effect, but are both the product of superior education. It is just as plausible, however, to argue that high verbal ability is linked with superior processing capacity, and it is the superior processing capacity that *allows* good strategies to be employed. There is some evidence to support this latter interpretation (Baddeley, Logie, Nimmo-Smith, & Brereton, 1985).

It is fairly clear that the strong version of the production deficiency hypothesis is hard to sustain. It lacks both intuitive plausibility and empirical support.

The weak production deficiency explanation

This version also claims that older people employ nonoptimal strategies but maintains that they are enforced by processing limitations rather than induced by cultural or educational factors. According to the weak production deficiency hypothesis, a reduction in processing capacity may dictate a shift to a less effortful strategy. Or, a weakness in any component operation may necessitate changing to a strategy that bypasses that particular operation. Thus age-related changes in processing are very likely to result in concomitant changes in strategy. If this is the case, the primary cause of age differences in text processing is the shortfall in processing capacity, and the use of an ineffective or inappropriate strategy is only a secondary cause. This weak version of the production deficiency explanation, although more plausible than the strong version, is not easy to distinguish empirically from a "pure" processing-capacity explanation because both predict that age differences will diminish only when processing demands are relaxed.

The processing capacity explanation

Several kinds of evidence can be advanced to support the claim that limitations in processing capacity are the primary cause of age-related defects in memory for text. Although not many studies of text memory were specifically designed as direct tests of the processing capacity explanation, relevant findings can be garnered from a variety of experimental paradigms. The processing capacity explanation generates three predictions. These predictions are:

(1) *Processing demands.* Experimental manipulations that reduce processing demands will reduce age effects, whereas those that increase processing demands will increase age effects.

(2) *Depth of processing.* Age-related deficits will be greatest for those aspects of the texts that require more or deeper processing and will be slight or absent for those aspects that require only shallow surface processing.

(3) *Individual differences.* Age differences in text comprehension and memory will not be apparent if young and old individuals do not differ in processing capacity. Age differences will appear when older individuals have lower processing capacity than young individuals.

What do we mean by processing capacity? Before we can see to what extent these predictions are confirmed, we need to specify both what is meant by processing capacity and how this capacity is employed in text processing. The term "processing capacity" is used inclusively in this chapter to encompass both working-memory capacity as described by Zelinski (this volume) and the factor that Zelinski calls processing resources and Zacks and Hasher (this volume) describe as general capacity.

In this chapter, three aspects of processing capacity that are particularly important in memory for text are identified.

(1) *Working memory.* The capacity of working memory is defined (Daneman & Carpenter, 1980) as the ability to hold information in temporary storage while simultaneously executing processes and storing the products of these processes. In this model, both the ongoing processes and the items of stored information compete for a limited capacity. Capacity may be exceeded by increases in either the number of items to be stored or the number or complexity of the processes to be performed.

(2) *Speed of processing.* With continuous sequential input, speed of processing is critically important. Two factors determine a minimum rate at which information must be processed: the rate of input and the rate of decay in working memory. If the rate of processing falls below the rate of input, some information will be lost or processed inadequately. If the rate of processing falls below the rate of decay, some items will decay before they are processed.

(3) *Processing resources.* Capacity also includes the power to execute multiple processes and to schedule and coordinate their execution. It is assumed (Kahneman, 1973, and Zacks and Hasher, this volume) that processing resources are consumed by effortful, attentional processes, but are not required by automatic processing. In the model of working memory developed by Baddeley (1981), processing resources reside in the central component of the working-memory system, the central executive, and are not differentiated from working-memory capacity as outlined in (1) above.

There is ample evidence for age-related differences in processing capacity. It is well established that the capacity of working memory tends to decline with age (Kausler, 1982) and that the rate of processing is slowed (Salthouse, 1980).

Current models of text processing and text memory allow us to specify how these aspects of processing capacity are involved. The operations required in processing text include lexical access, syntactic parsing, and semantic analysis; constructing inferences, elaborating and organizing the information; identifying and integrating logical and conceptual relationships within the text and between the text and prior knowledge stored in long-term memory. So how are these operations affected by processing capacity limitations?

The role of working memory is crucial. According to the model of text processing proposed by Kintsch and van Dijk (1978), text comprehension is a cyclical process. Working memory functions as a carry-over buffer store that maintains some of the propositions derived from analysis of a small local segment of the text. Propositions are selected for maintenance in the working-memory buffer on the basis of importance and recency, and these propositions are carried forward for recycling with the next segment of the text. Overlapping cycles of analysis produce a coherent text base that incorporates local relations between more or less adjacent propositions as well as a coherent higher-level macrostructure that reflects global relationships between propositions. The coherence of the text representation that is constructed is thus dependent on working-memory capacity. If fewer propositions can be maintained in working memory, the degree of integration and interrelationship between ideas in the text will be less accurately represented. Kemper (this volume) discusses the relationship of working memory and syntactic complexity, and Light and Albertson (this volume) describe the role of working memory in processes like anaphor resolution and anomaly detection that rely on cross-referencing propositions from different parts of the text.

Speed of processing is also important. Propositions need to be continually re-instated in the carry-forward buffer with each fresh cycle of analysis and eventually transferred to long-term memory. If processing is too slow, propositions may decay or be displaced before they can be reinstated or transferred. Both speed of process-ing and availability of processing resources determine how well text is understood and remembered. In text comprehension, lower-level processes like word recogni-tion are considered to be relatively automatic and therefore to make little demand on processing resources (Hasher & Zacks, 1979). Semantic analysis is considered to be more effortful, involving active constructive processes whereby the meaning is interpreted, inferred, elaborated, disambiguated, evaluated, and integrated with contextual information and prior knowledge. In effect, there is a trade-off between the amount of effort expended at encoding and the amount of effort required for retrieval because semantic representations that are more richly encoded are easier to retrieve. With rapid continuous input, any reduction in either processing resources or in the speed of processing is likely to curtail the depth and complexity of the se-mantic processing that can be carried out in the time available. Processing resources and rate of processing will therefore affect both the level of comprehension and the subsequent ability to recall information from texts.

One criticism that may be leveled at the processing capacity explanation is that it seems to be so broadly and loosely defined that it can explain anything and every-thing and so cannot be falsified. It is often difficult to form an accurate assessment of the processing demands inherent in a particular task or condition, and it is too easy, therefore, to attribute any and every observed age difference to the severity of the processing demands without good logical or empirical grounds for the claim. Nevertheless, there are many cases in which differences in the level of processing demands can be clearly identified and the processing capacity explanation can be tested by looking for the predicted age effects.

Processing demands

The first prediction following from the processing capacity explanation states that age differences will be larger when processing demands increase and will be smaller when processing demands are reduced. Processing demands can be increased or reduced by manipulations that affect the text, the presentation of the text, and the type of memory test. This section considers the effects of a variety of different ways of manipulating processing demands.

Levels effects. A so-called levels effect occurs in text processing whereby people typically recall more high-level superordinate propositions from a text than low-level specific details (e.g., Kintsch, Kozminsky, Streby, McKoon & Keenan, 1975; Meyer, 1977). Although age differences in the levels effect are not always found (see Hultsch & Dixon, 1984, for a review), elderly people are sometimes less successful in recalling high-level information (Meyer & Rice, in press). Whether this result is predicted by the processing capacity explanation depends on the particular definition of "level" that is adopted.

In Kintsch's (1974) analysis, high-level propositions are defined as those whose arguments are repeated in many other propositions in the text. This repetitive processing should confer an advantage on high-level propositions without imposing extra processing demands; thus elderly people should exhibit the same levels effect as young people. However, Meyer (1983) defines high-level propositions in terms of the logical relationships within the text. In this view, it is up to the reader or listener to search actively for the main ideas and to infer the relations between them. The identification of high-level propositions depends on judgments of importance and on analysis of logical relationships, and these processes are bound to consume resources. According to this account, an age-related deficit in recall of high-level information could arise from a shortfall in processing capacity. Such a deficit could, of course, be due to a production deficiency. Older people might have different views about what is important in a text.

The evidence generally favors the processing capacity explanation, since manipulations that make it easier to identify and extract the high-level information reduce or eliminate age differences in the levels effect. First, Meyer (1984) has demonstrated that old adults of high verbal ability are able to pick out the high-level propositions correctly when asked to underline them in a written text. In this self-paced task with no memory load, the elderly performed like the young. Second, Meyer (1975) has studied the effects of "signaling" on memory for texts. Signaling is a device for emphasizing the top-level structure of a text by inserting phrases like "in contrast," "as a result," or "on the other hand," so as to make the logical relationships explicit. Signals, and other forms of emphasis, are a way of cutting down the amount of processing required because high-level relationships are clearly delineated instead of having to be inferred by the reader or listener. The results reported by Meyer and Rice (in press) showed that older adults benefit more from signaling and have improved recall of high-level information. Meyer and Rice also noted that when no signals were supplied, the amount of high-level information recalled by elderly people varied inversely with the amount of specific detail in the text. When texts contained many details such as names, dates, and numbers, recall of global logical relationships was particularly poor. They concluded that the limited processing capacity of the elderly was absorbed by lower-level details. However, Meyer and Rice's data show that the effect of signaling is not simply to remedy a production deficiency by inducing a strategy of focusing on high-level information. Although improved recall of superordinate propositions was accompanied by a slight drop in recall of detail, the overall amount of information remembered was increased by signaling. Signaling frees processing resources so that they can be allocated more effectively.

Finally, several studies have reported that age differences in the levels effect are affected by organization. With clearly organized texts, age differences in recall of main ideas are minimal; when the main themes in the text are scrambled, interleaved, or randomly ordered, the elderly retain less information from the superordinate level (Byrd, 1981). The need to reorder propositions while holding them in memory clearly imposes demands on working memory that exceed available capacity.

Intonation and stress. Cohen and Faulkner (1986a) examined the effects of accentuated stress on the comprehension of spoken texts by elderly listeners. The placement of stress can serve to highlight the key words that are the semantic focus of a sentence, to bracket off the constituent parts of a sentence by demarcating syntactic boundaries to emphasize contrasts and logical relationships, and to disambiguate reference. Stress, like signaling, is an aid to processing because the message is delivered to the listener already partly decoded and the demands on processing capacity are thereby reduced. In this study, elderly listeners benefited from correctly placed accentuated stress more than young listeners and the beneficial effects of stress were more marked for some kinds of information than others. Within the elderly group, listeners who had heard a stressed version of a text answered questions that required inference construction or integration of information better than listeners who had heard an unstressed version. For questions that required only verbatim reproduction of information, there was no advantage for the stressed version. The facilitation afforded by accentuated stress benefits those aspects of the text that demand most processing and those listeners whose processing resources are most limited.

Topic familiarity. Processing demands can also be adjusted by varying the content of the text. It is well established that comprehension is easier when the topic is familiar and is clearly indicated (Cairns, Cowart, & Jablon, 1981). When the reader or listener has extensive prior knowledge of the topic, preexisting schemata are automatically accessed and guide the processing (Voss, Vesonder, & Spilich, 1980). Some of the information in the text may be redundant because it is duplicated in the schemata; inferences may be already explicit in the schemata and need not be constructed afresh; and schemata provide ready-made elaboration. Thus the overall effect of familiarity is to reduce processing demands. Hultsch and Dixon (1983) used biographical sketches of entertainers as texts. The entertainers were chosen so as to be more familiar to some age groups than others (e.g., Mary Pickford was well known to the old group, Steve Martin to the young group). The age differences in recall turned out to depend on the level of prior knowledge. When the material was highly familiar to them, the elderly recalled more than the young. Prior knowledge facilitates comprehension by reducing the amount of processing required and clearly compensates for any age-related deficit in processing resources.

Context. There is evidence that in some circumstances elderly adults fail to utilize contextual information. Simon (1979) found that young subjects recalled target words better if they were initially presented in a short sentence context and this sentence frame was used as a retrieval cue, but for old subjects recall was not facilitated by the sentence cue. However, as Burke and Light (1981) pointed out, it seems possible that this difference was due to the fact that the sentence was never encoded. Other studies have shown that old people do benefit from contextual support as much as or more than the young. Spilich and Voss (1983) tested recall of target sentences presented with either strongly related or weakly related context (e.g., the target sentence *Sue found worms in the tomatoes* was presented in a strongly related *garden pest* context versus a weakly related *shopping* context). Both young and old recalled target sentences better with the strong context as a retrieval cue.

Cohen and Faulkner (1983) examined the effects of context on word recognition. In a lexical decision task, visually presented target words were recognized faster when preceded by a sentence context (e.g., *Mary washed the dishes in hot WATER*) than when there was no prior context (e.g., *XXXX XXXXX XX XXX WATER*), and old subjects showed greater contextual facilitation than the young. Auditory word recognition was tested with target words spoken with or without sentence context in a background of white noise. Recognition was more accurate when context was provided, and the old subjects again showed superior contextual facilitation. The results showed a trend such that the old subjects benefited from the context more than the young as the level of white noise increased.

Word recognition normally occurs automatically and is therefore thought to make little demand on processing resources. However, Cohen and Faulkner's study showed that with high levels of noise or degradation, direct access fails, identification becomes difficult and effortful, and age differences increase. In accordance with the cohort model of word recognition (Marslen-Wilson & Welsh, 1978), the acoustic–phonetic signal produces parallel activation of a class of word candidates. As more of the signal is received, candidates that do not match drop out. Sentence context normally provides additional criteria for partitioning this initial cohort of candidates until a single choice remains. If the acoustic–phonetic information is degraded and no contextual information is available, fewer of the initial candidates can be eliminated. It is a reasonable assumption that, in these circumstances, word recognition demands more processing resources. The provision of sentence context effectively narrows down the choice and thus reduces the demands on processing resources and diminishes the age difference.

Distance. Processing demands can also be varied by manipulating the "distance" or amount of intervening material between related parts of a text. Light and Capps (1986) and Light and Albertson (this volume) tested the ability of young and old subjects to determine the correct antecedent of pronouns in text. This task requires complex processes involving lexical, syntactic, semantic, and pragmatic constraints. Light and Capps found that elderly subjects were able to use these constraints as well as young subjects, correctly choosing, for example, "John" as the referent of "he" in

(1a) Henry spoke at the meeting while John drove to the beach.
(1b) He brought along a surfboard.

and "Henry" as the referent in

(2a) Henry spoke at the meeting while John drove to the beach.
(2b) He lectured on the administration.

However, when additional material intervened between the first and second sentences of a pair, so increasing the memory load, older adults were less able to use constraints to resolve the anaphora, because they were unable to hold in mind the constraint-setting information conveyed in the initial sentence. Cohen (1979) also noted that errors of anaphoric reference are more common in elderly people. She reported that old subjects tended to attribute characteristics or actions to the wrong protagonists in recalling a story. Light and Capps's results indicate that this kind of error arises because working memory is overloaded.

Ordering. Instead of increasing the amount of material intervening between elements that have to be related, processing demands can also be made more severe by scrambling the order. Light, Zelinski, and Moore (1982) asked subjects to make true–false judgments about inferences derived from the three premises necessary to construct a four-term linear ordering, such as:

(3a)   The boys measured their heights.
(3b)   David was taller than Bob.
(3c)   Bob was taller than James.
(3d)   James was taller than Ron.

The load on working memory can be increased by varying the order in which the terms are presented. The problems are harder when adjacent premises do not share common terms because the information has to be mentally rearranged. The results of this study conformed to a processing capacity explanation. The size of the age deficit varied as a function of the size of the working-memory load. A similar effect has already been noted in connection with text structure. The elderly are penalized when the events in a story are presented in an order that does not correspond to the order of temporal occurrence (Mandel & Johnson, 1984), or when a two-episode story is presented with elements of the two episodes interwoven instead of one complete episode following another (Smith, Rebok, Smith, Hall, & Alvin, 1983). The extra work involved in carrying forward and reordering text components taxes the limited capacity of working memory in older people.

Rate of input. Stine, Wingfield, and Poon (in press) point out that "the comprehension of spoken language involves the rapid construction of meaning from a transitory acoustic signal which must be immediately interpreted." If processing capacity declines with age, the maximum rate at which speech can be processed effectively will decline with advancing age, and age differences in comprehension and memory can be expected to widen as speech rate is increased. Using time-compressed speech so as to produce rates varying from 200 to 400 words per minute, Stine et al. found that the age deficit in recall of sentences was larger at the faster rate. The elderly were especially penalized by the faster rate when the material to be recalled consisted of unstructured word-strings instead of grammatical sentences, as these offer no redundancy to compensate for the lack of processing time. The percentage of time-compressed propositions recalled by both old and young fell as the number of propositions presented per second increased, but this decline was steeper for the elderly.

Stine et al. (in press) also used a technique known as spontaneous segmentation whereby the listener is allowed to stop the speech input as often as necessary in order to recall each segment without error. The size of the segment chosen is a direct index of the capacity of working memory. The mean size of the segment chosen by the elderly was 7.6 words, as opposed to an average segment of 8.8 words chosen by the young. Both age groups used a similar strategy, choosing to terminate segments at syntactic boundaries, but the elderly needed more frequent pauses to unload. The segmentation method was also used with fast and slow speech rates. At the fast rate (350 wpm) the elderly adults worked with slightly longer segments than the young, but their recall was poorer, indicating that they had overestimated their capacity. All these findings point to an age-related slowing in the rate of on-line comprehension such that deficits appear when the system is pushed.

Cohen (1979) also found age deficits at fast speech rates. When the speech rate was increased from 120 wpm to 200 wpm, old subjects' ability to answer questions that required inferences deteriorated, although their ability to answer questions that needed only verbatim reproduction of stated facts was unimpaired. The increase in rate had no detrimental effects on the performance of the young subjects. Apparently, older people cannot carry out the extra processes required in constructing inferences when the speech rate is fast, and at the very high rates employed in Stine et al.'s study, even simple recall is affected.

Input modality. Is listening more demanding than reading? The relationship of input modality and processing is complex. In some ways, processing of written text is less demanding than processing of spoken text. Reading can be self-paced, and the reader can reduce the memory load by reviewing the material at will. On the other hand, according to some theories (e.g., Jackson & McClelland, 1979), reading may involve recoding the visual input to a phonemic form for storage in working memory. Spoken texts enter the system in the acoustic code and can be held in working memory without needing to be recoded. It is difficult, therefore, to decide whether listening or reading normally requires more processing capacity, and it is not surprising to find that the interaction of input modality, age, and text memory is a complex one.

For young adults, recall is generally superior after reading, but Dixon, Simon, Nowak, and Hultsch (1982) found that when immediate recall was tested, this was not true for old adults; and when recall was delayed, the old people remembered spoken material better. Dixon et al. surmised that the elderly failed to benefit from the visual presentation because they did not take full advantage of the opportunity to reread the written material. On the other hand, older people do sometimes benefit from written input. Cohen (1981) reported that both young and old found it easier to draw logical inferences when the premises were written, and the old group had particular difficulty with a spoken input. When the task is one, like inferential reasoning, that places a heavy load on working memory, the age differences are less marked if the material is presented in the visual modality so that it can be reviewed and reinstated as necessary.

Task factors. Processing demands may also vary according to the type of test that is used to interrogate comprehension and memory for text. Inadequate encoding is more likely to be exposed by free recall or question answering, whereas cued recall and recognition can sometimes be successful even when encoding is incomplete. Spilich and Voss (1983) found large age differences for free recall, smaller differences for cued recall, and no age differences for recognition. However, this relationship between age and type of test has not always emerged (e.g., Labouvie-Vief, Schell, & Weaverdyck, 1981). The difficulty of recognition relative to recall can vary greatly according to the number and type of distractors, and this may account for the discrepancies.

Depth of processing

The second prediction following from the processing capacity explanation concerns depth of processing and predicts that age deficits will be minimal for aspects of the text that require only shallow processing and will be larger for those that require deeper processing because deep processing consumes more resources. The concept of depth of processing, introduced by Craik and Lockhart (1972), allows us to define processing operations in terms of their level. At one end of a continuum, low-level, "shallow" processing is associated with early stages of analysis, with automatic operations that require little or no attention, and with relatively simple encoding of the surface form of language. At the other end of the continuum, "deep," or high-level, processing demands effort and attention and is concerned with complex analysis of meaning and constructive operations of elaboration, interpretation, and integration. Whether these distinctions are characterized as levels of processing or as domains of processing (Baddeley, 1982), they can be used to interpret age differences in memory for text. Craik and Simon (1980) and Craik and Rabinowitz (1984) have suggested that old people perform shallow processing operations adequately, but may fail to carry out deep processing. They argue that this age-related deficit in deep processing is the result of both diminished processing resources and faulty strategies. Hence it can be corrected only by relaxing processing demands (e.g., by slowing down the rate of input) and also by supplying instructions to specify the appropriate strategy.

The deep processing deficit. Studies of age effects in text processing have generated ample evidence confirming that age-related deficits can be described in terms of depth of processing. When the products of shallow processing are interrogated, age differences are slight. Cohen (1979) and Cohen and Faulkner (1983) found that there were no age differences in ability to answer "verbatim" questions after listening to texts. These questions require only straightforward reproduction of the surface form of parts of the text. With questions that require the listener to make inferences, a deeper level of processing is tapped, and these questions were more difficult for the older listeners.

In another study, Cohen and Faulkner (1981) asked subjects to listen to a spoken text and then detect changes in a written version. Some of the changes affected only the surface wording (these were shallow changes like *He published a book of poetry* for *He published a book of verse*). Others affected the meaning of the text (these were deep changes like *He quarreled with other writers* for *Other writers quarreled with him*). There were age differences in the ability to detect both kinds of changes, but these varied as a function of the retention interval. At delays of 10 and 25 seconds, young subjects were better than the old at detecting shallow changes, but by 40 seconds' delay the old and young were equally poor at detecting these changes. For deep changes, the age differences were larger and more persistent. After 40 seconds' delay the young could still detect 88% of the changes that affected the meaning, but the old detected only 33% of them. These results suggest that in old age processing resources are insufficient to produce the deeper levels of encoding that are necessary to support long-term retention. Interestingly, the type of change that the old subjects found most difficult to detect involved subject–object reversal (as in the example about quarreling with the writers). Memory of the relationship linking actors and actions appears to be particularly fragile.

As Craik suggests, age differences in depth of processing could be reflecting a production deficiency as well as, or instead of, a processing limitation. To test this, several researchers have employed orienting tasks. The rationale is that if the age deficit arises because old people do not spontaneously hit on deep processing strategies, the age differences should be eliminated when an orienting task forces them to employ the appropriate strategies. There is little support for this hypothesis. Orienting tasks have mostly been used in word list learning experiments (e.g., Eysenck, 1974) but have failed to remove the age effects. Dixon et al. (1982) studied age differences in text processing with four different orienting conditions designed to produce differing depth of processing. Subjects were asked to (1) mark spelling and grammatical errors in the text; (2) rate the content for interest, readability, etc.; (3) formulate advice for the people in the story; or (4) memorize the content. Whereas for young adults recall improved with the depth of the orienting task, older adults did not benefit from the deep orienting conditions. Because the age differences persisted in spite of the strategies being guided, processing limitations are a more likely explanation for inadequate depth of encoding.

For the older listener or reader, processing resources appear to be absorbed by low-level stages of surface structure analysis, leaving insufficient capacity available for the higher-level stages. To keep up with the input, the older person may be forced to skimp on semantic analysis and on the constructive and interpretive stages of comprehension. The consequences of this skimpy processing are evident when the memory task interrogates deeper levels of processing.

Inference construction. Making inferences during comprehension involves deep processing. In order to construct inferences or to understand what is implied but not stated, facts must be related to other facts presented in the text, or to facts acquired previously and stored in memory. Extra processes of integration and reasoning are required. A unified memory representation that integrates the relevant facts must be constructed either at encoding or at retrieval, so that inferences can be read off. Several experiments have demonstrated that old people are especially disadvantaged in answering questions or verifying conclusions that rest on inferences from the facts presented. In contrast with an age-related deficit in processing implicit information,

Cohen's studies showed that ability to comprehend and remember explicit information is relatively unimpaired (Cohen, 1979, 1981; Light et al., 1982; see also
Zacks & Hasher, and Light & Albertson, this volume, for a discussion of exceptions
to this finding). Light et al. (1982) studied the effects of various manipulations on age
differences in inference construction. Some of these manipulations were designed
to test the production deficiency hypothesis by guiding processing strategies. They
found that instructing the subjects that inferences would be tested did not eliminate
the age difference. Extended practice and attempts to induce semantic processing by
providing a story framework for the premises failed to benefit either young or old
significantly.

Light et al. also manipulated the processing demands of the task. They found
that the age difference was much less marked when the premises were presented
in the optimal order and did not have to be mentally rearranged. The influence of
processing limitations is also clearly indicated by Cohen's findings that old people
do construct inferences more effectively if the rate of input is slower (Cohen, 1979),
or if the presentation is written rather than spoken (Cohen, 1981). When the input is
too fast or when the facts have to be reordered in working memory, old people lack
the resources to construct the kind of unified representation that allows the inferences
to be read off. Light and Albertson (this volume) emphasize that age differences in
inference making seem to occur only when inference construction involves mental
gymnastics that impose a heavy load on working memory.

Integration. Text comprehension requires two kinds of integration: integration of
information within the text, and integration of the information in the text with prior
knowledge about the world. Cohen (1979) probed this latter type of integration by
asking subjects to detect anomalies in spoken texts. The anomalies took the form
of unlikely statements such as that a home near an airport was quiet and peaceful;
that a blind man was reading the newspaper; that a girl with a broken arm went
swimming. Old people were less successful at detecting these kinds of anomaly. It
might be argued that they did not understand what they were supposed to do, or that
they lacked the relevant prior knowledge, but both these explanations were unlikely.
Only the most commonplace knowledge was required to spot the anomalies and
the fact that all the subjects were able to identify some of the anomalies correctly
showed that they did understand the task. It is more likely that limited processing
resources did not always allow them to relate the input statements to their general
knowledge. Light and Albertson (this volume) found age deficits in this task only
when integration was hampered by introducing a topic shift between the propositions
that had to be related. When no topic shift occurred, their old subjects did the task as
well as the young. This discrepancy between the two studies is puzzling, but possibly
their subjects had a superior working-memory capacity or perhaps the conditions of
presentation were less demanding.

Further evidence for integration difficulties comes from the pattern of errors in
a study that Cohen and Faulkner (1984) reported. Multiple choices to questions
posed after a spoken text included the correct answer and two different kinds of
distractor. One of the distractors was classed as a *text intrusion,* that is, something
mentioned in the text that was not the answer to the question. The other distractor

was classed as a *frame intrusion,* that is, an answer that was plausible in the light of general knowledge about the topic, but which was not mentioned in the text. Old and young did not differ in the incidence of frame intrusions, which are essentially plausible guesses, but the old made substantially more text intrusion errors. So, in answering a question about who performed a particular action, for example, any of the persons mentioned in the text might be cited. These errors reflect a memory representation in which text elements have not been correctly integrated in a propositional network. The same failure to establish the correct linking relationships has already been noted in connection with the errors of anaphoric reference that Light and Capps (1986) found to be exacerbated by an increase in the distance (i.e., the number of intervening sentences) between referent and pronoun. Defective integration is also reflected in the tendency to transpose subject and object reported by Cohen and Faulkner (1981) and to confuse the protagonists in a story (Cohen, 1979). In contrast to these results, Zelinski (this volume) did not find any age deficit in integration, but in her experiment the demands on working memory were low because the to-be-integrated items were in adjacent sentences. When integration must be effected across larger spans of text, the age deficit in working memory becomes apparent.

Names. Some items of information in text appear to be harder to encode in memory than others and require more processing. Cohen and Faulkner (1981, 1984) have consistently found memory for proper names poorer than memory for other items. In one study, Cohen and Faulkner (1986b) presented short spoken texts consisting of fictional biographies. Each contained names (the name of a person, and the name of a place) and descriptions (the person's occupation and the person's hobby), as in *Charles Gibson is a printer who lives in Bolton and spends his spare time in rock-climbing.*

Recall of the proper names was much poorer than recall of the occupations or hobbies. A second presentation of the texts, giving the opportunity for further processing, improved recall of names so that for the young (ages 18–30), middle-aged (40–60), and young-old (60–70) groups the difference between the names and the descriptions was no longer significant. For the old-old (70+) group, however, recall of proper names was still 27% poorer than recall of the other information. It is unlikely that this age group was using a different strategy. Subjects knew what they had to remember and reported making special efforts to commit the names to memory. It seems more likely that proper names are particularly difficult to encode and need more processing than other items of information. As Kausler (1985) says, "effortful rehearsal is forced on us by the artificial or arbitrary nature of the to-be-memorized information" (p. 110). A second presentation allows younger people to complete the additional processing that is required, but older people need more repetitions before they can achieve an adequate level of recall.

Individual differences

The third prediction deriving from the processing capacity explanation states that when old and young individuals have equally high processing capacity, text memory will be relatively unimpaired by aging. This prediction proves more difficult to evaluate than the other two because there is, as yet, not a great deal of evidence that is directly relevant to it. Although the importance of individual differences in relation to the effects of aging on text memory is now well recognized, most studies have focused on education and verbal ability as the critical determinants. According to the arguments advanced here, the capacity of working memory and speed of processing should be at least as important, if not more so.

The significance of education and verbal ability have been amply demonstrated (e.g., Taub, 1979; Meyer & Rice, 1983), and in general, age deficits in text processing are less evident when verbal ability is high. Verbal ability is usually measured by performance on some kind of vocabulary test, so that high verbal ability reflects a rich and accessible store of lexical knowledge. Baddeley et al. (1985) found that scores on a vocabulary test correlated negatively with lexical decision time and positively with reading comprehension. If high verbal ability individuals are better readers, it is not surprising that they perform well on tests of text comprehension and memory. Verbal ability may also be associated with a variety of other skills and abilities. Hultsch, Hertzog, and Dixon (1984) attempted to clarify the relationship between age, verbal ability, and text memory by analyzing the influence of a set of intellectual abilities including general intelligence, and some aspects of verbal ability such as verbal productive thinking, verbal comprehension, and associative memory. An extremely complex pattern of results was obtained. Verbal comprehension did not affect age differences in text memory, and verbal productive thinking and associative memory had only small and transient effects. Whereas general intelligence was found to predict performance for young adults, it did not determine the performance of the elderly. These findings are not much help in clarifying the role of verbal ability in text memory.

Some evidence has already been cited showing that high verbal ability is associated with the use of hierarchical organization strategies. Dixon, Hultsch, Simon, and von Eye (1984) found that young, middle-aged, and old adults of high verbal ability all exhibited a similar levels effect but that the typical preferential recall of high-level information was less likely to be shown by old adults of low or average verbal ability. This finding appears to support a production deficiency account of age differences. It looks as if adults of high verbal ability know how to set about processing a text and employ the right strategies. However, it is quite possible that high verbal ability is also linked with superior processing capacity that allows optimal strategies to be implemented. The correlation of vocabulary score with working-memory capacity reported by Baddeley et al. (1985) lends support to this interpretation.

A few studies have related text memory to memory span as an index of working-memory capacity. Daneman and Carpenter (1980) reported strong correlations between sentence span and text memory as measured by fact retrieval and recall of pronoun referents. Spilich (1983) tested a young group with a mean score on the Wechsler Memory Scale of 68, a normal elderly group with a mean score of 55, and a memory-impaired elderly group with a mean score of 42. The average number of propositions recalled from texts for each group was 31, 14, and 2, respectively.

Using the methods devised by Kintsch and van Dijk (1978), Spilich estimated the capacity of the working-memory buffer store during text processing. For the young group, the number of propositions held in the buffer was estimated at 4, and for the normal elderly it was 2. These groups did not differ according to which propositions were selected for loading into the buffer. Both groups used the same strategy of selecting on the basis of thematic importance, but the normal elderly group carried forward fewer propositions. In contrast, the memory-impaired elderly group were selecting propositions for storage in the buffer at random. It is clear that the young and normal elderly differed in working-memory capacity, but not in strategy. In the impaired group it appears likely that the strategy had broken down as a consequence of a further reduction in working memory.

A similar relationship between memory capacity and recall of information from texts was also noted by Cohen and Faulkner (1986a) who found a correlation of .46 between digit span and question-answering scores. However, Light and Anderson (1985) failed to find any evidence that working-memory capacity predicts age differences in text memory. Hartley (this volume) found that working-memory capacity as measured by sentence span did not decline with age but was nevertheless strongly correlated with text recall for old and middle-aged groups. It is not clear yet how these discrepancies can be accounted for.

It is worth noting, though, that very low memory capacity can produce a total breakdown of text organization. When Cohen (1979) asked subjects to recall a spoken story, a few of the old subjects turned out to be too severely memory-impaired for inclusion in the experimental group. When these people, who had digit spans of 3 or 4, attempted to recall the story, they produced totally unstructured lists of items mentioned in the story (e.g., "There was something about an island – there was a man – I think there was some talk about fishing – I can't remember any more"). It is tempting to claim, on the basis of these cases, that without the binding and cohesive operations of working memory a text turns into a list; some of the items are retained, but the structure is lost.

The age-related decline in speed of processing is generally reflected in a slower reading rate. Hartley (this volume) discusses the relationship between individual differences in various measures of processing speed and text recall, and her study identifies speed of processing as a powerful predictor of memory for text.

Conclusions

Of the three predictions that follow from the processing capacity explanation, the first two are well supported by the evidence. Age differences are commonly observed when processing demands are high and persist until they are relaxed. The third prediction has less support, but the available evidence is as yet rather sparse. Taken together, the findings point strongly to the conclusion that age differences in text comprehension and memory are caused by an age-related reduction in processing capacity. Several aspects of processing capacity are involved, and these are clearly interdependent. For example, the inadequacy of processing resources may be exposed only when the memory load is heavy or the rate of input is high. In general, the processing capacity explanation for age differences in memory for text is much more convincing than the strong version of the production deficiency hypothesis. The weak version, whereby age differences reflect differences in strategy which are in turn determined by processing capacity, is more difficult to reject, but, in this case, processing capacity still emerges as the primary determinant of text comprehension and memory.

References

Baddeley, A. D. (1981). The concept of working memory: A view of its current state and probable future development. *Cognition, 10,* 17–23.

Baddeley, A. D. (1982). Domains of recollection. *Psychological Review, 89,* 708–729.

Baddeley, A. D., Logie, R., Nimmo-Smith, I., & Brereton, N. (1985). Components of fluent reading. *Journal of Memory and Language, 24,* 119–131.

Burke, D. M., & Light, L. L. (1981). Memory and aging: The role of retrieval processes. *Psychological Bulletin, 90,* 513–546.

Byrd, M. (1981). *Age differences in memory for prose passages.* Unpublished doctoral dissertation, University of Toronto, Toronto.

Cairns, H. S., Cowart, W., & Jablon, A. D. (1981). Effects of prior context upon the integration of lexical information during sentence processing. *Journal of Verbal Learning and Verbal Behavior, 20,* 445–453.

Cohen, G. (1979). Language comprehension in old age. *Cognitive Psychology, 11,* 412–429.

Cohen, G. (1981). Inferential reasoning in old age. *Cognition, 9,* 59–72.

Cohen, G., & Faulkner, D. (1981). Memory for discourse in old age. *Discourse Processes, 4,* 253–265.

Cohen, G., & Faulkner, D. (1983). Word recognition: Age differences in contextual facilitation effects. *British Journal of Psychology, 74,* 238–251.

Cohen, G., & Faulkner, D. (1984). Memory for text: Some age differences in the nature of the information that is retained after listening to texts. In H. Bouma & D. Bouwhuis (Eds.), *Attention and performance X: Control of language processes* (pp. 501–513). Hillsdale, NJ: Erlbaum.

Cohen, G., & Faulkner, D. (1986a). Does 'elderspeak' work? The effects of intonation and stress in comprehension and recall of spoken discourse in old age. *Language and Communication, 6,* 91–98.

Cohen, G., & Faulkner, D. (1986b). Memory for proper names: Age differences in retrieval. *British Journal of Developmental Psychology, 4,* 187–197.

Craik, F. I. M., & Lockhart, R. S. (1972). Levels of processing: A framework for memory research. *Journal of Verbal Learning and Verbal Behavior, 11,* 671–684.

Craik, F. I. M., & Rabinowitz, J. C. (1984). Age differences in the acquisition and use of verbal information. In H. Bouma & D. Bouwhuis (Eds.), *Attention and performance X: Control of language processes* (pp. 471–499). Hillsdale, NJ: Erlbaum.

Craik, F. I. M., & Simon, E. (1980). Age differences in memory: The roles of attention and depth of processing. In L. W. Poon, J. L. Fozard, L. S. Cermak, D. Arenberg, & L. W. Thompson (Eds.), *New directions in memory and aging: Proceedings of the George A. Talland Memorial Conference* (pp. 95–112). Hillsdale, NJ: Erlbaum.

Daneman, M., & Carpenter, P. A. (1980). Individual differences in working memory and reading. *Journal of Verbal Learning and Verbal Behavior, 19,* 450–466.

Dixon, R. A., Hultsch, D. F., Simon, E. W., & von Eye, A. (1984). Verbal ability and text structure effects on adult age differences in text recall. *Journal of Verbal Learning and Verbal Behavior, 23,* 569–578.

Dixon, R. A., Simon, E. W., Nowak, C. A., & Hultsch, D. F. (1982). Text recall in adulthood as a function of level of information, input modality, and delay interval. *Journal of Gerontology, 37,* 358–364.

Eysenck, M. W. (1974). Age differences in incidental learning. *Developmental Psychology, 10,* 936–941.

Grant, E. A., Storandt, M., & Botwinick, J. (1978). Incentive and practice in the psychomotor performance of the elderly. *Journal of Gerontology, 33*, 413–415.

Hasher, L., & Zacks, R. T. (1979). Automatic and effortful processes in memory. *Journal of Experimental Psychology: General, 108*, 356–388.

Hultsch, D. F., & Dixon, R. A. (1983). The role of pre-experimental knowledge in text processing and adulthood. *Experimental Aging Research, 9*, 17–22.

Hultsch, D. F., & Dixon, R. A. (1984). Memory for text materials in adulthood. In P. B. Baltes & O. G. Brim (Eds.), *Life-span development and behavior* (Vol. 6, pp. 77–108). New York: Academic Press.

Hultsch, D. F., Hertzog, C., & Dixon, R. A. (1984). Text processing in adulthood: The role of intellectual abilities. *Developmental Psychology, 20*, 1193–1209.

Jackson, M. D., & McClelland, J. L. (1979). Processing determinants of reading speed. *Journal of Experimental Psychology: General, 108*, 151–181.

Kahneman, D. (1973). *Attention and effort*. Englewood Cliffs, NJ: Prentice-Hall.

Kausler, D. H. (1982). *Experimental psychology and human aging*. New York: Wiley.

Kausler, D. H. (1985). Episodic memory: Memorizing performance. In N. Charness (Ed.), *Aging and human performance* (pp. 101–141). New York: Wiley.

Kintsch, W. (1974). *The representation of meaning in memory*. Hillsdale, NJ: Erlbaum.

Kintsch, W., Kozminsky, E., Streby, W. J., McKoon, G., & Keenan, J. M. (1975). Comprehension and recall of text as a function of content variables. *Journal of Verbal Learning and Verbal Behavior, 14*, 196–214.

Kintsch, W., & van Dijk, T. A. (1978). Toward a model of text comprehension and production. *Psychological Review, 85*, 363–394.

Labouvie-Vief, G., Schell, D. A., & Weaverdyck, S. E. (1981). *Recall deficit in the aged: A fable recalled*. Unpublished manuscript, Wayne State University, Department of Psychology, Detroit.

Light, L. L., & Anderson, P. A. (1985). Working-memory capacity, age, and memory for discourse. *Journal of Gerontology, 40*, 737–747.

Light, L. L., & Capps, J. L. (1986). Comprehension of pronouns in young and older adults. *Developmental Psychology, 22*, 580–585.

Light, L. L., Zelinski, E. M., & Moore, M. (1982). Adult age differences in reasoning from new information. *Journal of Experimental Psychology: Learning, Memory, and Cognition, 8*, 435–447.

Mandel, R. G., & Johnson, N. S. (1984). A developmental analysis of story recall and comprehension in adulthood. *Journal of Verbal Learning and Verbal Behavior, 23*, 643–659.

Marslen-Wilson, W. D., & Welsh, A. (1978). Processing interactions and lexical access during word recognition in continuous speech. *Cognitive Psychology, 10*, 29–63.

Meyer, B. J. F. (1975). *The organization of prose and its effects on memory*. Amsterdam: North Holland Publishing.

Meyer, B. J. F. (1977). What is remembered from prose: A function of passage structure. In R. O. Freedle (Ed.), *Discourse processes: Advances in research and theory* (Vol. 1, pp. 307–336). Norwood, NJ: Ablex.

Meyer, B. J. F. (1983). Text structure and its use in studying comprehension across the adult life span. In B. A. Hutson (Ed.), *Advances in Reading Language Research* (Vol. 2, pp. 9–54). Greenwich, CT: JAI Press.

Meyer, B. J. F. (1984). Text dimensions and cognitive processing. In H. Mandl, N. Stein, & T. Trabasso (Eds.), *Learning and comprehension of text* (pp. 3–51). Hillsdale, NJ: Erlbaum.

Meyer, B. J. F., & Rice, G. E. (1981). Information recalled from prose by young, middle and old readers. *Experimental Aging Research, 7*, 253–268.

Meyer, B. J. F., & Rice, G. E. (1983). Learning and memory from text across the adult life span. In J. Fine & R. O. Freedle (Eds.), *Developmental studies in discourse* (pp. 291–306). Norwood, NJ: Ablex.

Meyer, B. J. F., & Rice, G. E. (in press). Prose processing in adulthood: The text, the reader, and the task. In L. W. Poon, D. C. Rubin, & B. A. Wilson (Eds.), *Everyday cognition in adulthood and later life*. Cambridge: Cambridge University Press.

Salthouse, T. A. (1980). Age and memory: Strategies for localizing the loss. In L. W. Poon, J. L.

Fozard, L. S. Cermak, D. Arenberg, & L. W. Thompson (Eds.), *New directions in memory and aging: Proceedings of the George A. Talland Memorial Conference* (pp. 47–65). Hillsdale, NJ: Erlbaum.

Schaie, K. W., & Labouvie-Vief, G. (1974). Generational versus ontogenetic components of change in adult cognitive behavior: A fourteen year cross-sequential study. *Developmental Psychology, 10,* 305–320.

Simon, E. (1979). Depth and elaboration of processing in relation to age. *Journal of Experimental Psychology: Human Learning and Memory, 5,* 115–124.

Smith, S. W., Rebok, G. W., Smith, W. R., Hall, S. E., & Alvin, M. (1983). Adult age differences in the use of story structure in delayed free recall. *Experimental Aging Research, 9,* 191–195.

Spilich, G. J. (1983). Life-span components of text processing: Structural and procedural differences. *Journal of Verbal Learning and Verbal Behavior, 22,* 231–244.

Spilich, G. J., & Voss, J. F. (1983). Contextual effects upon text memory for young, aged-normal and aged-impaired individuals. *Experimental Aging Research, 9,* 45–49.

Stine, E. L., Wingfield, A., & Poon, L. W. (in press). Speech comprehension and memory through adulthood: The roles of time and strategy. In L. W. Poon, D. C. Rubin, & B. A. Wilson (Eds.), *Everyday cognition in adulthood and late life.* Cambridge: Cambridge University Press.

Taub, H. A. (1979). Comprehension and memory of prose materials by young and old adults. *Experimental Aging Research, 5,* 3–13.

Voss, J. F., Vesonder, G. T., & Spilich, G. J. (1980). Text generation and recall by high knowledge and low knowledge individuals. *Journal of Verbal Learning and Verbal Behavior, 19,* 651–667.

11 Episodic memory and knowledge interactions across adulthood

Gary Gillund and Marion Perlmutter

In this chapter we explore possible adulthood changes in the contributions of knowledge to acquisition of new information into memory (episodic memory). In particular, we are interested in the ways that prior knowledge may compensate for a loss of processing resources associated with increasing age. We begin with the assumption that there is a decline in the efficiency of cognitive resources with increasing age. Although this assumption is not universally accepted, there is much evidence of age deficits on tasks varying in range of complexity from simple reaction time (see Salthouse, 1985a) to complex problem solving (e.g., Denney, 1982). In the area of memory, recent research has been directed at characterizing these declines. Alternatives commonly discussed include a loss of processing speed (Salthouse, 1985b), reduction in attentional resources (Craik & Byrd, 1982), deficit in retrieval (Burke & Light, 1981), and reductions in information-processing capacity (Hasher & Zacks, 1979).

In this chapter we describe memory tasks in which age deficits are commonly observed and discuss when and how prior knowledge seems to compensate at least partially for loss of processing resources. We suggest that equalization of prior knowledge of materials tends to ameliorate, but not eliminate, age differences in memory performance. We attempt to specify when variables related to knowledge would or would not be expected to reduce age differences. The review does not cover all aspects of memory. Instead, it focuses on episodic memory. Episodic memory is used in the heuristic sense; episodic memory tasks are ones in which satisfactory levels of performance cannot be obtained without recent presentation of the stimulus material.

The review of the literature that follows is based upon three major assumptions. The first is that *memory is a resource-limited system* (Hasher & Zacks, 1979; Schneider & Shiffrin, 1977). This assumption implies that there are limits in how effectively the memory system can function. The limits are determined by such fac-

Work on this chapter was supported by BRSG Grant No. S07 RR07092 to the first author from the Biomedical Research Support Grant Program, Division of Research Resources, National Institutes of Health at the University of Utah, and by a fellowship to the second author from the Brookdale Foundation. Correspondence should be directed to Gary Gillund, Department of Psychology, University of Utah, Salt Lake City, Utah 84112.

tors as the time required to complete mental processes and ability or capacity to divide attention.

The second assumption is that *resource limits are not static but are variable*. The two most relevant factors that influence resources are age and knowledge. Much evidence indicates that information-processing resources decrease with increasing age (e.g., Craik & Byrd, 1982; Hasher & Zacks, 1979; Salthouse, 1985b). In addition, it appears that various forms of knowledge, ranging from advance warnings of a task, to practice with it, or schematic knowledge relevant to it, may reduce limits on the memory system (e.g., Johnston & Dark, 1986; Schneider & Shiffrin, 1977).

The third assumption is that *various tasks place differential demands on the memory system*. For example, tasks may be categorized as automatic or controlled (effortful). The former, automatic type of task places very few demands on the cognitive system. The latter, effortful type of task places many demands on the cognitive system.

The three assumptions have implications for age differences in memory performance. In particular, such differences are expected to be small when the task places few demands on the memory system, and large when it places extensive demands on the system. For example, on the one hand, in forward three-letter memory span tasks, which are well within the capacity of normal adults, age differences are virtually nonexistent. On the other hand, in more demanding tasks age deficits are evident. Yet, variations in knowledge of the material to be remembered or in knowledge of the task itself often leads to changes in the pattern of age differences.

Types of knowledge relevant to age deficits in memory performance

Knowledge may take many forms, but in this chapter we limit our discussion to types of knowledge that previously have been considered to be relevant to aging. These are briefly introduced below.

Knowledge of the materials

It appears that prior knowledge of to-be-remembered material facilitates memory performance (e.g., Chiesi, Spilich, & Voss, 1979; Crowder, 1976; Mandler, 1967). For example, as Salthouse (1985b) has succinctly summarized results of research in this area, "it appears that the amount and organization of information possessed by the individual affects the efficiency with which material can be entered and retrieved from the long-term storage system" (p. 101).

Prior knowledge of materials may range from varying degrees of exposure to it, to different amounts and organization. These factors produce several positive effects on memory performance. First, material that is familiar may be processed quickly (Poon & Fozard, 1978) and therefore places less demand on the memory system than unfamiliar material. Second, material that is deeply processed is interpreted "by some richly structured knowledge base and the integration of the new information with that knowledge base" (Craik & Lockhart, 1986). Thus, for material to be deeply processed (Craik & Lockhart, 1972) it must be meaningful. This processing does not require fewer resources than does shallow processing; in fact, it may require more. However, given a particular amount of processing resources, better memory will result when information is processed deeply. Finally, complex knowledge structures, such as scripts and schemata, facilitate encoding, free up resources for encoding of novel or unexpected material, and serve as important guides to retrieval (e.g., Bower, Black, & Turner, 1979; Hasher & Griffin, 1978; Johnson & Kieras, 1983).

Knowledge of the task

Knowledge of the task refers primarily to practice with the task. Evidence from a variety of tasks and domains indicates that practice improves performance and that it does so, at least in part, by reducing the processing requirements of the task (Anderson, 1985). In fact, the development of an automatic process is critically dependent on extensive practice with a task that employs the process (Schneider & Shiffrin, 1977). Practice appears to reduce the cognitive resources required to complete the task.

Strategic knowledge and mnemonics

Strategies and mnemonics may greatly facilitate memory performance, although in particular situations or for certain tasks some mnemonics are more effective than others (see Poon, 1985). Strategies do not appear to reduce the amount of cognitive resources required in a task and may in fact increase the requirements. However, if sufficient resources are available to employ an effective strategy, memory performance is improved by utilization of strategies.

Metamemory

Metamemory refers to knowledge about the functioning of one's own memory system. Such knowledge is considered important for decisions about which strategy should be employed in a given situation (see Cavanaugh & Perlmutter, 1982, for a critical review). If one has poor metamemorial knowledge, one may not employ strategies even in situations where it would be beneficial to do so.

Age deficits in memory performance have been attributed to age-related deficits in each of these types of knowledge. That is, it has been argued that older adults perform more poorly than young adults because the materials used in typical memory experiments are more meaningful to younger adults, and younger adults have had more recent practice with memory tasks, employ more strategies, and have better metamemorial skills. In general, such explanations have not fared well (see Burke & Light, 1981; Salthouse, 1982). It appears that acknowledgment of some sort of processing resource difference is also needed to account for knowledge effects.

All four of the types of knowledge described here can aid memory performance. An important point is that increased knowledge in any of these areas improves memory performance of younger as well as older adults. It is not the case that increased knowledge necessarily reduces age-associated differences in performance.

Age-associated differences are expected to be reduced under three conditions. First, if younger adults are already at ceiling levels of performance, their performance cannot be improved further. In contrast, increased practice can improve performance of the older subjects and thus reduce the age-associated differences. Problems of ceiling effects are well documented and need not concern us further.

Second, it is possible that performance on a given task may be data-limited for younger but not older adults. In that case, knowledge-related variables that increase the resources available to subjects would improve performance of the older adults only (Norman & Bobrow, 1975). This effect is very similar to the ceiling effect except that in this instance performance is not perfect. That is, in certain tasks increased resources or increased efficiency may not improve performance because performance is limited by other factors. For example, if words for a memory task were presented at a rate of one word every 20 msec, no strategy or amount of resources would improve performance because the limits of the visual system are not such that the task could be completed.

Third, if, because of increased knowledge, the task changes from one that is dependent primarily on processing resources to one that is dependent primarily on knowledge, a reduction in age deficits would be expected. The reduced deficit in this case is dependent on equivalent relevant knowledge by younger and older adults.

Finally, even in cases where age-associated differences would be expected to be reduced, they might not be eliminated because the use of knowledge in the acquisition of new information can, in itself, require processing resources. For example, Britton and Tesser (1982) have shown that people with well-developed knowledge bases in a particular domain require more resources to process related material than people without such knowledge. Salthouse (1980) has demonstrated that older adults may not be able to use a given strategy as well as younger adults because they cannot process information as quickly as younger adults. Similarly, it may be that the effort required to practice a given task and to monitor one's memory performance may differentially affect older and younger adults.

Review of the literature

Analysis of age-related differences in performance involves consideration of the resources required for given tasks and the amount and type of prior knowledge available to both younger and older subjects. In this section we review literature on episodic memory performance with these factors in mind. The review is not meant to be comprehensive. Instead, we focus on tasks in which age differences are commonly observed and variables related to prior knowledge are manipulated. The variables we discuss are age specificity of materials, strength of preexisting word associations, categorical materials, depth of processing and forewarning of test, domain-specific knowledge, verbal ability, and mnemonic training programs. For each variable we provide an analysis based on the stated framework and then evaluate research relevant to the analysis.

Age specificity of materials

Many studies demonstrate age differences in memory for verbal materials ranging from unrelated lists of words to texts. In general, this literature suggests that as long as the lists exceed memory span, relatively large age differences are found (see Kausler, 1982, and Poon, 1985, for reviews). Therefore, memory for verbal material is an appropriate area in which to examine the influence of knowledge on memory.

One way to examine the influence of knowledge on memory performance is to manipulate the materials such that older adults are more knowledgeable about one set of materials and younger adults are more knowledgeable about another. Both sets of materials can then be presented for study and recall to both younger and older adults. A number of predictions about performance in this situation are possible. First, the material for which a group has superior prior knowledge should be better remembered than the less familiar or less meaningful material. That is, older adults should remember the "old" material better than the "young" material, and younger adults should remember the "young" material better than the "old" material. This effect should occur because the familiar or meaningful material is processed more quickly and more deeply, given a constant amount of cognitive resources. Second, because younger adults are expected to have superior processing resources, they should perform better on the "young" materials than the older adults perform on the "old" materials. Similarly, younger adults would be expected to perform better on the "old" materials than older adults perform on the "young" materials. Finally, the above-stated factors, when combined, lead to the prediction that age differences favoring the younger adults should be very large on "young" materials, and age differences should be very small on "old" materials.

It should be noted that younger adults would be expected to outperform older adults on both sets of materials, unless the materials were so extremely biased that the "old" materials were essentially nonwords to younger adults. A number of studies have been carried out with this design. When the words are chosen to be extremely biased (i.e., when younger adults know very little about the "old" items and older adults know very little about the "young" items), younger adults perform better than old adults on the "young" materials and older adults perform better than young adults on the "old" materials (e.g., Barrett & Watkins, 1986; Barrett & Wright, 1981).

However, younger adults perform better than older adults when the groups are compared on either age-appropriate or age-inappropriate materials. When the materials are chosen to be less age biased, so that both age groups have some knowledge of both sets of materials, age differences are typically smaller for "old" materials than for either "young" or standard materials, but younger adults are better in all conditions (e.g., Howell, 1972; Hultsch & Dixon, 1983). That is, younger adults remember more material than older adults do across all types of materials, but the age differences are smallest when the materials are biased in favor of older adults.

Strength of preexisting word associations

Large age differences are found on paired-associate recall tasks with arbitrarily paired words (see Kausler, 1982; Salthouse, 1982). Good performance on a paired-associate task requires that the words be linked together to form a meaningful pair or interacting image (see Kausler, 1982). At retrieval, in order for the memory to be retrieved, the cue must reinstate the link. Because both encoding and retrieval demand cognitive resources, large age deficits would be expected. In addition, older adults are much less likely than younger adults to employ the useful strategy of producing mediators between pairs of words. For example, Hulicka and Grossman (1967) found that younger adults spontaneously employed mediators for 68% of the pairs in their study whereas older adults employed mediators for only 36%. If the pairs are highly associated prior to the experiment, age differences are greatly reduced or eliminated (e.g., Kausler & Lair, 1966; Ruch, 1934; Shaps & Nilsson, 1980). For example, when older and younger adults' performance has been compared on high (preexperimentally associated words like *dream–sleep*) versus low associates (e.g., *river–stove*), age differences are much greater for low associates.

The two most common explanations of this pattern are that older adults *do not* use strategies as often as young adults (a production deficiency) or that older adults *cannot* use strategies as often (a processing deficiency). It is not entirely clear why older adults would not use strategies, but typical explanations argue that older adults are not tested for memory performance very often and so have not maintained relevant strategies. The argument that older adults cannot use strategies as well is based on the idea that the linking of pairs of words demands processing resources that older adults do not have. The fact that when the pairs are preexperimentally associated age differences are eliminated or significantly reduced seems to fit best with the resource explanation of age differences. Preexperimentally associated words require less effort to encode because a good association between the words already exists in memory. Moreover, preexperimentally associated words require less effort to retrieve because they have been recalled together in other situations. Therefore, given preexperimentally associated words, resource limitations are not likely to play a large role in overall performance. More important in determining the level of performance is the preexperimental strength of association between words. If these associations are equivalent for older and younger adults, and, if they are strong, age differences should be very small.

It is possible that strong associates do not require strategies, or that older adults' poorer strategic or metamemorial knowledge is responsible for the age deficit. Rabinowitz, Craik, and Ackerman (1982) attempted to test this account. Younger and older adults were given a series of words and asked to generate either unique or common associates to them. At retrieval, subjects were asked to recall the same words and were cued either with the words they generated in the first phase of the experiment or the category name associated with a word. Because the generation of unique or common associates did not interact with retrieval cue or age, this factor will be ignored in the following discussion. There were two major findings relevant to the present concerns. First, younger adults performed better when given their own generated word as a cue than when given the category cue, whereas older adults performed equally well with either cue. Second, the difference between younger and older adults was much smaller in the category-cue condition than in the generated-cue condition. These results suggest that both younger and older adults processed the general category relationships (preexperimental knowledge). The fact that only the younger adults significantly benefited from their own generated cues suggests that only the younger adults employed effective unique encodings in addition to processing existing associations.

Thus far the results can be interpreted within either the production deficiency or processing resource framework. However, if the processing resource explanation is correct, then if the resources available to younger adults are reduced, younger adults should perform much like the older adults. The authors (Rabinowitz, Craik, & Ackerman, 1982) tested this prediction by having a group of younger adults perform an arithmetic task concurrently with the generation task. The results were as predicted. Specifically, in the divided-attention condition there was no difference in the effectiveness of generated cues and general category cues. Thus, under conditions of reduced processing resources, younger adults performed much like older adults.

Categorical materials

Categorical information is of interest in memory research and aging because it is a form of knowledge that is assumed to be equally available to younger and older adults. Categorizing items at encoding and using category cues at retrieval facilitate memory performance (Mandler, 1967; Tulving & Pearlstone, 1966). Furthermore, the fact that emphasizing category relationships at encoding and making category cues available at test facilitate performance suggests that the effective employment of categorical information requires effort.

Given this background, three predictions are possible. First, if younger and older adults are compared on categorical information, an age deficit should be observed. This result would be expected because processing categorical information is demanding, and younger adults have more resources available. Second, if the demands of the task are reduced by provision of category cues at encoding or retrieval, age differences should be reduced. Third, if memory for categorical information is compared to memory for information that is not easily categorized, age differences in performance would be expected to be smallest for the category materials. These latter predictions are based on the assumption that performance in the category conditions is less dependent on cognitive resources than on preexisting knowledge.

The prediction that age-associated differences will be found on tests of categorical information can be examined in a study by Hultsch (1975). Hultsch presented three age groups of adults 40 words composed of 4 words from each of 10 categories. The oldest group performed worse than the youngest group in terms of total number of items recalled, number of categories recalled, and number of items per category recalled. We attribute this age difference in performance to the superior resources available to younger adults.

A study by Smith (1977) supports the idea that if the resource requirements of the task are reduced and performance is made to depend more on prior knowledge, age differences will be reduced. Smith presented young, middle-aged, and old adults with 20 words, each from a different taxonomic category and each starting with a different letter of the alphabet. Subjects were given letter cues, category names, or nothing before the words were studied. Then they were given a free-recall test, which was followed by a cued-recall test where either the letters or category names served as cues. Smith found that category cues presented at input facilitated both cued- and free-recall performance and that this effect was especially pronounced for older adults. When the category cues were presented before study, there were no age differences in either cued or free recall. When the category cues were not presented at study, there were age differences favoring the young.

If the effects were due simply to a strategy difference, the same pattern would be expected with the letter cues. That is, there would be large age effects when the cues were not presented before study and no age effects when the cues were presented for study. Age deficits were found favoring the youngest group in both conditions and across cued and free recall. This finding suggests that older adults do not have the resources to use letter cues as effectively as younger adults. Presumably because information is organized by meaning in memory, the category but not letter cues were effective in narrowing the search set. If younger adults are faster or in some other way more efficient in searching memory, age differences should be larger with the larger search sets (letter cues).

Laurence (1967) compared older and younger adults on lists of 12 words that belonged either to a single category or to different categories. She found that age differences were reduced but not eliminated in the single-category list. This finding suggests that when memory performance is made less dependent on processing resources and more dependent on prior knowledge, age differences are reduced.

Domain-specific knowledge

The amount and organization of information available to an individual is perhaps most pronounced with highly specialized domains of knowledge. Domain-specific knowledge has been shown to facilitate processing of information related to the domain. For example, in several domains it has been demonstrated that experts have especially good memories for domain-related but not other information (see Anderson, 1985). Much of this facilitation is presumed to come from the integration of new information with well-organized, domain-specific knowledge. However, integrating new information with knowledge is a resource-demanding task (Britton & Tesser, 1982). Therefore, predictions for this type of task are very similar to those for tasks with other materials. First, if memory for domain-specific knowledge is compared to memory for less organized material, age differences should be smaller in the domain-related area. Second, because the task is demanding of resources even within the domain, age differences would be expected even within the domain of expertise. Third, if older adults have and use domain-specific knowledge, they should show a pattern of recall much like that of younger adults with similar domain-specific knowledge.

Unfortunately, we know of no research that has compared older and younger experts for memory of material related to the domain of their expertise as well as for material not related to the domain. However, Charness (1981) equated older and younger adults in chess ability and measured their memory for briefly presented game boards. Even though chess ability was equated, the younger adults had superior memory for the chess positions. This finding suggests that the memory task was resource demanding and that older adults have fewer resources.

A study by Light and Anderson (1983) examined patterns of recall on material for which subjects had complex prior knowledge. In a first experiment the investigators had subjects generate scripts for routine activities like going grocery shopping. The scripts generated by older and younger adults were very similar, suggesting that both age groups had similar knowledge regarding these activities. In a second experiment both age groups were asked to recall and recognize particular instantiations of these activities. Younger adults performed better than older adults. More interesting, perhaps, older and younger adults exhibited the same pattern of recall across typical, average, and atypical actions within the scripts.

The above finding is interesting because it suggests that older and younger adults possessing similar knowledge for particular complex but common materials employ similar strategies. In addition, the study indicates that age differences are not due to differential integration of new information with existing knowledge. Nor does it appear that older adults concentrate solely on general knowledge or typical actions. If either of these explanations were correct, older adults would remember atypical actions differentially worse than other actions. In fact, performance was best on such actions for both age groups, and the difference between younger and older adults was approximately the same across the different types of items. Light and Anderson suggested that the deficit older adults exhibited was the result of older adults' smaller processing capacity, which made it more difficult for them to simultaneously maintain old knowledge and new information in memory.

Azmitia and Perlmutter (1987) conducted a similar study. Older and younger subjects rated objects as typical or atypical for various settings such as bedrooms, kitchens, and garages. Then other groups of older and younger adults were asked to recall and recognize particular objects from pictures of these settings that contained both typical and atypical objects. As in the Light and Anderson study, younger adults outperformed older adults. In addition, the age differences were largest for the atypical objects. At first this finding may seem counter to Light and Anderson's findings, but there are some hints that the same sorts of factors account for both results. In the Azmitia and Perlmutter study, all subjects recalled more typical than atypical objects, whereas the reverse was true in the Light and Anderson study. In addition, recall performance in the Azmitia and Perlmutter study was less than half that in the Light and Anderson study. If the reasonable assumption is made that the Azmitia and Perlmutter task was more demanding of processing resources than the Light and Anderson task, the results make sense. When demands on processing are high, less information is remembered. If typical objects are noticed and processed first, atypical objects will be processed only if sufficient time is available. If more time is available, more atypical objects will be processed, and, because of their distinctiveness, they will be remembered better than the typical objects. In the Light and Anderson study, we assume that subjects had time to process the unexpected events and thus recalled them better. In the Azmitia and Perlmutter study, sufficient time generally was not available and thus typical objects were studied first. Younger adults were more likely to have extra time to process the unexpected items, and they therefore performed differentially better on the atypical items.

Depth of processing and forewarning of memory test

The idea that depth of processing is important for determining memory performance of both younger and older adults has been suggested at several points in this chapter. There has been considerable research directed at depth of processing and aging. In a typical study, older and younger subjects are asked to perform a number of orienting tasks or simply to remember material. The various orienting tasks are designed to guide processing to different levels, ranging from acoustic or physical to semantic. By comparing younger and older adults' memory after these various tasks, age-related processing deficits are expected to be located. When the memory test is one of free recall, age differences are usually found to increase with increasing depth of the task, whereas when the memory test involves recognition, the results are quite mixed and no general statement can be made (see Burke & Light, 1981, for a review of the literature).

Most often research on levels of processing is discussed within the framework of processing or production deficits. A *processing deficit* is a *loss in the ability* to analyze information at a deep level. A *production deficit* is a *failure to carry out* a process even though the capability to do so is present. Thus, if older adults have a processing deficit they cannot process information deeply, whereas if they have a production deficit they simply do not process information deeply, although presumably they have the ability to do so.

Recent evidence from semantic priming studies suggests that older and younger adults process semantic information in very similar ways, although older adults may be slower in some aspects of processing (see Burke & Harrold; Howard, this volume). This evidence suggests that older adults can process information deeply. Burke and Light (1981) have reviewed the memory literature and have suggested that the age deficit requires some sort of processing deficit account.

If it is the case that the age deficits obtained in depth of processing studies are due to the fewer resources available to older adults, the results are somewhat confusing. For example, it is not clear why different patterns emerge on recall and recognition tests or why there is such variability of findings across studies. At first glance, consideration of knowledge might not seem to add clarity. However, if one makes the reasonable assumptions that both older and younger adults possess enough knowledge to answer the orienting questions (which is suggested by the fact that performance on such questions usually is equivalent), and that only processes required to answer the questions are carried out, then minimal age differences would be expected. The age differences should be small because the tasks usually are not speeded or otherwise very demanding and therefore should require relatively few resources for either age group. If extra processing is permitted, larger age differences would be expected. The age differences should be larger because extra processing places extra demand on the system and younger adults are more likely to have cognitive resources available to carry out extra processing.

Perlmutter and Mitchell (1982), in an analysis of previously published experiments that manipulated level of processing, examined whether memory tests were expected or not. Expectation of a memory test is important because only if subjects expect a memory test is there reason to process beyond the level required to answer the orienting question. If a memory test is expected, additional processing might be carried out. They found that when orienting tasks were combined with expectation of a memory test, age differences averaged 13% across 12 experiments involving free recall and 12% for recognition. However, when a memory test was not expected, age differences averaged only 5% for both recall and recognition. It was argued (Perlmutter & Mitchell, 1982) that when memory tests were expected, the primary difference between younger and older adults was in use of strategies. When the tests were not expected, age differences were quite small and usually not significant. Perlmutter and Mitchell attributed the differential use of strategies to a processing resource reserve in younger adults.

Verbal ability

Another means of examining the role of knowledge on unrelated lists is to compare performance of individuals who are high or low in verbal knowledge. High verbal ability may be linked to good memory performance for at least four reasons. First, high verbal ability individuals may be faster at certain component processes related to verbal processing. For example, Hunt (1985) found that individuals high in verbal ability were faster at lexical access, naming, symbol manipulation, and sentence verification. Second, high verbal ability subjects may possess more meaningful information about verbal material than low verbal ability subjects, as indicated by their superior vocabulary scores. Third, high verbal ability subjects, because they possess good verbal skills, may use those skills more often and benefit from the practice (Rice, 1986; Rice & Meyer, 1985). Finally, because of reduced time necessary for basic verbal operations, greater amount of verbal information available, and more practice with verbal material, high verbal ability subjects may employ more strategies than low verbal ability subjects (Rice & Meyer, 1985).

High verbal ability subjects would be expected to exhibit superior memory for verbal material, regardless of age. Whether age interacts with verbal ability is more difficult to predict. Most studies of verbal ability employ vocabulary as the criterion variable and show little, if any, age-related decline in performance until very late in life, or improvement in vocabulary scores with age into the 60s (Horn & Cattell, 1966, 1967; Schaie & Labouvie-Vief, 1974). This finding is important because vocabulary size is a good predictor of other factors that make up verbal intelligence (e.g., Matarazzo, 1982). However, older adults often show a significant decline on verbal measures that tap verbal fluency and/or on tasks that are timed (see Hartley; Salthouse, this volume).

The above findings suggest that loss of resources will play a role in older adults' performance on some tasks. On the one hand, older individuals of high verbal ability who maintain their vocabulary scores, exhibit a reduced loss of speed, and employ useful strategies because of practice with verbal material, would be expected to perform similarly to high verbal ability younger adults, and both groups should outperform low verbal ability subjects of both ages. On the other hand, older adults of lower verbal ability should be at a relatively large disadvantage. In fact, in a number of studies these results have been obtained with material as varied as simple lists of words (Bowles & Poon, 1982), television programs (Cavanaugh, 1983), and texts (Taub, 1979; Till, 1985). That is, older adults of high verbal ability perform very much like younger adults of high verbal ability. There is essentially no age-related decline in performance. In addition, low verbal ability adults perform more poorly than high verbal ability adults, and there is a pronounced age decline for the "low verbal" older group.

Conclusions that can be made from studies of verbal ability are not without problems. For example, verbal ability usually is analyzed in a post hoc fashion. That is, although verbal ability is measured in all subjects, it is only after the experiment is completed that subjects are divided into high and low verbal groups, and the division is usually made on the basis of some arbitrary criterion. Much stronger evidence would be obtained if age and vocabulary were covaried. A second major problem is that it is not clear whether older individuals labeled "low verbal" have always been low verbal, or whether they simply are showing earlier declines in verbal ability than the individuals labeled "high verbal." Third, the definition of verbal ability is not always well justified. Verbal ability actually may include many abilities (see Hartley, this volume). Given these problems it is not surprising that there are exceptions to the pattern described above (e.g., Meyer & Rice, 1983). Perhaps more surprising is the large number of studies in which precisely that pattern has been found.

Mnemonic training

It is clear that older adults employ strategies less often than younger adults, and that when they use strategies they tend not to be effective strategies (Sanders, Murphy, Schmitt, & Walsh, 1980). It is also clear that older adults can improve their memory with the use of mnemonics (e.g., Poon, Walsh-Sweeney, & Fozard, 1980). Two important questions are why older adults do not use strategies more often, and whether mnemonic training reduces age differences in memory performance.

The analysis presented in this chapter predicts that age differences will not disappear with training except in restricted cases. The reasons for this are that mnemonics, in general, are very demanding of processing resources, and older adults have fewer resources than younger adults. Only when perfect performance is possible, or when the mnemonic is very simple (as in making judgments about whether a stimulus is pleasant) and no other processes are carried out, will age differences be eliminated. However, there is very little research that explicitly tests these hypotheses.

A number of explanations have been posed to account for the findings that older adults are less likely to employ effective strategies. For example, it has been suggested that older adults have not had recent practice in using strategies required for laboratory tasks and so are "rusty" (Treat, Poon, & Fozard, 1981). In addition, it may be that older adults do use strategies, but only for materials frequently encountered in everyday life (Perlmutter, 1986). In general, there is not much support for the idea that practice alone eliminates age differences in strategy use. Whereas Treat, Poon, and Fozard (1981) found that age differences were reduced after 2 weeks of practice, other researchers have found that both age groups improve with practice and that age differences are maintained across practice sessions (e.g., Robertson-Tchabo, Hausman, & Arenberg, 1976). In addition, Poon (1985) has suggested that not all mnemonic techniques facilitate older adults' performance, and maintenance of learned techniques has not been demonstrated over time.

Another explanation of older adults' strategy deficit is that mnemonic techniques require too many processing resources. If processing resources decline with age, age-related declines in the efficiency of such mnemonic techniques as rehearsal would be expected (e.g., Salthouse, 1980). In addition, strategies are most likely to be employed when enough processing resources are available to complete the task. Thus, because older adults have fewer processing resources available, they would be expected to employ strategies less often.

Finally, knowledge of the material or tasks used may sometimes allow strategies to be employed in cases where if knowledge were not available they could not be employed. The finding of approximately equivalent performances of younger adults on "young" materials and older adults on "old" materials (e.g., Barrett & Wright, 1981) and the finding of equivalent or near equivalent performance of "high verbal" younger and older adults support this notion. If knowledge is considered in terms of everyday activities, then the notion that knowledge allows for the use of strategies is consistent with Perlmutter's (1986) notion that older adults use strategies to deal with environmental press.

Summary

We have presented evidence from a number of studies to suggest that knowledge facilitates memory performance for both younger and older adults. Knowledge of various types appears to facilitate performance by reducing the resources required in a task, by allowing for deeper processing to occur, and by facilitating effective encoding and retrieval. Age differences tend to be reduced in situations where older and younger adults have approximately equal amounts and types of knowledge, and where effective performance depends primarily on prior knowledge.

It is interesting to note that when knowledge is equated for younger and older adults, older adults often appear strategic. Conversely, on very demanding tasks, or when little knowledge is available, older adults do not appear to employ strategies. A plausible explanation of these results is that older adults do not use strategies and appear to have poor metamemorial knowledge on tasks in which processing demands are high and in which the employment of strategies and metamemorial knowledge is extremely difficult.

Additional considerations

In this section we briefly discuss three additional issues that are relevant to the discussion of knowledge effects on the acquisition of new information.

Difficulty

Several researchers have argued that difficulty is an important variable in determining age differences (e.g., Craik, 1968). This point is of interest because age differences are often found to be most pronounced on difficult tasks (see Salthouse, 1982). The problem with this argument is that there is usually no independent measure of difficulty.

Our analysis suggests that difficulty is determined in large part by processing requirements and knowledge of the task. Overall, difficulty is determined by the interaction of these two factors. We believe that this is a better way to frame the issue of difficulty because knowledge and processing demand can be measured independently. Processing demands can be measured by dual-task procedures, for example, by requiring subjects to perform a second task simultaneously. In this situation, a decrease in performance of the first task that is caused by the second task is taken as evidence that the second task depleted resources. The greater the demands on resources of the second task, the greater the drop in performance. In addition, processing demand can be manipulated, for example, by making almost any task a speeded task. Knowledge can be examined separately in several ways, including standardized tests, priming, typicality ratings, and generating schemata. Measuring processing demands and knowledge concurrently should lead to a better understanding of what determines difficulty and how age is influenced by various forms of difficulty.

Knowledge across the life-span

It is interesting to note that many of the same arguments regarding knowledge and processing resources that we have discussed also apply to the developing child. For example, increases in factual knowledge appear to be a major factor in improvements in memory performance across childhood (e.g., Lindberg, 1980; Perlmutter, 1986; Perlmutter & Myers, 1979). It may be that within a given task differences among children of various ages are largest when knowledge affects processing (Naus & Ornstein, 1977). In addition, procedural knowledge, strategies, and metamemorial abilities seem to develop across childhood (e.g., Brown, 1975; Brown & De-Loache, 1978). Although it is difficult to determine the direction of causality, at least some of the increase in strategy use appears to be due to increases in factual knowledge (Chi, 1978).

Knowledge undoubtedly is important for memory performance across the life-span. For children, an increase in knowledge appears to allow processing resources to reach their potential, and in old age knowledge may compensate for a loss of basic processing resources. A life-span investigation of the influence of knowledge on memory would be useful. For example, it would highlight the role of knowledge at the extremes, that is, when knowledge is relatively limited (e.g., in children) and probably maximal (i.e., in older adults).

The very old

The research on aging that we have summarized has been conducted with older adults in their 60s and 70s, with the oldest age group typically averaging 70 or less. There is very little research available on adults older than this age, but what research exists suggests that previous findings may not generalize to the very old. For example, thus far research suggests that whereas vocabulary may increase across adulthood to age 70, it generally declines after 70 (Schaie & Labouvie-Vief, 1974). The reasons for this decline are not clear, but one possibility is that a decline in processing resources in the very old is so severe that compensation by knowledge is not possible.

Conclusions

We have suggested that knowledge is a very important factor in determining memory performance of any age group. In addition, we have argued that knowledge may compensate for a loss of processing resources in older adults, and reduce age-related deficits found on many memory tasks. Factual knowledge appears to facilitate performance by reducing the time necessary to process information, by increasing depth of processing, and by making use of existing memory structures to facilitate encoding and retrieval of new information. All of these factors are likely to increase the probability that strategies are used and thus improve performance even more. In addition, practice with tasks and strategies is likely to make some aspects of tasks easier and again to decrease processing demands.

References

Anderson, J. R. (1985). *Cognitive psychology and its implications* (2nd ed., pp. 232–260). San Francisco: Freeman.

Azmitia, M., & Perlmutter, M. (1987). *Age differences in adults' scene memory: Knowledge and strategy interactions.* Unpublished manuscript, University of Michigan, Institute of Gerontology, Ann Arbor.

Barrett, T. R., & Watkins, S. K. (1986). Word familiarity and cardiovascular health as determinants of age-related recall differences. *Journal of Gerontology, 41,* 222–224.

Barrett, T. R., & Wright, M. (1981). Age-related facilitation in recall following semantic processing. *Journal of Gerontology, 36,* 194–199.

Bower, G. H., Black, J. B., & Turner, T. J. (1979). Scripts in memory for text. *Cognitive Psychology, 11,* 177–220.

Bowles, N. L., & Poon, L. W. (1982). An analysis of the effect of aging on recognition memory. *Journal of Gerontology, 37,* 212–219.

Britton, B. K., & Tesser, A. (1982). Effects of prior knowledge on use of cognitive capacity in three complex cognitive tasks. *Journal of Verbal Learning and Verbal Behavior, 21,* 421–436.

Brown, A. L. (1975). The development of memory: Knowing, knowing about knowing, and knowing how to know. In H. W. Reese (Ed.), *Advances in child development and behavior* (Vol. 10, pp. 103–152). New York: Academic Press.

Brown, A. L., & DeLoache, J. S. (1978). Skills, plans, and self-regulation. In R. S. Siegler (Ed.), *Children's thinking: What develops?* (pp. 3–36). Hillsdale, NJ: Erlbaum.

Burke, D. M., & Light, L. L. (1981). Memory and aging: The role of retrieval processes. *Psychological Bulletin, 90*, 513–546.

Cavanaugh, J. C. (1983). Comprehension and retention of television programs by 20- and 60-year olds. *Journal of Gerontology, 38*, 190–196.

Cavanaugh, J. C., & Perlmutter, M. (1982). Metamemory: A critical examination. *Child Development, 53*, 11–28.

Charness, N. (1981). Visual short-term memory and aging in chess players. *Journal of Gerontology, 36*, 615–619.

Chi, M. T. H. (1978). Knowledge structures and memory development. In R. S. Siegler (Ed.), *Children's thinking: What develops?* (pp. 73–96). Hillsdale, NJ: Erlbaum.

Chiesi, H. L., Spilich, G. J., & Voss, J. F. (1979). Acquisition of domain related information in relation to high and low domain knowledge. *Journal of Verbal Learning and Verbal Behavior, 18*, 257–273.

Craik, F. I. M. (1968). Types of error in free recall. *Psychonomic Science, 10*, 353–354.

Craik, F. I. M., & Byrd, M. (1982). Aging and cognitive deficits: The role of attentional resources. In F. I. M. Craik & S. Trehub (Eds.), *Aging and cognitive processes* (pp. 191–211). New York: Plenum.

Craik, F. I. M., & Lockhart, R. S. (1972). Levels of processing: A framework for memory research. *Journal of Verbal Learning and Verbal Behavior, 11*, 671–684.

Craik, F. I. M., & Lockhart, R. S. (1986). CHARM is not enough: Comments on Eich's model of cued recall. *Psychological Review, 93*, 360–364.

Crowder, R. G. (1976). *Principles of learning and memory* (pp. 322–352). Hillsdale, NJ: Erlbaum.

Denney, N. W. (1982). Aging and cognitive changes. In B. B. Wolman (Ed.), *Handbook of developmental psychology* (pp. 807–827). Englewood Cliffs, NJ: Prentice-Hall.

Hasher, L., & Griffin, M. (1978). Reconstructive and reproductive processes in memory. *Journal of Experimental Psychology: Human Learning and Memory, 4*, 318–330.

Hasher, L., & Zacks, R. T. (1979). Automatic and effortful processes in memory. *Journal of Experimental Psychology: General, 108*, 356–388.

Horn, J. L., & Cattell, R. B. (1966). Age differences in primary mental ability factors. *Journal of Gerontology, 21*, 210–220.

Horn, J. L., & Cattell, R. B. (1967). Age differences in fluid and crystallized intelligence. *Acta Psychologica, 16*, 107–129.

Howell, S. C. (1972). Familiarity and complexity in perceptual recognition. *Journal of Gerontology, 27*, 364–371.

Hulicka, I. M., & Grossman, J. L. (1967). Age-group comparisons for the use of mediators in paired-associate learning. *Journal of Gerontology, 22*, 46–51.

Hultsch, D. F. (1975). Adult age differences in retrieval: Trace-dependent and cue dependent forgetting. *Developmental Psychology, 11*, 197–201.

Hultsch, D. F., & Dixon, R. A. (1983). The role of pre-experimental knowledge in text processing in adulthood. *Experimental Aging Research, 9*, 17–22.

Hunt, E. (1985). Verbal ability. In R. J. Sternberg (Ed.), *Human abilities: An information-processing approach* (pp. 31–58). San Francisco: Freeman.

Johnson, W., & Kieras, D. (1983). Representation-saving effects of prior knowledge in memory for simple technical prose. *Memory & Cognition, 11*, 456–466.

Johnston, W. A., & Dark, V. J. (1986). Selective attention. *Annual Review of Psychology, 37*, 43–75.

Kausler, D. H. (1982). *Experimental psychology and human aging*. New York: Wiley.

Kausler, D. H., & Lair, C. V. (1966). Associative strength and paired-associate learning in elderly subjects. *Journal of Gerontology, 21*, 278–280.

Laurence, M. W. (1967). A developmental look at the usefulness of list categorization as an aid to free recall. *Canadian Journal of Psychology, 21*, 153–165.

Light, L. L., & Anderson, P. A. (1983). Memory for scripts in young and older adults. *Memory & Cognition, 11*, 435–444.

Lindberg, M. A. (1980). Is knowledge base development a necessary and sufficient condition for memory development? *Journal of Experimental Child Psychology, 30*, 401–410.

Mandler, G. (1967). Organization and memory. In K. W. Spence & J. T. Spence (Eds.), *The psychology of learning and motivation* (Vol. 1, pp. 327–372). New York: Academic Press.

Matarazzo, J. D. (1972). *Wechsler's measurement and appraisal of adult intelligence* (5th ed.). Baltimore: Williams & Wilkins.

Meyer, B. J. F., & Rice, G. E. (1983). Learning and memory from text across the adult life-span. In J. Fine & R. O. Freedle (Eds.), *Developmental studies in discourse* (pp. 291–306). Norwood, NJ: Ablex.

Naus, M. J., & Ornstein, P. A. (1977). Developmental differences in the memory search of categorized lists. *Developmental Psychology, 13*, 60–68.

Norman, D. A., & Bobrow, D. G. (1975). On data-limited and resource-limited processes. *Cognitive Psychology, 7*, 44–64.

Perlmutter, M. (1986). A life span view of memory. In P. B. Baltes, D. Featherman, & R. Learner (Eds.), *Advances in life-span development and behavior* (Vol. 7, pp. 272–313). Hillsdale, NJ: Erlbaum.

Perlmutter, M., & Mitchell, D. B. (1982). The appearance and disappearance of age differences in adult memory. In F. I. M. Craik & S. E. Trehub (Eds.), *Aging and cognitive processes* (pp. 127–144). New York: Plenum.

Perlmutter, M., & Myers, N. A. (1979). Development of recall in 2 to 4 year olds. *Developmental Psychology, 15*, 73–83.

Poon, L. W. (1985). Differences in human memory with aging: Nature, causes and clinical implications. In J. E. Birren & K. W. Schaie (Eds.), *Handbook of the psychology of aging* (2nd ed., pp. 427–462). New York: Van Nostrand Reinhold.

Poon, L. W., & Fozard, J. L. (1978). Speed of retrieval from long-term memory in relation to age, familiarity, and datedness of information. *Journal of Gerontology, 33*, 711–717.

Poon, L. W., Walsh-Sweeney, L., & Fozard, J. L. (1980). Memory skill training for the elderly: Salient issues on the use of imagery mnemonics. In L. W. Poon, J. L. Fozard, L. S. Cermak, D. Arenberg, & L. W. Thompson (Eds.), *New directions in memory and aging: Proceedings of the George A. Talland Memorial Conference* (pp. 461–484). Hillsdale, NJ: Erlbaum.

Rabinowitz, J. C., Craik, F. I. M., & Ackerman, B. P. (1982). A processing resource account of age differences in recall. *Canadian Journal of Psychology, 36*, 325–344.

Rice, G. E. (1986). The everyday activities of adults: Implications for prose recall – Part I. *Educational Gerontology, 12*, 173–186.

Rice, G. E., & Meyer, B. J. F. (1985). Reading behavior and prose recall performance of young and older adults with high and average verbal ability. *Educational Gerontology, 11*, 57–72.

Robertson-Tchabo, E. A., Hausman, C. P., & Arenberg, D. (1976). A classical mnemonic for older learners: A trip that works! *Educational Gerontology, 1*, 215–226.

Ruch, F. L. (1934). The differentiative effects of age upon human learning. *Journal of General Psychology, 11*, 261–268.

Salthouse, T. A. (1980). Age and memory: Strategies for localizing the loss. In L. W. Poon, J. L. Fozard, L. S. Cermak, D. Arenberg, & L. W. Thompson (Eds.), *New directions in memory and aging: Proceedings of the George A. Talland Memorial Conference* (pp. 47–65). Hillsdale, NJ: Erlbaum.

Salthouse, T. A. (1982). *Adult cognition: An experimental psychology of human aging*. New York: Springer-Verlag.

Salthouse, T. A. (1985a). Speed of behavior and its implications for cognition. In J. E. Birren & K. W. Schaie (Eds.), *Handbook of the psychology of aging* (2nd ed., pp. 400–426). New York: Van Nostrand Reinhold.

Salthouse, T. A. (1985b). *A theory of cognitive aging*. New York: Elsevier Science.

Sanders, R. E., Murphy, M. D., Schmitt, F. A., & Walsh, K. K. (1980). Age differences in free recall rehearsal strategies. *Journal of Gerontology, 35*, 550–558.

Schaie, K. W., & Labouvie-Vief, G. (1974). Generational versus ontogenetic components of change in adult cognitive behavior. *Developmental Psychology, 10*, 305–320.

Schneider, W., & Shiffrin, R. M. (1977). Controlled and automatic human information processing: I. Detection, search and attention. *Psychological Review, 84*, 1–66.

Shaps, L. P., & Nilsson, L. (1980). Encoding and retrieval operations in relation to age. *Developmental Psychology, 16*, 636–643.

Smith, A. D. (1977). Adult age differences in cued recall. *Developmental Psychology, 13*, 326–331.

Taub, H. A. (1979). Comprehension and memory of prose materials by young and old adults. *Experimental Aging Research, 5*, 3–13.

Till, R. E. (1985). Verbatim and inferential memory in young and elderly adults. *Journal of Gerontology, 40*, 316–323.

Treat, N. J., Poon, L. W., & Fozard, J. L. (1981). Age, imagery, and practice in paired-associate learning. *Experimental Aging Research, 7*, 337–342.

Tulving, E., & Pearlstone, Z. (1966). Availability vs. accessibility in memory for words. *Journal of Verbal Learning and Verbal Behavior, 5*, 381–391.

12   The disorder of naming in Alzheimer's disease

F. Jacob Huff

Alzheimer's disease is a degenerative disease of unknown etiology, the incidence of which increases with advancing age. Neurons are affected in many brain regions, but the distribution of degenerative changes is not random. The hippocampus and amygdala, which are known to be involved in learning, and areas of the frontal, temporal, and parietal lobes known to be involved in language and related processes are typically affected intensely by the pathological process of Alzheimer's disease (Brun & Englund, 1981). Disorders of memory and language are accordingly clinical features of the disease, which is characterized by an insidiously progressive dementia. Patients consistently develop an impairment of naming, or *anomia*, as a prominent feature of their language disorder. In this chapter, the general features of Alzheimer's disease are described, followed by a discussion of the language disorder, emphasizing research on anomia and its associated cognitive deficits. The chapter concludes with presentation of an experimental investigation in which an effort was made to establish the importance of a visual, semantic, and word-retrieval deficits in accounting for anomia in Alzheimer's disease.

Neuropathological features of Alzheimer's disease

Although a presumptive diagnosis of Alzheimer's disease can be made clinically (McKhann et al., 1984), the diagnosis can be made definitively only by histopathological examination. Abundant intracellular tangles of neurofilaments and extracellular plaques composed of degenerating neuronal cell processes and deposits of amyloid protein are diagnostic of Alzheimer's disease. These abnormalities are associated with loss of neurons in the cerebral cortex and several subcortical nuclei. The degenerative changes just described are also observed in association with normal aging, but are limited both in intensity and distribution relative to cases of Alzheimer's disease (Terry & Katzman, 1983).

This work was supported by NIH grant AG00232. The experimental study described was performed at the Massachusetts Institute of Technology Clinical Research Center. The author thanks Suzanne Corkin, Ph.D., and John H. Growdon, M.D., for providing the research environment and subjects for this study, Ann Carr for statistical analyses, and Darlene Bumford for typing the manuscript.

Clinical course of Alzheimer's disease

Patients with Alzheimer's disease undergo steadily progressive intellectual deterioration. Plateau periods of slowed progression may be observed, but remissions do not occur. The most common initial symptom of the disease is impaired recent memory. However, in some cases the first symptom may be a language disorder (Kirshner, Webb, Kelly, & Wells, 1984), a visuospatial deficit (Crystal, Horoupian, Katzman, & Jotkowitz, 1982), or a change in personality such as irritability, apathy, or depression (Reding, Haycox, & Blass, 1985).

The clinical course has been divided into three stages by some investigators (Cummings & Benson, 1983; Sjögren, 1952). In the first stage, new learning is defective, remote recall is impaired, spatial and temporal disorientation develop, word-finding pauses occur in conversation, and patients may exhibit poor judgment, difficulty in reasoning through problems, carelessness in grooming and work habits, or a change in personality. The second stage of illness usually supervenes between 2 and 10 years after the initial symptoms, and is marked by definite syndromes of amnesia, aphasia, agnosia, and apraxia. The initial apathy may be replaced by restlessness with frequent pacing, agitation, and delusional thinking. The third, terminal stage typically develops 8–12 years after onset of symptoms. All intellectual capacities are impaired, and spontaneous activity diminishes to an eventual bed-ridden state that leads to intercurrent illnesses such as pneumonia, which is frequently the direct cause of death.

Clinical features of the language disorder in Alzheimer's disease

A disorder of language is consistently present by the middle of the clinical course, ranging from 2 to 10 years after onset of dementing symptoms (Cummings & Benson, 1983; Sjögren, 1952). On standardized tests designed for evaluation of aphasia, patients with Alzheimer's disease are impaired in both expressive and receptive language functions (Appell, Kertesz, & Fisman, 1982), and have a prominent deficit in naming ability. Semantic and pragmatic aspects of language are disturbed, whereas phonological and morphosyntactic aspects of language are relatively preserved (Emery & Emery, 1983; Irigaray, 1973). Syntactic function is not normal, however, and use of complex linguistic forms is impaired, as is discussed by Emery (this volume). The typical pattern of progression of the language disorder in Alzheimer's disease is summarized in Table 12.1.

In the early phase of the disease, speech is typically fluent, with normal prosody and articulation. Difficulty in finding substantive words is apparent in pauses and in circumlocutory discourse, where general vocabulary is used in an effort to refer to objects, concepts, or people whose name or specific designation cannot be recalled (Goodman, 1953). Phonemic (e.g., *log* for *dog*) or semantic (e.g., *cat* for *dog*) substitution errors (paraphasias) are rarely produced spontaneously. However, if the listener suggests words to the patient that are semantically related to the target word, off-target suggestions such as *sister* for *daughter* or *table* for *chair* are often accepted as correct, although phonemic substitutions are rejected (Schwartz, Marin, & Saffran, 1979).

Table 12.1. *Typical progression of language disorder in Alzheimer's disease*

Early symptoms
Circumlocutory discourse
Word-finding pauses
Difficulty in naming objects
Late symptoms
Paraphasias
Simplified syntax
Impaired comprehension
Final symptoms
Meaningless repetition of words
Repetition of nonsense sounds
Mutism

As the disease progresses, this impairment in differentiating between semantically related words becomes more pronounced. Phonemic and semantic paraphasias occur more frequently. Verbal expressions typically become briefer and less elaborate syntactically, although errors in syntax do not generally occur. Writing deteriorates, characterized by spelling errors and omission or repetition of words (Folstein & Breitner, 1981). Comprehension of language, both aural and written, also deteriorates. Patients usually are able to repeat utterances and to read aloud with normal prosody, correctly pronouncing irregularly spelled words (Nelson & O'Connell, 1978). In the advanced stages of the disease, speech is often reduced to meaningless repetition of words or nonsense sounds, and many patients become mute (Cummings & Benson, 1983).

Anomia and associated cognitive deficits

Although anomia, the impairment in naming, is recognized as a prominent clinical feature of Alzheimer's disease, there remains considerable disagreement regarding the cognitive disorder underlying this symptom. Anomia in a broad sense refers to difficulty in producing names in spoken discourse, but it is commonly documented by asking patients to name visually presented objects or pictures of objects. One explanation of anomia is that it results from impaired visual perception of the object to be named. Another hypothesis is that lexical–semantic information necessary for selecting the correct name is lost. A third explanation is that lexical–semantic information is preserved, but an impairment in word retrieval results in anomia. These three hypotheses are discussed in sequence.

Lawson and Barker (1968) reached the conclusion that visual impairment causes anomia after observing that naming improved when demented patients were allowed to handle objects, and when the use of the objects was demonstrated to them. Rochford (1971) reported that demented patients were accurate in naming body parts indicated on the examiner but not in naming line drawings of objects, whereas aphasics with focal brain lesions were equally impaired with both types of stimuli. Reasoning that body parts are visually familiar and therefore easy to recognize, he concluded that naming errors in demented patients result from failures of visual recognition. Kirshner, Webb, and Kelly (1984) presented objects at four levels of perceptual difficulty: the actual object, a photograph of the object, a line drawing of the object, and a line drawing masked by superimposed lines. Although perceptual difficulty influenced naming performance both in patients with Alzheimer's disease and in healthy, age-matched control subjects, performance was more affected in the patients, particularly those with severe dementia. Thus, impaired visual perception may become a more frequent cause of naming errors as dementia progresses. Enhanced sensitivity to perceptual difficulty does not, however, imply that visual impairment is the cause of all confrontation naming errors in patients with Alzheimer's disease. Moreover, although visual impairment may explain some confrontation naming errors, it does not account for word-finding difficulty in spoken discourse.

Impaired access to, or loss of, semantic information is another possible cause of the naming disorder in Alzheimer's disease. Warrington (1975) studied three patients with progressive dementia, all of whom had difficulty naming pictured objects. She evaluated their ability to recognize the lexical superordinate category (e.g., *animal*) and various attributes of both pictured objects and the corresponding written names. Patients were able to assign objects correctly to categories, but were unable to specify the attributes that distinguished among objects within a category. Difficulty distinguishing among members of a category has been observed in several other studies of dementia (Martin & Fedio, 1983; Schwartz et al., 1979). Whether this symptom results from disruption of lexical information, or of a conceptual semantic system that underlies use of lexical information, is not clear. The expression *lexical–semantic impairment* is used to reflect this uncertainty about the nature of the disorder, and the term *semantic* is understood as an abbreviated term for "lexical–semantic."

A third possible cause of impaired confrontation naming in Alzheimer's disease is a word-retrieval deficit, characterized by inability to name an object that has been successfully identified. According to this hypothesis, lexical–semantic information is intact, and the patient can correctly identify the name if it is presented in a list of alternative names. Word-retrieval ability may be evaluated by fluency tests, in which the subject is requested to list members of categories such as animals, or words beginning with a specified letter. Patients with Alzheimer's disease produce fewer words than do normal subjects on fluency tests (Miller & Hague, 1975; Rosen, 1980), and Benson (1979) has reported that this deficiency precedes the development of impaired confrontation naming. These observations suggest that a word-retrieval deficit may be responsible for object-naming failures.

The perceptual and semantic accounts of anomia in Alzheimer's disease have been compared by analyzing errors on object-naming tasks and contrasting the number of errors that could be attributed to misperception or misrecognition of the object (e.g., *snake* for a picture of a pretzel) with the number of errors that reflect semantic confusion (e.g., *potato chip* for the same picture). Rochford (1971) reported that the majority of errors in demented patients were attributable to misrecognition. Other investigators found that semantic errors occurred more frequently than misrecognition errors in demented patients, although both types of error occur more often than in healthy adults (Bayles & Tomoeda, 1983; Martin & Fedio, 1983). Inspection of naming errors frequently does not permit distinction between the perceptual and semantic hypotheses, however, because many errors are similar to the target both visually and semantically (e.g., *hippopotamus* for a picture of a rhinoceros). The perceptual and semantic accounts of anomia therefore cannot be differentiated conclusively by analysis of error types, the technique used by Bayles and Tomoeda (1983) and Martin and Fedio (1983). Research that attempts to avoid this problem is described below.

Investigation of anomia in Alzheimer's disease

In an effort to evaluate the relative contributions of impairments in lexical retrieval, semantic discrimination, and visual processing to the anomia of Alzheimer's disease, an experiment was designed to compare performance on tests of all these abilities in patients with early symptoms of Alzheimer's disease and age-matched control subjects. (The results of this study have been summarized in Huff, Corkin, and Growdon, 1983, and in Huff and Corkin, 1984.) Tests were selected that measured lexical retrieval independently of visual processing, semantic impairment independently of lexical retrieval, and visual discrimination independently of semantic processing. By comparing performance on these tests with one another and with confrontation naming, inferences were drawn regarding which cognitive deficits were sufficient to produce anomia, and about the relationships among these deficits in Alzheimer's disease.

A model of the cognitive processes involved in naming is presented in Figure 12.1. The naming act may be prompted by visual or verbal stimuli that are processed through a system of lexical–semantic knowledge. The naming act may consist of retrieval and production of a word (name), or recognition of the correct word in a multiple-choice list. Confrontation naming requires retrieval of a word in response to a visual stimulus. Other tasks used in this experiment were designed to measure cognitive components of the confrontation naming task. The specific cognitive components assayed by each task are mentioned with the description of the task.

Materials and procedure

The following tests were given in the order in which they are described.

Boston Naming Test. This test (Kaplan, Goodglass, & Weintraub, 1978) was used as a quantitative measure of anomia. In this test, a series of line drawings of objects were presented to the subject. The subject was allowed 20 seconds to name each object. If the correct word was not produced in that time, a semantic cue (e.g., "something that grows outdoors" for "tree") was given, and an additional 20 seconds was allowed for response. Correct responses during the uncued and semantically cued conditions were combined in calculating the test score. Two equivalent subtests, each consisting of 42 items from the original 85-item Boston Naming Test

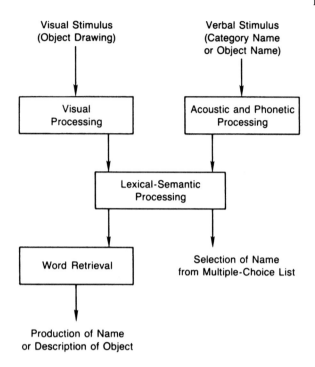

Figure 12.1. Model of the cognitive processes involved in naming.

(BNT), have been developed (Huff, Collins, Corkin, & Rosen, 1986). The correlation between scores on the two forms was 0.97 in subjects who took both forms. The data presented here are the mean scores on the two forms for each subject (maximum score, 42).

Multiple-choice naming task. A multiple-choice version of each 42-item form of the BNT was designed for this experiment and was administered after the standard version. In this test, five words were printed below each line drawing. One word was the correct response (e.g., *tree*). Another was a semantically related distractor (e.g., *vine*). A third was a phonemic distractor containing the same initial phoneme as the correct name (*tray*), and the remaining two distractors were concrete nouns unrelated to the correct response, but matched with it in word frequency. The choices were randomly ordered for each item. The subject was required to read aloud the choices for each item, and reading errors were corrected by the examiner as they occurred. The subject then selected the name corresponding to the line drawing. The mean score for the two forms of the test is presented (maximum score, 42).

This task involves the same visual discrimination and lexical–semantic processes as the confrontation naming task (Fig. 12.1), but rather than requiring word retrieval in the response it requires selection of the correct word from a list. Selection of semantic distractors on this test by patients with normal visual processing suggests an impairment in lexical–semantic processes that are also involved in confrontation naming. Normal performance on this test in a patient with impaired confrontation naming suggests that the confrontation anomia is due to a word-retrieval deficit.

Category fluency task. The subject listed words aloud from a category of natural objects specified by the examiner. Four categories were tested: vegetables, vehicles, tools, and clothing. One minute was allowed for each category, and the examiner wrote the patients' responses as they were produced. The test score is the sum of the correct responses given for all four categories. This task involves the lexical–semantic processing and word retrieval components of confrontation naming (Fig. 12.1), but does not involve visual processing.

Form discrimination task. The stimuli for this test were modified from LaBerge and Lawrence (1957), and consisted of sixteen 12-sided, irregular polygons that differed quantitatively from each other. On each of 24 trials, two polygons were presented in a vertical array. Subjects were asked to decide whether the two forms were "exactly the same or different." Half of the items required a "same" response, and half required a "different" response. The 12 "different" items included 4 at each of three levels of difficulty, based on the similarity between the paired polygons. The score reported here is the number correct out of 24 items. This task requires visual processing, but not lexical–semantic processing. Many objects can be identified by their silhouetted contours (Rosch, Mervis, Gray, Johnson, & Boyes-Braem, 1976), and performance on form discrimination was therefore assumed to require visual processing that is involved in confrontation naming.

Subjects. Seventeen patients with a clinical diagnosis of Alzheimer's disease were tested. These patients were diagnosed on the basis of a history of progressive dementia with insidious onset, and exclusion of other causes of dementia by physical examination and accessory studies. The patients ranged in age from 52 to 77 (mean 64.0), and in years of education from 10 to 20 (mean 13.9). The degree of dementia in each case was rated as "mild," "moderate," or "severe" on the basis of the patient's performance in activities of daily living. Twenty-eight healthy control subjects were tested. An effort was made to match these subjects with the patients on the basis of age (range, 53–84; mean, 66.6) and years of education (range, 7–19; mean, 14.3). The control group comprised 9 spouses and 1 sibling of patients, 7 World War II veterans with peripheral nerve injuries and 3 of their spouses, and 8 ambulatory nursing-home residents. None of the control subjects were clinically demented.

Results and discussion

Patients were grouped according to their performance on three tests, each probing for a cognitive deficit possibly causing anomia: (1) number correct on category

Table 12.2. *Summary of test performance: Mean scores (standard deviation)*

Tasks	Healthy control group ($n = 28$)	Alzheimer's disease groups		
		Word-retrieval deficit ($n = 5$)	Word-retrieval and semantic deficits ($n = 6$)	Word-retrieval, semantic, and visual deficits ($n = 4$)
Category fluency	52.6 (9.6)^c	28.8 (4.1)^d	15.0 (11.5)^e	7.0 (6.6)^e
Correct responses on multiple-choice naming^a	41.2 (0.9)^c	40.8 (1.1)^c	31.3 (11.6)^d	22.0 (8.9)^e
Semantic errors on multiple-choice naming^a	0.5 (0.6)^c	0.6 (0.6)^c	6.6 (6.0)^d	10.4 (2.7)^d
Visual form discrimination^b	21.9 (1.6)^c	21.0 (1.6)^c	21.5 (1.4)^c	16.2 (1.5)^d
Boston Naming Test^a	34.8 (4.6)^c	30.2 (8.0)^c	17.0 (13.6)^d	7.8 (4.8)^d

^{a}Maximum possible score = 42.
^{b}Maximum possible score = 24.
^{c,d,e}For each test, group means indexed by different letters are significantly different by Duncan's Multiple Range Test, alpha level = .05.

fluency, a measure of word retrieval; (2) number correct and number of semantic errors on multiple-choice naming, a measure of lexical–semantic processing; and (3) number correct on form discrimination, a measure of visual processing. Patients whose performance fell outside the range of normal subjects on one of these tests were grouped together; those abnormal on a specific pair of tests, and those abnormal on all three tests were also grouped together. Of the possible 7 patient groups based on this procedure, only 3 groups were actually represented among the patients. In addition, two patients performed normally on all the tests. The 3 groups are indicated in Table 12.2, which also indicates mean test scores for each group. Duncan's Multiple Range Test was performed across groups for each test, in order to determine which groups differed significantly with respect to each test variable.

Patients whose only deficit was on the category fluency task performed normally on the multiple-choice naming task. The mean BNT score for this group was not significantly lower than that for the healthy control group, although one patient had a BNT score that was three standard deviations below the control group mean. If the category fluency task is accepted as a valid measure of word-retrieval processes involved in confrontation naming (Fig. 12.1), this result indicates that a word-retrieval deficit alone rarely results in confrontation anomia in Alzheimer's disease.

Category fluency is in fact probably more sensitive to word-retrieval deficits than is confrontation naming, because in the latter task each name is prompted by a pictured object, whereas category fluency requires retrieval and production of multiple object names in response to each category name. In addition to requiring word retrieval, category fluency performance involves other cognitive processes attrib-

Table 12.3. *Analysis of error types on Boston Naming Test*

Response type	Percentage of total errors ($n = 393$) in patients with Alzheimer's disease ($n = 17$)
Errors	
Omission	55
Semantic	30
Superordinate	9
Coordinate	19
Subordinate	2
Visual	8
Visual or semantic	6
Phonemic	1
Correct descriptive comment	19

uted to frontal lobe function, such as the ability to suppress dominant responses in order to produce additional responses on a task (Perret, 1974). Benson (1979) suggested that a verbal fluency deficit occurs earlier in the course of dementia than does confrontation anomia. Consistent with this suggestion, several recent studies have indicated that fluency tests are useful in early diagnosis of Alzheimer's disease (Eslinger, Damasio, Benton, & Van Allen, 1985; Storandt, Botwinick, Danziger, Berg, & Hughes, 1984). Impaired category fluency corresponds to anomia in the broad sense that includes occurrence of word-finding pauses in free speech, as well as difficulty naming objects (Table 12.1).

Although patients with only a word-retrieval deficit detected by the category fluency task did not generally have confrontation anomia, patients with a lexical–semantic deficit, defined by the number of semantic errors on the multiple-choice naming task, all had abnormal performance on the BNT. This was true in 6 patients with normal visual processing, measured by the form discrimination task, as well as in 4 patients with impaired visual processing (Table 12.2). A lexical–semantic deficit thus appears to be sufficient to produce confrontation anomia, whereas a visual processing deficit is not. This result supports the conclusion of Bayles and Tomoeda (1983) and Martin and Fedio (1983), and contradicts that of Lawson and Barker (1968) and Rochford (1971), who argued that a visual impairment is the cause of confrontation anomia.

All 4 patients with visual processing deficits were moderately demented, whereas the group with word-retrieval and semantic deficits but normal visual processing consisted of 3 mild and 3 moderate cases. This pattern suggests that visual impairment may become a more prominent cause of anomia as dementia progresses, and is consistent with the results of Kirshner et al. (1984). There were no differences in age between the patient and control groups, or among the different patient groups. Age differences thus cannot account for the pattern of deficits observed.

An analysis of error types on the BNT (Table 12.3) indicated that the majority of errors (55% of the total) were omissions, in which no naming response was produced. Semantic errors were more common (30%) than both visual errors (8%) and instances that were ambiguous between semantic and visual errors (6%), although many errors classified as "semantic" could arguably have been assigned to the "ambiguous" category. Among the semantic errors, the most common types were substitution of a coordinate member of the same category (e.g., *brush* for a picture of a comb) or substitution of the category name (e.g., *an animal* for a picture of a rhinoceros). Substitution of the name for a subordinate part of the picture (e.g., *paints* for a picture of a palette) occurred infrequently. These results suggest that the semantic deficit in Alzheimer's disease involves an impairment in the ability to distinguish among objects that belong to the same semantic category, perhaps because the specific information required to make such distinctions is lost or inaccessible.

In 19% of incorrect naming trials on the BNT (Table 12.3), the patient spontaneously supplied correct descriptive information about the object (e.g., "a thing you look out of" for a telescope, or "you pour liquid through that" for a funnel). This phenomenon corresponds to the circumlocutory discourse that has been noted early in the course of Alzheimer's disease (Table 12.1), which probably represents an adaptation to anomia.

Phonemic errors comprised only 1% of total errors on the BNT, indicating the rarity of such errors in Alzheimer's disease. Similarly, on the multiple-choice naming task, patients selected the phonemic distractor on only 17% of incorrect trials, which is lower than the chance rate, whereas they selected the semantic distractor on 56% of incorrect trials. Patients with mild to moderate dementia due to Alzheimer's disease thus appear to retain normal phonological processing of words despite having impairments in word retrieval and lexical–semantic processing.

General discussion

The study just described was based upon the assumption that lexical–semantic processing and word retrieval are distinct cognitive processes. This distinction was supported by the observation that some patients had impaired word retrieval, defined by impaired category fluency, but had normal lexical–semantic processing, defined by multiple-choice naming. Two patients in this group had been demented for more than 10 years, and their overall dementia was rated as "moderate," suggesting that a word-retrieval deficit may exist independently of the confusion among semantically related objects that characterizes "lexical–semantic" impairment in Alzheimer's disease.

On the other hand, it may be argued that a word-retrieval deficit represents merely a mild form of a lexical–semantic deficit. This view is suggested by the observation that no patient had a lexical–semantic deficit without a word-retrieval deficit. Category fluency performance was in fact significantly worse in patients with semantic deficits than in those with only a word-retrieval deficit (Table 12.2). In addition, the correlation between performance on category fluency and semantic errors on multiple-choice naming was substantial ($r = .77$), consistent with the suggestion that a common mechanism underlies deficits on both tests.

Another issue that is unresolved by the study just described is the nature of the lexical–semantic deficit in Alzheimer's disease. Whether this deficit is manifested in semantic errors on multiple-choice naming, or in word retrieval tasks as was just suggested, it remains to be determined whether the deficit results from a loss of semantic information or from difficulty accessing semantic information. The latter alternative implies that semantic information is preserved, but that access to it is impaired. Butterworth, Howard, and McLaughlin (1984) have reported evidence that the semantic impairment in patients with aphasia associated with focal brain lesions is due to intermittent failure of access to information. They studied the patterns of errors when naming was tested on two occasions with the same set of object drawings. Patients made errors on different items in the two test sessions, suggesting that the impairment was due to unreliable access to semantic information, rather than to loss of information, which would have resulted in consistent failure to name specific items in the two test sessions. Similar studies of error patterns on repeated testing in patients with Alzheimer's disease may clarify this aspect of their semantic impairment.

Because the brain pathology in Alzheimer's disease is widely distributed, it is reasonable to expect qualitative differences between the semantic impairments in patients with Alzheimer's disease and those with focal brain lesions. Studies that contrast features of the semantic impairments in these two types of brain disorder may yield insights into the mental representation of lexical–semantic processing. Because impaired lexical–semantic processing is strongly associated with anomia, such insights would be relevant to understanding this clinical symptom of Alzheimer's disease.

References

Appell, J., Kertesz, A., & Fisman, M. (1982). A study of language functioning in Alzheimer patients. *Brain and Language, 17*, 73–91.

Bayles, K. A., & Tomoeda, C. K. (1983). Confrontation naming impairment in dementia. *Brain and Language, 19*, 98–114.

Benson, D. F. (1979). Neurologic correlates of anomia. In H. Whitaker & H. A. Whitaker (Eds.), *Studies in neurolinguistics* (Vol. 4, pp. 293–328). New York: Academic Press.

Brun, A., & Englund, E. (1981). Regional pattern of degeneration in Alzheimer's disease: Neuronal loss and histopathological grading. *Histopathology, 5*, 549–564.

Butterworth, B., Howard, D., & McLaughlin, P. (1984). The semantic errors in auditory comprehension and picture naming. *Neuropsychologia, 22*, 409–426.

Crystal, H. A., Horoupian, D. S., Katzman, R., & Jotkowitz, S. (1982). Biopsy-proved Alzheimer disease presenting as a right parietal lobe syndrome. *Annals of Neurology, 12*, 186–188.

Cummings, J. L., & Benson, D. F. (1983). *Dementia: A clinical approach*. Boston: Butterworths.

Emery, O. B., & Emery, P. E. (1983). Language in senile dementia of the Alzheimer's type. *The Psychiatric Journal of the University of Ottawa, 8*, 169–178.

Eslinger, P. J., Damasio, A. R., Benton, A. L., & Van Allen, M. (1985). Neuropsychologic detection of abnormal mental decline in older persons. *Journal of the American Medical Association, 253*, 670–674.

Folstein, M. F., & Breitner, J. C. S. (1981). Language disorder predicts familial Alzheimer's disease. *Johns Hopkins Medical Journal, 149*, 145–147.

Goodman, L. (1953). Alzheimer's disease: Clinico-pathologic analysis of twenty-three cases with a theory on causation. *Journal of Nervous and Mental Health Diseases, 117*, 97–130.

Huff, F. J., Collins, C., Corkin, S., & Rosen, T. J. (1986). Equivalent forms of the Boston Naming Test. *Journal of Clinical and Experimental Neuropsychology*, *8*, 556–562.

Huff, F. J., & Corkin, S. (1984). Recent advances in the neuropsychology of Alzheimer's disease. *Progress in Neuropsychopharmacology and Biological Psychiatry*, *8*, 643–648.

Huff, F. J., Corkin, S., & Growdon, J. G. (1983). Anomia in Alzheimer's disease: Associated cognitive deficits. *Society for Neuroscience Abstracts*, *9*, 94.

Irigaray, L. (1973). *Le langage des déments*. The Hague: Mouton.

Kaplan, E., Goodglass, H., & Weintraub, S. (1978). *The Boston Naming Test* (experimental edition). Boston, MA.

Kirshner, H. S., Webb, W. G., & Kelly, M. P. (1984). The naming disorder of dementia. *Neuropsychologia*, *22*, 23–30.

Kirshner, H. S., Webb, W. G., Kelly, M. P., & Wells, C. E. (1984). Language disturbance: An initial symptom of cortical degeneration and dementia. *Archives of Neurology*, *41*, 491–496.

LaBerge, D. L., & Lawrence, D. H. (1957). Two methods for generating forms of graded similarity. *Journal of Psychology*, *43*, 77–100.

Lawson, J. S., & Barker, M. G. (1968). The assessment of nominal dysphasia in dementia: The use of reaction-time measures. *British Journal of Medical Psychology*, *41*, 411–414.

Martin, A., & Fedio, P. (1983). Word production and comprehension in Alzheimer's disease: The breakdown of semantic knowledge. *Brain and Language*, *19*, 124–141.

McKhann, G., Drachman, D., Folstein, M., Katzman, R., Price, D., & Stadlan, E. M. (1984). Clinical diagnosis of Alzheimer's disease: Report of the NINCDS–ADRDA work group under the auspices of Health and Human Services Task Force on Alzheimer's Disease. *Neurology*, *34*, 939–944.

Miller, E., & Hague, F. (1975). Some characteristics of verbal behavior in presenile dementia. *Psychological Medicine*, *5*, 255–259.

Nelson, H. E., & O'Connell, A. (1978). Dementia: The estimation of premorbid intelligence levels using the New Adult Reading Test. *Cortex*, *14*, 234–244.

Perret, E. (1974). The left frontal lobe of man and the suppression of habitual responses in verbal categorical behavior. *Neuropsychologia*, *12*, 323–330.

Reding, M. D., Haycox, J., & Blass, J. (1985). Depression in patients referred to a dementia clinic: A three-year prospective study. *Archives of Neurology*, *42*, 894–896.

Rochford, G. (1971). A study of naming errors in dysphasia and in demented patients. *Neuropsychologia*, *9*, 437–443.

Rosch, E., Mervis, C., Gray, W., Johnson, D., & Boyes-Braem, P. (1976). Basic objects in natural categories. *Cognitive Psychology*, *8*, 382–439.

Rosen, W. (1980). Verbal fluency in aging and dementia. *Journal of Clinical Neuropsychology*, *2*, 135–146.

Schwartz, M. F., Marin, O. S. M., & Saffran, E. M. (1979). Dissociations of language function in dementia: A case study. *Brain and Language*, *7*, 277–306.

Sjögren, H. (1952). Clinical analysis of morbus Alzheimer and morbus Pick. *Acta Psychiatrica et Neurologica Scandanavica* (Suppl. 82), 68–115.

Storandt, M., Botwinick, J., Danziger, W. L., Berg, L., & Hughes, C. P. (1984). Psychometric differentiation of mild senile dementia of the Alzheimer type. *Archives of Neurology*, *41*, 497–499.

Terry, R. D., & Katzman, R. (1983). Senile dementia of the Alzheimer type. *Annals of Neurology*, *14*, 497–506.

Warrington, E. K. (1975). The selective impairment of semantic memory. *Quarterly Journal of Experimental Psychology*, *27*, 635–657.

13   Language and memory processing in senile dementia Alzheimer's type

Olga B. Emery

Persons over 65 years of age have increased more than eight fold since 1900, from approximately 3.1 million persons to 26 million in 1980. This represents a rise from 4.1% to 11.3% of the total population (U.S. Department of Health and Human Services, 1984). The U.S. Bureau of Census (1980) projects that the number of persons over age 65 may reach 36.6 million by the year 2000, accounting for 13% of the total population. Further, the proportion of old people who will survive beyond the age of 75, the "old-old" age stratum, will account for 43.3% of the total aged population in the year 2000. In 1970 and 1940, the figures were 38.2% and 29.5%, respectively (Wang, 1977).

Senile dementia Alzheimer's type (SDAT) is a major pathology of old age (Emery, 1985; Pincus & Tucker, 1985; Shamoian, 1984). Estimates of the prevalence of dementia from population studies in Europe and the United States range from 3.9% to 22%; the mean estimate tends to be around 7% across age, rising to more than 22% in the age stratum of 80 years and older (Kay & Bergmann, 1980; Nielson, 1963; Pincus & Tucker, 1985; Primrose, 1962; Woods & Britton, 1985).

Given the increasing number of older people in our society, understanding the nature and causes of SDAT must rank high on research priorities. My goal in this chapter is to elucidate one aspect of SDAT, the deterioration of higher-order cortical processes which is at the center of the symptom complex that characterizes senile dementia Alzheimer's type (Emery, 1984, 1985). Thus, to understand the dementing process in SDAT, one must understand the process of dissolution of higher cortical functions. The research to be presented in this chapter probes the structure of dissolution of language and memory in elderly persons, aged 75 and over, with Alzheimer's dementia. The data to be presented are part of a larger ongoing research project investigating the deterioration of higher cortical functions, as well as possible distal causation, in normal elderly persons and in the elderly with Alzheimer's dementia; normal pre–middle-aged persons serve as the normative baseline.

The language deficit in senile dementia Alzheimer's type

In the original description of the dementing syndrome which subsequently was named after him, Alzheimer (1906) noted a language disorder along with impaired memory and personality changes. Most notably, Alzheimer described single paraphasic disturbances as part of this dementing illness (Alzheimer, 1906). Despite this

221

original emphasis on a language disorder as part of the symptomatology of Alzheimer's disease, most descriptions of the syndrome, until very recently, focused on global cognitive deficits and/or memory impairment, with no recognition of the language deficit which is an integral part of this disease process (Emery, 1985; Emery & Emery, 1983; for exceptions, see DeAjuriaguerra, Gainotti, & Tissot, 1969, and Schwartz, Marin, & Saffran, 1979).

This lack of awareness of the language dimension in the higher-order cortical deterioration of Alzheimer's disease is reflected in the fact that the first edition (1952) and second edition (1968) of the *Diagnostic and Statistical Manual of Mental Disorders (DSM)* of the American Psychiatric Association (APA) made no mention of abnormal language structure or function in characterizing senile dementia. More recently, however, the *DSM-III* (1980) does give a brief description of language deficits in SDAT. Unfortunately, the description is global and impressionistic. Language is described as being vague, stereotyped, and imprecise with long circumlocutory phrases. Further, *DSM-III* states that language might show specific signs of aphasia, such as difficulty in naming objects, and in defining words and concepts (p. 107). The *DSM-III-R* (1987) description of language impairment in primary degenerative dementia of the Alzheimer type (SDAT) is essentially the same as that found in the *DSM-III*.

It is understandable that the *DSM-III/DSM-III-R* descriptions of language disorder in Alzheimer's senile dementia are vague because there has been a paucity of systematic data on language disturbance in Alzheimer's (Yudofsky, 1984). Although there have been descriptions of language disorder in the context of the single case study, as well as important informal observations of language disturbance (Barker & Lawson, 1968; Critchley, 1933; Cummings, Benson, Hill, & Read, 1985; Ernst, Dalby, & Dalby, 1970; Stengel, 1964), studies using systematic linguistic analysis have been rare (Appell, Kertesz, & Fisman, 1982; Emery, 1982, 1985; Huff & Corkin, 1984; Irigaray, 1973; Kirshner & Freemon, 1982).

Most of the studies of the language disorder in Alzheimer's disease have been limited in focus to the level of lexical function. These studies are concerned with how the Alzheimer patient processes words. Included here are studies of *anomia* (i.e., problems in naming objects or pictures) in the Alzheimer syndrome (for extensive discussion of anomia in Alzheimer's disease, see Huff, this volume). Data from studies focused at the word level of analysis consistently show that Alzheimer's disease involves poverty of speech and/or restricted vocabulary, impaired word production and comprehension, altered patterns of word association, word finding difficulty, and the related confrontation naming disorder (Barker & Lawson, 1968; Bayles & Tomoeda, 1983; Cummings et al., 1985; Ernst et al., 1970; Gewirth, Shindler, & Hier, 1984; Martin & Fedio, 1983; Miller & Hague, 1975; Pearce & Miller, 1973). There is nevertheless a significant difference between the "anomia" manifested by patients with focal lesions and "the dilapidation of speech associated with diffuse organic changes in the hemispheres" in senile dementia (Critchley, 1964, p. 3; see also Joynt, 1984; Rochford, 1971; and Stengel, 1964). Thus, the term "anomic aphasia" is not descriptive of the language disorder found in Alzheimer's disease.

Although almost all research on language impairment in Alzheimer's disease has been limited to inquiry at the lexical level, there are a few studies that have also investigated syntactic and/or semantic levels. Appell et al. (1982) found that all language functions, not just the lexical, were impaired to some extent in SDAT. Further, when compared to age-matched normal controls, the greatest impairment did not occur at the lexical–morphological level. *Information,* a semantic processing task that extends to the level of the phrase/sentence, was relatively more impaired, when the SDAT group was compared to the normal group, than was *naming,* a lexical–morphological task. The information task used by Appell and colleagues was embedded in a broader test of spontaneous speech and was thus relatively unstructured. It consisted of the seven items *How are you today?, Have you been here before?, What is your name?, What is your address?, What is your occupation?, Tell me a little about why you are here?,* and *Describe this picture.* The naming task, which consisted of the four subtests Object Naming, Word Fluency, Sentence Completion, and Responsive Speech, was more extensive and structured than was the information task. Also, in a comparison of Alzheimer patients with stroke patients and a general aphasic sample, the Alzheimer group had the lowest number of persons classified as having anomic aphasia. In contrast, the Alzheimer patients were represented heavily in the receptive aphasic categories.

Similarly, Kirshner and Freemon (1982) emphasized wide-ranging language deficits in Alzheimer's disease which extend beyond the lexical–morphological level into syntax and semantic processing at the level of the phrase or sentence. Kirshner, Webb, Kelly, and Wells (1984) used the Boston Diagnostic Aphasia Examination (Goodglass & Kaplan, 1972) to analyze the deficits of six persons with Alzheimer's dementing illness. They found that repetition was relatively well preserved in all cases, but four persons showed generalized decrement in all other language functions, and two persons showed disproportionate decrement on semantic processing tasks at the level of the phrase or sentence, especially on the auditory comprehension task, whereas naming was accurate.

A primary goal of my research is to provide a systematic, comprehensive investigation of the structure of language deficits in SDAT. To understand the nature and meaning of the language disorder in SDAT (or any kind of dementia), it is important to supplement analysis of lexical function with analyses of word-internal morphology (such as inflection), syntax, and semantics; vocabulary studies need to be supplemented with investigation of how variables of sentence structure and meaning are dealt with. Otherwise, analysis occurs at too circumscribed a level, so that although certain details may be perceived, the broader pattern cannot be discerned. The research described in this chapter involves the investigation of language in comparison groups of elderly adults with SDAT, normal elderly adults, and normal pre–middle-aged adults who provided a normative baseline. The research was designed within the ordered hierarchical framework of the semiotic system (deSaussure, 1966; Emery, 1982, 1985; Newmeyer, 1980; Yngve, 1986), through which it is possible to compare phonological, lexical–morphological, word-internal morphological, syntactic, and semantic ranks.

The specific goals of the present research were (1) to analyze normative linguistic patterning at two age points in the adult segment of the life cycle, pre–middle-age and old age; (2) to determine if a shift in linguistic patterning occurs between pre–middle-age and old age, and to analyze the structure of the shift; (3) to analyze the structure and sequence of linguistic deficits in SDAT; (4) to determine if linguistic deterioration in normal aging is qualitatively as well as quantitatively distinct from SDAT; and (5) to examine the relation between linguistic patterning and measures of other cognitive processes such as memory.

Method

The research comparison groups consisted of 20 elderly adults with SDAT, 20 optimally healthy elderly adults, and 20 healthy pre–middle aged-adults. Each sample of 20 persons consisted of 10 men and 10 women. Age was controlled, with the elderly with SDAT and the normal elderly encompassing approximately the same age range (75–91 years, with the exception of one 71-year-old in the Alzheimer sample; and 75–93 years for the normal sample), and having roughly the same mean (80.25 years for the Alzheimer sample and 83.35 years for the normal sample). The normal pre–middle-aged adults were between the ages of 30 and 42, with a mean age of 36.4 years. All subjects were Caucasian and had graduated from high school; none had attended college. Variables of native birth, native language, native birth and language of parents, and occupation were controlled. Literate socialization and current reading habits also were controlled (Csikszentmihalyi & Emery, 1979; Emery & Csikszentmihalyi, 1981).

Subjects with SDAT were selected from a population having been first diagnosed at age 65 or more. Excluded from the SDAT sample were persons with multi-infarct history, history of stroke, high blood pressure, cardiovascular abnormality of any kind, left–right impairment, space-occupying tumors, and endocrine or metabolic disease. A source of confounding interaction in the selection of SDAT samples is institutionalization, which blurs the distinction between organic and functional disorders (Kahn & Miller, 1978); thus, subjects with SDAT were found who resided with relatives and/or with paid personnel in private homes.

Previous studies cited above describe their patient populations as having "senile dementia" without specifying which kind of senile dementia and without adequate exclusionary criteria to permit inference that the patient populations studied are, in fact, ones with senile dementia of the Alzheimer type; the patient populations are confounded heavily with both multi-infarct dementia and Pick's disease among others. Further, it is not even certain whether early-onset Alzheimer's disease and late-onset Alzheimer's disease represent a continuous disease entity, or whether they represent disparate disease processes. Thus, the fact that most of the studies analyzing language deficits in Alzheimer's disease lack a control for the variable of age of onset of disease is of potential significance in terms of validity of findings. Such problems, and there are many of them, lead to an ambiguity in knowledge.

In the elderly, depression can manifest itself as a full-blown organic disorder, a syndrome that has been termed "pseudodementia" (McAllister, 1983; Pincus & Tucker, 1985; Post, 1975) or most recently "Type I cognitive–affective disorder"

(Reifler, personal communication, 1986) or depression cognitive-type (Emery, in press). This psychopathology, although organic in appearance, is considered to be psychogenic in etiology (Clayton & Barrett, 1982; Grunhaus, Dilsaver, Greden, & Carroll, 1983). It was therefore essential to distinguish between persons having SDAT and those with pseudodementia. Differential diagnostic procedures included the Langner Depression Scale, Hamilton Depression Scale, Twenty-two Item Symptom List, Kahn–Kodish–Emery Interview for Psychosis, Kahn–Goldfarb Mental Status Questionnaire, and the Face–Hand Test (Emery, 1982, 1985; Kahn & Miller, 1978; Kahn, Goldfarb, Pollack, & Peck, 1960). Additionally, SDAT was ascertained through the criteria of Eisdorfer and Cohen (1980) with especial attention to evidence for gradual progressive mental deterioration. Thus, SDAT was determined operationally by negative scores on tests for affect, positive scores on tests of cognitive function, and the extended medical history and examination.

Severity of dementia was established through the Kahn–Goldfarb Mental Status Questionnaire and the Face–Hand Test. The Mental Status Questionnaire is used extensively in the evaluation of mental function in the elderly, and consists of 13 questions, 5 testing orientation for place and time, and 8 testing simple items of general information. No or mild brain dysfunction is indicated by 9–13 correct; moderate dysfunction, by 4–8 correct; and severe brain dysfunction, by 0–3 correct. The Face–Hand Test consists of 16 trials of tactile stimulation applied in various combinations to the cheeks and hands. The patient's task is to indicate which areas are stimulated. Although normal persons may make errors on the first few trials, only persons with organic brain dysfunction make persistent errors (Kahn, 1971; Kahn & Miller, 1978; Kahn, Zarit, Miller, & Niederehe, 1975; Kahn et al., 1960). Mild organic brain dysfunction is indicated by 9–13 correct; moderate dysfunction, by 4–8 correct; and severe organic brain dysfunction, by 0–3 correct.

Cognitive measures/Linguistic data

The linguistic measures represented different levels of the hierarchical semiotic system of ranks; thus they tested phonological, morphological, syntactic, and semantic aspects of language ranging from simple to more complex units of speech. All tasks were chosen to be of equal familiarity to all cohorts represented. To this end, I chose and/or developed tasks that incorporated traditional grammatical forms representing a point of common socialization for the represented cohorts; all subjects were drawn from populations educated prior to the permissive modernization trend in American education, after which traditional grammar was not always taught rigorously and systematically. Similarly, memory tasks were chosen which would be of equal familiarity for all subjects.

Token Test. The Token Test, designed by DeRenzi and Vignolo (1962) and later adapted by Spreen and Benton (1969), consists of 39 verbal instructions that are brief, simple, and of increasing linguistic complexity, in which the persons must process relationships between tokens of varying color, size, and shape. Increasing linguistic complexity is attained primarily through the use of prepositions, which are relatively complex forms and have the concomitant property of late acquisition in language development (Brown, 1973; Chomsky, 1979; Dale, 1976; Luria, 1973, 1980). The Token Test is divided into six sections which are weighted for difficulty, increasing directly with linguistic complexity, for a test total of 163 points. Sample items are *Show me a circle, Show me a blue circle,* and *Put the white circle in front of the blue square.*

For purposes of our research, we added to the Token Test the requirement that subjects first repeat the instruction after the examiner. In this way, we provided a phonological linguistic task as an addition to the test, as well as a control for memory. It is a consistent research finding that memory decrements occur in SDAT (Kahn et al., 1975; Kral, 1962; Wilson, Bacon, Fox, & Kaszniak, 1983). For this reason, controls for memory were incorporated in both the Token Test and the Test for Syntactic Complexity. The Token Test provided data at phonological, syntactic, and semantic levels of linguistic operations.

Test for Syntactic Complexity. The Test for Syntactic Complexity (TSC) is a 36-item instrument designed by Emery (1982, 1986). The test has a 36-point total (1 point per item) and consists of five sections. Four sections test comprehension of various syntactic relations that are complex and relatively late to develop, namely:

(1)   Prepositions of time sequence, for example: *Do you put on your stockings after your shoes? What season comes before spring and after autumn?*
(2)   Passive subject–object discrimination, for example: *The dog was bitten by the cat; which animal bit the other and which was bitten? The woman is seen by the man; who is seen and who did the seeing?*
(3)   Possessive relations of a reversible construction, for example: *What is the relationship of your mother's sister to you? Your sister's mother? Your uncle's daughter? Your daughter's uncle?*
(4)   Communication of narrative actions events that are concrete and/or alogical, versus communication of abstract and/or logical relations of the same number of words per sentence, for example: *John and Mary run to the hospital really fast* versus *John runs faster than George but slower than Hamilton.*

This syntactic section consists of four pairs of communications of equal word-length per sentence, thus controlling for memory as an intervening variable. Memory was controlled further by the requirement, in all sections of the test, that the subject first repeat each sentence after the interviewer, prior to answering the question. A fifth section tests for word-internal morphology, permitting comparison of subject performance at morphological and syntactic levels of the semiotic hierarchy.

Chomsky Test of Syntax. Chomsky described four grammatical forms that approach normative adult levels by the age of 10, but which are absent in the grammar of 5-year-olds (1979). This late acquisition is directly correlated with linguistic complexity. The Chomsky Test of Syntax (1979) consists of four subtests; each subtest is based on one of the four syntactic conditions under which maximal complexity occurs. These four conditions are as follows:

(1)   The true grammatical relations that hold among the words in a sentence are not expressed directly in its surface structure, for example: The subject is presented with a blindfolded doll and asked, "Is this doll easy to see or hard to see?"

(2) The syntactic structure associated with a particular word is at variance with a general pattern in the language, for example: The subject is presented with figures of Donald Duck and Mickey Mouse and instructed, "Mickey tells Donald to hop up and down; make him hop," or "Mickey promises Donald to stand on his head; make him do it."

(3) A conflict exists between two of the potential syntactic structures associated with the complement verb "to do," a violation of the minimal distance principle, for example: The subject is asked a series of questions ending in "Ask him what to do" or "Tell him what to do."

(4) Pronominalization/restriction on a grammatical operation applies under certain limited conditions only, for example: The subject is shown figures of Donald Duck and Mickey Mouse and is asked to point to the figure to which the pronoun in the sentence refers. Items include "Donald knew that he was tired; who was tired and who knew it?" "He found out that Mickey had won the race; who won the race and who found out?"

These Chomsky subtests were used in our research. The Chomsky Test of Syntax has a 100-point total. The questions are constructed so that the answer of the participant depends on the processing of the complex syntactic forms; no semantic cues are given outside the syntactic structures being tested. For more details of this test, as well as other tests, see Emery (1985).

Boston Diagnostic Aphasia Examination. The Boston Diagnostic Aphasia Examination (BDAE; Goodglass & Kaplan, 1972) provides phonological, lexical–morphological, and semantic data, but contains no specifically syntactic tests. The tests used to provide phonological data were Oral Agility and Repetition of Sounds and Words. A rote lexical–morphological test used in the research was Automatized Sequences. The lexical–morphological tests were Body-Part Identification, Word Discrimination/Auditory, Word Reading, Symbol and Word Discrimination, Phonetic Word Recognition, and Comprehension of Oral Spelling. Semantic processing at the level of the sentence/paragraph was tested through Paragraph Comprehension. The standardization populations for the BDAE did not include the Alzheimer population. For this reason, our data provide useful and little-known information regarding the relation between classically defined forms of aphasia and the language disturbance in senile dementia Alzheimer's type.

Cognitive measures/memory

Wechsler Memory Scale. Our research utilized six tests from the updated Wechsler Memory Scale (Wechsler, 1973; Wechsler & Stone, 1979). Test 1 is comprised of six simple questions of personal and current information, whereas Test 2 consists of five simple questions for immediate orientation. Test 3, labeled Mental Control, consists of the three tasks of saying the alphabet, counting backward from 20 to 1, and counting by threes. Test 4 (Logical Memory) is one of paragraph recall. Test 5 is the memory span for digits forward and backward. Test 6 is associate learning, with 10 paired associates, some easy and some difficult.

We dropped the standard time limits and administered the test in an unpaced manner because of the well-known psychomotor slowing with age (Botwinick, 1984;

Table 13.1. *Comparison of test means by sample*

Sample	Maximal score possible	Pre–middle-aged	Normal elderly combined	Normal elderly, younger half	Normal elderly, older half	Alzheimer elderly
Mean age		36.4	83.4	78.5	88.2	80.2
Face–Hand Test	16	16.0	16.0[c]	16.0	16.0	3.5
Mental Status Questionnaire	13	13.0	13.0[c]	13.0	13.0	2.9
Token Test[a]	163	159.9	129.8	142.4	117.3	26.4
Test for Syntactic Complexity	36	33.1	24.4	26.2	22.5	5.4
Chomsky Test of Syntax	100	90.4	58.0	68.5	47.4	13.2
Wechsler Memory Scale[b]	82	62.0	47.1	52.0	42.2	11.7

[a]Dichotomous scoring; no partial credits.
[b]No age corrections in scoring; no time limits imposed.
[c]Only normal elderly with perfect scores were accepted as part of the study.
Source: Emery (1985), p. 29.

Troll, 1985); we did not wish to have the variable of increased response time interact with the specific parameters of interest, thus confounding results. The results
reported for the Wechsler Memory Scale are based on raw scores without age corrections. The updated Wechsler Memory Scale incorporates an age correction based
upon the fact that older persons do less well than younger persons. Because it was
age differences, in and of themselves, that we were interested in, we did not make
the age corrections.

Results and discussion

This section is organized around the following points which are central to the research goals outlined in the introduction of this chapter.

(1) There is a significant drop in performance from pre–middle-age to old age on most
    tasks but proportionately even greater impairment in SDAT.
(2) Performance in SDAT is related to organic damage as indexed by the Face–Hand
    Test.
(3) Analysis of the pattern of deficits in SDAT shows a direct correlation between
    deficits and linguistic complexity across the semiotic hierarchy; that is, there is
    relatively more impairment in syntactic than phonological or morphological pro-
    cessing.
(4) There are qualitative as well as quantitative differences in the pattern of decrement
    in SDAT compared to normal aging.
(5) The pattern of deficits in SDAT is unlike that of any of the classically defined
    aphasias.

Comparisons of performance in pre–middle-age, normal old age, and SDAT

The results given in Table 13.1 show that there is a drop in performance from pre–
middle-age to old age on most tasks, but there is proportionately even greater impairment in SDAT. There were significant differences between the pre–middle-aged and

Table 13.2. *Distribution of raw scores on Face–Hand Test by elderly with Alzheimer's dementia*

Occupation	Age	Face–Hand Test	Mental Status Questionnaire	Token Test	Test for Syntactic Complexity	Chomsky Test of Syntax	Wechsler Memory Scale
Maximal score possible		16	13	163	36	100	82
Street department worker	71	10	8	78	18	40	26
Croquet factory worker	78	9	4	62	11	43	24
Truck driver	79	9	5	72	5	10	20
Stage agency clerk	76	7	5	30	9	31	19
Accountant	85	7	3	62	6	12	18
Foreman, saw mill	75	6	4	30	11	12	22
Physical therapist	80	6	6	49	5	11	17
Owner, notions store	84	6	4	27	14	22	20
Nurse	76	5	7	5	4	19	18
Housewife	91	4	5	32	4	9	10
Dry goods clerk	83	1	2	12	2	8	6
Paralegal	75	0	0	9	3	0	0
Housewife	75	0	1	35	8	10	12
Store manager	78	0	0	4	1	0	3
Teacher, 5th gr.	79	0	0	2	0	16	0
Banker	80	0	1	7	3	6	6
Gym teacher	80	0	0	5	3	0	6
Housewife	84	0	2	4	0	16	6
Housewife	86	0	0	3	0	0	0
Drummer, band	90	0	0	0	0	0	0

Source: Emery (1985), p. 37.

the normal elderly samples on the Token Test, the Test for Syntactic Complexity, the Chomsky Test of Syntax, and the Wechsler Memory Scale. However, as discussed below, there were no significant differences between the two groups on the BDAE. The differences between the Alzheimer elderly and the normal elderly were highly significant on all tests.

The normal elderly were subdivided into younger and older halves with mean ages of 78.5 and 88.2, respectively. Comparisons of the performance of these two groups on the four tests in Table 13.1 consistently showed significantly higher performance for the younger half than the older half. In each case the pre–middle-aged still had reliably better performance than the younger half. Thus the analyses of the pre–middle-aged and the normal elderly point to an inverse relation between linguistic performance and age. Further, our data corroborate the established inverse relation between age and memory function (Botwinick, 1984; Kral, 1962; Troll, 1985).

The relation between performance and organic brain damage in SDAT

As can be seen in Table 13.1 the deficit in SDAT is proportionately greater than the deficit of normal aging. There is a strong relation between organic brain damage in SDAT, as indexed by the Face–Hand Test, and performance on the cognitive measures administered (see Table 13.2). The Pearson correlations between number of correct answers on the Face–Hand Test and number of correct answers on the Token

Table 13.3. *Comparison of test means for SDAT subjects by Face–Hand Test severity category*

Severity category	Maximum possible	Mild (9–13 correct)	Moderate (4–8 correct)	Severe (0–3 correct)
Face–Hand Test	16	9.33	5.85	.10
Mental Status Questionnaire	13	5.66	4.88	.60
Token Test	163	70.66	33.57	8.10
Test for Syntactic Complexity	36	11.33	7.57	2.00
Chomsky Test of Syntax	100	31.00	16.57	5.60
Wechsler Memory Scale	82	23.33	17.71	3.95

Test, Test for Syntactic Complexity, Chomsky Test of Syntax, and Wechsler Memory Scale were all significant, with values of .87, .76, .73, and .93, respectively. Subjects were assigned to severity categories on the basis of performance on the Face–Hand Test (FHT) with "mild" having 9–13 correct; "moderate," 4–8 correct; and "severe," 0–3 correct. These groups were compared within each measure by t tests, and all comparisons reached statistical significance at either $p = .01$ or $.001$ levels (see Table 13.3).

The importance of the relationship between FHT severity categories and performance on the cognitive measures administered is evidenced throughout the data. Nine persons in the FHT impairment category of "severe" received a score of zero on the Face–Hand Test; these nine persons, together, received a total of only 69 points on the Token Test. This group total is in striking contrast to one subject in the "mild" category, a street department worker with a score of 10 on the Face–Hand Test, who received 78 points on the Token Test himself alone. In other words, one person with 10 correct responses on the Face–Hand Test received more points on the Token Test than nine subjects, with a score of zero on the Face–Hand Test, put together. This pattern held true across tests. Further, the Alzheimer elderly showed a large standard deviation on all tests. The standard deviations for the Token Test, Test for Syntactic Complexity, Chomsky Test of Syntax, and Wechsler Memory Scale were 25.72, 5.05, 12.67, and 8.92, respectively; it appears that a large amount of the variance can be accounted for by the variable of organic deficit.

The correlation between the Face–Hand Test and the Mental Status Questionnaire was .86. Further, the correlations between the Mental Status Questionnaire and all measures discussed above were significant. We choose to put primary emphasis on the Face–Hand Test as our measure of organic decrement because of the apparent conceptual independence of the contralateral tactile stimulation tasks of the Face–Hand Test from the cognitive measures given. In contrast, the Mental Status Questionnaire has some overlap with both form and content of cognitive measures administered. The strong convergence between the Face–Hand Test and Mental Status Questionnaire in establishing a significant positive relation between organic deficit and poor processing of linguistic and memory tasks is a sign of internal validity; there appears to be a true relation between organicity and performance on tasks administered.

Table 13.4. *Boston Diagnostic Aphasia Examination (BDAE) standardized mean subtest scores compared to mean subtest scores of sample of Alzheimer elderly*

	Maximum possible score	Mean subtest scores			
		Goodglass & Kaplan BDAE[a]	Normal pre– middle-aged	Normal elderly	Alzheimer subjects
Oral Agility/Repetition	14	8.1[b]	14.0	14.0	13.7
Repetition of Sounds and Words	10	7.5	10.0	10.0	8.8
Automatized Sequences	8	4.9	8.0	8.0	6.1
Body-Part Identification	20	14.0	20.0	18.5	15.5
Word Reading/Oral	30	19.0[b]	30.0	30.0	23.8
Phonetic Word Recognition	8	6.3	8.0	8.0	5.5
Word Discrimination/Auditory	72	55.0[b]	72.0	70.2	42.0
Symbol and Word Discrimination	10	8.5	10.0	10.0	4.6
Comprehension of Oral Spelling	8	3.5	8.0	7.3	4.3
Paragraph Comprehension	10	4.8	10.0	9.5	2.0

[a]Mean scores for aphasia standardization sample.
[b]BDAE incorporates speed/time as part of the score whereas our research does not. See text.
Source: Emery (1985), p. 45.

Pattern of deficits in senile dementia Alzheimer's type

At no level of the semiotic hierarchy was the performance of the SDAT group comparable to the normal elderly or the normal pre–middle-aged. Nevertheless, the performance of the SDAT group varied markedly on different tasks; there was considerable gradation in performance corresponding to the semiotic ranks. The data suggest there is an inverse relation between SDAT performance and complexity in tasks, and a direct relation between good performance and early acquisition of a linguistic form in the developmental sequence of language.

First, on the BDAE, the best performance of the SDAT group was at the most simple, least complex level of the semiotic hierarchy, the phonological level (see Table 13.4). The Alzheimer mean percentages of correct responses on phonological tasks, – that is, Oral Agility (98%) and Repetition of Sounds and Words (88%) – were significantly higher than the mean percentages of correct answers on mor-phological tasks – that is, Body-Part Identification (78%), Word Reading (79%), Phonetic Word Recognition (69%), Word Discrimination (58%), Symbol and Word Discrimination (46%), and Comprehension of Oral Spelling (54%). Further, the mean percentages of correct answers on these phonological tasks were significantly higher than the mean percentage for the semantic processing task at the level of the sentence/paragraph in the Paragraph Comprehension task (20%), as were the mean percentages of correct answers on the morphological tasks.

The Test for Syntactic Complexity, a test for repetition wherin the subject re-peated all 36 items, one at a time, without regard to meaning, preceded the task of syntactic processing. The mean of the Alzheimer group on the repetition task was 12.7, reliably higher than the syntactic processing mean of 5.35 (Table 13.1).

This significant difference between repetition without regard to meaning and the syntactic processing of items was found also on the Chomsky Test of Syntax, where the Alzheimer group mean for syntactic processing was 13.25 (Table 13.1) and the phonological mean was 31.84.

This gap between the capability of the Alzheimer elderly to repeat phrases and sentences and to process the same items syntactically is of interest also for our analysis of memory in SDAT. The task of repeating each item immediately after the interviewer was used as an indicator of immediate memory. Thus, the relatively superior ability of the SDAT group to repeat in contrast to process syntactically would imply that deterioration of complex syntactic processing is more severe than, and/or occurs prior to, deterioration of immediate memory. We make this statement even though the SDAT literature emphasizes memory decrement, and even though memory decrement is more visible upon usual clinical inspection than is decrement in complex syntactic tasks. We consider this finding on the relation between memory and syntactic processing to be important, although it will require additional research to ferret out the full meaning of this finding.

At the morphological level, which represents greater linguistic complexity than does the phonological level, the Alzheimer elderly did worse than at the phonological level; however, performance was better at the morphological level than it was at the syntactic level. There are eight items of word-internal morphology on the Test for Syntactic Complexity; items include *The woman cries every night, she did the same last night; last night the woman_____?, John swims every Sunday, next Sunday John_____?*. The Test for Syntactic Complexity has a 36-point total. Across the 20 subjects this represents a maximum of 720 points. Out of this possible maximum of 720 points, the Alzheimer elderly garnered 107 points. These 107 points were distributed across the five sections of the TSC as follows: Prepositions of Time Sequence (28 points), Passive Subject–Object Discrimination (4 points), Possessive Relations of Reversible Construction (8 points), Communication of Relations versus Communication of Events (14 points), Word-Internal Morphology (53 points); the maximal number of points possible for the 20 subjects per section were 120, 120, 160, 160, 160, respectively. By far the best performance of the Alzheimer elderly was on the word-internal morphological items, and this was statistically greater than performance on all syntactic sections.

At the syntactic rank of the hierarchy, the research shows unequivocally that elderly with Alzheimer's disease are incapable of processing syntactic complexities. The Alzheimer elderly answered incorrectly most items of syntax, receiving very few points on syntactic processing tasks. On the passive subject–object discrimination tasks of the TSC, the Alzheimer elderly were totally unable to make correct passive subject–object discriminations, consistently imposing an active-voice interpretation on passive-voice constructions. Not one single person had more than one correct response in processing passive-voice constructions; 4 subjects had one correct response, and 16 subjects had no correct responses. Even the highest scorers on the Face–Hand Test were unable to process this syntactic complexity of constructions in the passive voice. This inability was demonstrated again on the Chomsky "Easy To See Test," in which a blindfolded doll was presented to the subject with the question "Is this doll easy to see or hard to see?" Only 4 persons in the SDAT sample made the correct discrimination; 5 failed to give any relevant answer; and 11 stated that the doll was "hard to see" because *she* couldn't see with the bandana around her eyes, thus discriminating erroneously in terms of the subject and object of the verb *to see*. Interestingly, 6 normal elderly processed this syntactic complexity incorrectly, whereas no pre–middle-aged participant gave the "hard to see" response.

Further, the SDAT elderly were incapable of processing the communications of logical relations on the TSC, for example: "Mary is paler than Louise who is paler than Judy." Not one single SDAT subject processed correctly any question of communication of relations. In contrast, 14 correct responses were given to communications of concrete action events, for example: "John ran to the store and Mary ran to the store." In the TSC section requiring comprehension of reversible possessive relations, the inability of the Alzheimer elderly to process syntactically mediated logical relations was demonstrated again as there were only 8 correct answers out of a possible total of 160. Several Chomsky subtests showed yet another syntactically complex task which the Alzheimer elderly could not do, that of pronominal reference wherein the participant was called upon to make subtle syntactic distinctions revolving around the referents of pronouns (see Chomsky, 1979, or Emery, 1985). The syntactic data from both the Test for Syntactic Complexity and Chomsky Test of Syntax converge in the finding that there is an inverse relation between SDAT performance and syntactic complexity; the Alzheimer elderly are not able to process post–Stage II syntactic forms (Brown, 1973; Chomsky, 1979; Dale, 1976) which include the syntactic constructions that constitute the Chomsky Test of Syntax and the Emery Test for Syntactic Complexity. In contrast, there is a relative preservation of the simpler syntactic forms.

Shifting our attention now to the semantic rank of the semiotic hierarchy, semantic processing involves comprehension or analysis of meaning. Semantic processing may be analyzed either at the level of the word or at the level of larger units such as the phrase or sentence, and thereby overlaps the morphological and syntactic ranks, respectively; despite this overlap, however, semantics constitutes a separate rank because of its specified focus on meaning, whereas morphology and syntax involve many dimensions besides meaning (see Emery, 1985). Semantic processing at the level of larger units such as the phrase or sentence constitutes a more complex linguistic task than semantic processing at the level of the word (Brown, 1973). The data from the BDAE and the Token Test converge to show there is an inverse relation between SDAT performance and semantic complexity. As discussed earlier in this chapter, the Alzheimer elderly did consistently better on all the lexical–morphological tasks on the BDAE than they did on the semantic processing task at the larger unit of the paragraph on the paragraph comprehension task (Table 13.4); because this latter task constitutes a linguistic task more complex than that of comprehension at the level of the word (i.e., the lexical–morphological tasks), it can be concluded from the data of the BDAE that the Alzheimer elderly do better at the simpler semantic processing tasks than they do on the more complex semantic processing tasks. Similarly, the principle of cumulative complexity (Brown, 1973) underpins the Token Test. The Token Test consists of 39 instructions representing a continuum of complexity, in which the last 16 items are the most complex with the concomitant property of late acquisition in language development. The Alzheimer elderly did significantly worse on this last section, as compared with previous less complex sections. Of 320 possible correct responses (16 items × 20 SDAT patients) in this complex section, only 33 responses were correct, these responses being made exclusively by the subjects in the "mild" and a few in the "moderate" categories of the Face–Hand Test. No participant, irrespective of Face–Hand Test performance, showed consistent semantic integration in the last section of the Token Test. Further, the simpler, the more concrete (as opposed to abstract) the task, the better the SDAT performance. When a semantic task converges in being simple, concrete, as well as personal, SDAT performance is maximized; thus the SDAT patient does relatively well at body-part identification (Table 13.4) and similar tasks. Finally, there is a direct relation between SDAT performance and redundancy, the more redundancy the better the performance; when the SDAT subject is required to process meaning in the context of structured linguistic cues only, with no redundancy, performance is adversely affected.

To conclude, our data have shown that linguistic patterning in senile dementia Alzheimer's type is not random; rather, there is a definitive and predictable pattern. It appears there is an inverse relation between SDAT linguistic performance and complexity, both within and across the semiotic hierarchy, with the associated negative relation between performance and abstractness. The Alzheimer elderly showed their best performance on tasks requiring only simple repetition; this principle held true across all tests. SDAT patients no longer capable of processing ordinary linguistic complexities were still able to meet the requirements of simple repetitions.

A similar set of principles emerged from the findings on the Wechsler Memory Scale. The two tasks that the Alzheimer elderly were able to perform consistently were repetition of digits forward and the automatized alphabet sequence, although their performance was qualitatively and quantitatively inferior to the normal elderly. On the repetition of digits forward, 15 subjects were able to perform to some degree, with one person attaining a two digit span forward, 3 persons with five digits, 4 with six digits, and 1 person with a span forward of seven digits. On the digit span backward, which requires more active thought processing, as well as a greater concentration and integration of thought than does the task of simple repetition which is required in the span forward, 10 subjects gave a response, with 8 persons doing a two digit span backward, and 2 people able to reverse three digits. No SDAT patient was able to exceed three digits in this more complex task. Analysis of data from the automatized alphabet sequence shows that 7 people were able to say the alphabet from beginning to end, 3 got half-way through the sequence, 1 gave five letters in sequence, and 3 SDAT patients were able to say "A, B, C." Automatized sequences and/or rote tasks require a less active and less integrated use of thought in the verbal production of mental representations than do less rehearsed sequences. In sum, the data indicate an inverse relation between SDAT performance and the integrative requirements of memory tasks.

Analysis of differences in decrement profile between SDAT and normal aging

In addition to the highly significant quantitative differences in performance of SDAT and normal elderly on all cognitive tasks discussed above, there were also qualitative differences between the two groups. The most extreme contrast was at the semantic rank of the semiotic hierarchy. Unlike the normal elderly who all showed equivalence in code (denotation) and commonality in context (connotation) (Jakobson, 1964), only six of the SDAT sample showed both consistent equivalence in denotation and commonality in connotation; these six subjects were in the "mild" and "moderate" severity categories of the Face–Hand Test. Equivalence of code or denotation occurs when both speaker and listener know and understand the lexical units being used, their grammatical forms, and the syntactic rules of their combination. Thus, to demonstrate equivalence in code on the Token Test item, "Show me a blue circle," the SDAT patient must share with the interviewer understanding of the words *show, me, a, blue, circle;* further, the SDAT patient must share with the interviewer knowledge of conjugation of the verb *to show,* declension of the pronoun *I,* and meaning derived from the syntactic variable of word order. However, meaning emanating from a common code is not enough, there must be a commonality in context between the encoder and the decoder. Thus, when asked to respond to the above item, the SDAT patient must understand that the context is one of a test with structured questions for which there is an expectation of an answer. An example of a response given by an SDAT subject who showed equivalence in code but not commonality in context is provided by a woman patient who pointed to the circles under her eyes when asked to "show a blue circle"; she was unable to share the test context with the interviewer and answered all questions with idiosyncratic personalized associations. Of our SDAT sample, three persons showed equivalence in code but consistently interjected highly personal meaning into the context, demonstrating an inability to share in normative connotation. Further examples include an 80-year-old former physical therapist, who clearly evidenced denotative knowledge, but showed deficit in the connotative dimension; when asked who was the president of the United States she replied, "It's a peach…and I like it, too." Similarly, an 85-year-old accountant who demonstrated knowledge of code, replied in answer to the same question of who was president, "Well, it isn't me…it's the one who was straight up." Of the three individuals showing consistent equivalence in code, but idiosyncratic use of context, two were in the "moderate" category, whereas one was in the "severe"; thus of the nine persons showing equivalence in code, eight were either mildly or moderately impaired organically.

Shifting our attention to the "severe" category, a 90-year-old man who was at one time a band drummer received a Face–Hand Test score of zero correct, as well as a score of zero on all other tests. This man was capable of neither equivalence in code nor commonality in context; his responses were syllabic sounds not related to questions asked. Much of the time he would say, "What, what, what…she blows, she blows, she blows." Although this individual was active in sound production, he could not use language in a consensually validated form; it was as though socialized patterns of communication had broken down. It was this kind of evidence that led us to think that the dementing process of Alzheimer's disease is also a process of desocialization because it strips the person of the capability of interacting according to socially prescribed patterns. The inability of 11 members of the Alzheimer sample to use code and context in a normative manner represents a qualitative difference between the SDAT and normal elderly samples in decrement profile.

How can one begin to understand this qualitative difference between the two populations? First, the data show that there is a direct relation between normative denotation/connotation and organic integrity as indexed by the Face–Hand Test. Concomitantly, there is an inverse relation between organic integrity and personalized, inconstant use of language. As Alzheimer's dementing degeneration progresses, the patient's capability for common code and context deteriorates, but before reaching a mute end state the use of language becomes personal, idiosyncratic, and lacking in constancy.

In looking for other differences in decrement profile between the SDAT group and the normal elderly, one is struck by the differential mediation of the age variable in the two samples. In the normal elderly, there is a consistent, highly significant negative relation between age and test score. The Pearson correlations between age in the combined normal samples (pre–middle-aged and elderly) and Token Test, Test for Syntactic Complexity, Chomsky Test of Syntax, and Wechsler Memory Scale were $-.73$, $-.79$, $-.86$, and $-.71$, respectively. When one excludes the pre–middle-aged sample from the analysis, the Pearson correlations between age and test score for the 20 normal elderly are $-.48$, $-.70$, $-.61$, and $-.43$ for the Token Test, Test for Syntactic Complexity, Chomsky Test of Syntax, and Wechsler Memory Scale, respectively; three of these correlations are still statistically significant, despite the severely restricted range represented by the normal elderly. For the elderly with SDAT, however, the Pearson correlations between age and test scores on the Token Test, Test for Syntactic Complexity, Chomsky Test of Syntax, and Wechsler Memory Scale are $-.28$, $-.49$, $-.41$, and $-.41$, respectively; only the correlation between age and Test for Syntactic Complexity ($-.49$) reached statistical significance ($p = .05$).

Thus for the SDAT sample, in addition to the factor of restricted range, it appears that although chronological age explains some of the variance in the higher cortical decline of SDAT, the predominant variable is that of the degenerative dementing process which has a critical impact on the biological aging of persons such that their chronological age ceases to be a valid and reliable indicator of their organismic and/or biological age. Although the SDAT pattern basically parallels the pattern of decline of the normal aged, it appears to represent an accelerated version of the normal aging pattern. Thus, the description of primary degenerative dementia as an accelerated aging of the brain (APA, 1980) is evidenced in our data. The dementing process in Alzheimer's disease appears to effect a separation between biological age and chronological age through accelerated aging of the brain, thus rendering chronological age a less valid indicator of the biological age of the individual. Using the method of extrapolation, it would seem that the normal aging process would have to continue beyond the time frame of normative species longevity to reach the modal

Table 13.5. *Alzheimer elderly aphasic Z-score profile compared to Z-score profiles of major known aphasia types*

		Aphasia type					
BDAE subtest	SDAT	Broca's	Wernicke's	Anomic	Conduction	Trans- cortical sensory	Trans- cortical motor
Oral Agility/Repetition	+1.00	− .50	omitted	+1.00	0	omitted	+1.00
Repetition of Sounds and Words	+ .50	0	−2.25	+ .75	+ .25	+ .50	+1.00
Automatized Sequences	+ .50	− .25	−1.75	+ .50	+ .75	+ .50	− .25
Body-Part Identification	+ .25	0	−2.25	+ .25	+1.25	−1.00	0
Word Reading/Oral	+ .25	+ .25	−1.75	−1.75	+ .25	−1.75	+ .25
Phonetic Word Recognition	− .50	+ .50	−2.75	−1.50	+ .75	−2.25	+ .50
Word Discrimination/Auditory	− .75	+ .50	−2.50	− .25	+1.00	−1.75	+ .50
Symbol and Word Discrimination	−1.75	+ .50	−2.50	−1.00	+ .50	−2.25	+ .50
Comprehension of Oral Spelling	+ .25	− .25	−1.25	−1.50	+1.25	−1.25	− .25
Paragraph Comprehension	−1.00	+1.00	−1.50	−1.25	+1.25	−1.50	+1.00

Source: Based on Z-score profile data of Goodglass and Kaplan (1972).

decrement point found in SDAT. One can argue that quantitative differences that extend beyond what is possible, normatively speaking, become qualitative. In any event, the mediating variable of primary degenerative dementing intervenes between age and cognitive function to create both quantitative and qualitative differences between the decrement profiles of normal aging and SDAT.

The aphasic profile of senile dementia Alzheimer's type

There are many systems for the classification of aphasia, indicating lack of consensus as to the form, content, and boundaries of the problem. Currently, there are eight patterns of aphasia that are well recognized: Broca's, Wernicke's, anomic, conduction, transcortical, global, semantic, and modality-specific aphasias (Kertesz, 1979). These classes of aphasia were derived on the basis of sampling from populations of brain-injured accident, war, stroke, and tumor victims; elderly persons with Alzheimer's disease have not been part of the populations used in developing aphasia typology. For this reason, it should not be surprising that we found a lack of goodness-of-fit between the structure of language deficit in SDAT and the classical aphasic types. Goodglass and Kaplan (1972) developed a subtest mean aphasia profile, as well as the related Z-score profile of aphasic performance on subtests of the BDAE. The standardization sample consisted of 207 aphasia patients who were hospitalized for focal lesions; aphasia type and severity level of aphasia were controlled, and a generalized set of aphasia subtest means (Table 13.4) were developed which cut across both aphasia type and severity level. Using these generalized aphasic subtest means as the reference point, Goodglass and Kaplan delineated Z-score profiles descriptive of five classical aphasia types (Table 13.5) by analyzing differing subtest scoring clusters correlated with type (see also Kertesz, 1979, for profiles of these five aphasia types). We can look now at the Z-score profiles of our SDAT sample and compare them with these five aphasia types (Table 13.5).

Broca's aphasia (Broca, 1861) has been referred to, in modern nomenclature, as expressive or motor aphasia and represents an agrammatism characterized by comparative preservation of nouns compared to syntactic forms. Short nouns are more likely to remain intact than any of the other linguistic forms, including verbs. Although several of the SDAT patients showed a relative preservation of nouns in combination with agrammatic communication, the overall Z-score profile of SDAT does not fit the Z-score profile of Broca's aphasia (Table 13.5). Broca's aphasia involves poor to mean repetition, poor automatized sequences, mean body-part iden-tification, good auditory word discrimination, poor comprehension of oral spelling, good oral word reading, and good to very good paragraph comprehension (the des-ignates of "good," "poor," "very good," "very poor" are based on whether the Z-score is above or below the mean and the degree to which it is so; i.e., "good" and "poor" are within one standard deviation of the mean, whereas "very good" and "very poor" are more than one standard deviation from the mean). In contrast to Broca's Z-score profile, the SDAT Z-score clusters showed good to very good repetition, good automatized sequences, above mean body-part identification, poor auditory word discrimination, above mean comprehension of oral spelling, good oral word reading, poor phonetic word recognition, very poor symbol word dis-crimination, and poor to very poor paragraph comprehension. In sum, it would be inaccurate to state that the linguistic deficits in SDAT correspond to Broca's aphasia.

Wernicke's aphasia involves impaired auditory comprehension (even evident at the one-word level) and fluently articulated but paraphasic speech. In extreme cases, auditory comprehension might be totally absent, whereas paraphasia is so pervasive as to produce meaningless jargon. Goodglass and Kaplan (1972) pointed out that in Wernicke's there is usually a free use of complex verb tense, embedded subordinate clauses, and other complex grammatical forms. The major features of Wernicke's do not correspond sufficiently with major features in SDAT. Careful analysis shows a lack of goodness-of-fit between the two patterns. The preserved capacity of the SDAT patient for repetition is in fundamental contradiction to the key defining feature of Wernicke's: that of impaired auditory comprehension evident even at the one-word level. This point is borne out in the data on Table 13.5. Although Goodglass and Kaplan omitted a Wernicke value for oral agility/repetition, the Wernicke Z-score of −2.25 for repetition of sounds and words clearly indicates the Wernicke patients' difficulty with repetition, whereas the SDAT subjects' Z-score for oral agility/repetition is +1.00 and the Z-score for repetition of sounds and words is +.50. Other Z-score differences indicate that the two patterns are dissimilar.

Turning now to anomic aphasia, one finds a "prominence of word-finding dif-ficulty in the context of fluent, grammatically well-formed speech" (Goodglass & Kaplan, 1972, p. 61). Although superficial appraisal would appear to indicate us-age of grammatical forms that are complex, more careful analysis shows that in SDAT grammatical forms are severely misused, and that the SDAT sample cannot be regarded as having grammatically well-informed speech. Our results show that

SDAT involves great syntactic difficulties with a regression in syntactic usage from complex to simplest forms when criteria of correct usage are applied. Further, to label the SDAT population as "fluent" is inaccurate; our SDAT group had variable fluency, with fluent persons tending to use words in an arbitrary way, with words lacking in normative denotation and connotation. The data in Table 13.5 show that although there is some overlap between anomia and SDAT in direction of deficits on some measures, degree and direction of deficits on other measures differ; the two patterns are not coterminous. The data indicate that it is not correct to describe the language deficit of SDAT with the term "anomia," although anomic components may exist in the broader pattern of deficits of SDAT.

It was possible to eliminate conduction aphasia quickly, because the defining feature of comprehension which is disproportionately superior to repetition is not descriptive of the SDAT profile; indeed, there is an opposite effect in SDAT wherein repetition is disproportionately superior to comprehension. In transcortical aphasia or echolalic aphasia, the clinical picture is the opposite of conduction aphasia: Repetition is preserved out of proportion to other language functions. This category was subdivided by Wernicke into transcortical motor aphasia, which is characterized by poor fluency, good repetition, and good comprehension, and transcortical sensory aphasia, which is characterized by very good fluency, good repetition, and poor comprehension. These categories are coextensive with Broca's and Wernicke's aphasias with the difference of good repetition. We have indicated above that the Z-score profile of SDAT differs from Broca's and Wernicke's aphasias. Further, the quality of repetition in SDAT is poorer than in the transcortical aphasias. The SDAT subjects were competent in and even enthusiastic about, repetition of sounds and words and did significantly better on the repetition of complex, lengthy sentences than they did on the syntactic and/or semantic processing of those same sentences. Nonetheless, the repetition of the SDAT group is inferior to the repetition of transcortical aphasic subjects in terms of length and complexity of repetition. And indeed, why should one expect the diffuse organic deterioration of SDAT to result in patterns of decrement identical to those produced by focal lesions?

We also considered three aphasic profiles described by Kertesz (1979) but not standardized on the BDAT by Goodglass and Kaplan (1972), namely, single-modality aphasia, semantic aphasia, and global aphasia. We could at once eliminate single-modality aphasia (pure aphasia) as being characteristic of our sample because the Alzheimer elderly showed decrement in several modalities. Semantic aphasia, described initially by Head (1926), refers to a disorder of impaired word-meaning relationships. More recently, Luria (1973) conceptualized semantic aphasia as a deficit of simultaneous synthesis in which comparative constructions, interrelated subordination of words, and propositional relations were impaired. Our findings do show that the word-meaning relation is impaired in SDAT. However, the term "semantic aphasia" is inadequate for the description of linguistic deficits of SDAT because it is too narrow and incomplete. Our data show that the structural deficits in SDAT involve the morphological and syntactic levels of the semiotic system, as well as the semantic level. Thus, the use of the term "semantic aphasia" for characterization of the pattern in SDAT is not sufficient. Finally, it is our view that global or total aphasia should not be included in aphasia typologies because it is on a different level of analysis than the other types; global aphasia is descriptive of a quantitative end state of deterioration rather than a specified sequence of deficits. Although such an end state is descriptive of the last stage of SDAT, the term nevertheless denotes a severity state rather than a deficit pattern.

To conclude, we have analyzed eight patterns of aphasia and have found that none of them describe accurately the structure of language decrement which is part of the diffuse organic deterioration of SDAT. In consequence, we shall provisionally outline an additional pattern of language disorder based on the configuration of deficits found in SDAT; this ninth pattern is termed *regressive aphasia*. The terminology underscores the finding that SDAT involves a process of regression, a reversion due to organic and not psychological causes, in which there is linguistic reversion to earlier, less advanced, less complex forms. SDAT involves a linguistic dedifferentiation such that the capacity for use of late-developing linguistic forms (post–Stage II forms; see Brown, 1973; Chomsky, 1979; Dale, 1976), which are more complex, relational, and abstract than earlier forms, is compromised. There is a regression from later to earlier and, relatedly, from more complex to simpler automatized language usage. The term "regressive aphasia" is descriptive of this process, although it awaits further validation.

Future directions

The research described in the foregoing discussion continues. In addition to our attempt to replicate the findings that we have reported in this chapter, we are comparing Alzheimer's disease late and early onsets, SDAT and pseudodementia (depression cognitive-type), a major depression and pseudodementia, and SDAT and multi-infarct dementia in demographically controlled, age-matched populations. To date, it appears that the patterns described in this chapter will be replicated. Further, it appears that Alzheimer's disease early and late onsets involve the same patterns of cognitive deficit, although the disease process in Alzheimer's early onset follows an accelerated course when compared to SDAT. Although it is too early to discriminate with any certainty definitive patterns of similarity and contrast, the trends emerging from the group with depression cognitive-type suggest that the pattern of decrement in pseudodementia is less constant and less stable than that found in SDAT. Finally, it appears that the regressive model of cognitive deficits outlined in this chapter which is characteristic of SDAT does not fit multi-infarct dementia; the latter appears to be better described with the oft-used term "patchy," whereby one finds patchy deterioration in both complex and early developing cognitive functions. The ongoing research underscores the idea that focal lesions do not produce patterns of decrement identical to those produced by diffuse organic degeneration such as is found in Alzheimer's disease.

Future research also includes trying to disentangle further the relations between language, memory, and thought. As discussed in this chapter, it appears that linguistic problems are among the first to appear in Alzheimer's disease, and that given an immediate memory recall task and a comprehension task using the same sentences, there is greater decrement in the comprehension task than there is in the immediate recall task. The meaning of this finding awaits further clarification in future research. These issues are difficult to disentangle because, just as the specialist in intelligence testing has difficulty creating a language-free test, it is difficult to devise tasks wherein language, memory, and thought are not confounded. Nevertheless, although we feel we have to a great extent controlled for these design problems in the present research, we need to focus on the more specific questions that have emerged from the research already done.

While researching the patterns of cognitive deficit in our comparison populations, we are ever mindful of the question of etiology, with especial interest in the distal causation of Alzheimer's disease. The question of etiology proves elusive. As we go over the medical histories of our subjects, we have begun to wonder if the model of diathesis/stress will not prove relevant for Alzheimer's syndrome. Diathesis is constituted by genetic vulnerability in the patient, and stress is constituted of environmental variables inclusive of viral invasion of tissue. In our Alzheimer subjects we have found a significantly higher incidence of herpes simplex, varicella zoster, cytomegalovirus, and meningeal infections than in control populations. Whether this higher incidence will continue to manifest itself as our research continues, it is too soon to say.

To conclude, we have discussed some of our findings and some of our future plans for research. The findings presented constitute a good foundation for the understanding and elucidation of the research goals outlined in this chapter. Future research will clarify and detail some of the models of cognitive decrement we have begun to develop.

References

Alzheimer, A. (1906). Uber eine artige Erkrankieng der Hirmrinde. *Psychgerichtlich Medicine, 64,* 146–148.

American Psychiatric Association. (1952). *Diagnostic and statistical manual of mental disorders* (1st ed.). Washington, DC: Author.

American Psychiatric Association. (1968). *Diagnostic and statistical manual of mental disorders* (2nd ed.). Washington, DC: Author.

American Psychiatric Association. (1980). *Diagnostic and statistical manual of mental disorders* (3rd ed.). Washington, DC: Author.

American Psychiatric Association. (1987). *Diagnostic and statistical manual of mental disorders* (3rd ed. rev.). Washington, DC: Author.

Appell, J., Kertesz, A., & Fisman, M. (1982). A study of language functioning in Alzheimer's patients. *Brain and Language, 17,* 73–91.

Barker, M., & Lawson, J. (1968). Nominal aphasia in dementia. *British Journal of Psychiatry, 114,* 1351–1356.

Bayles, K., & Tomoeda, C. (1983). Confrontation naming impairment in dementia. *Brain and Language, 19,* 98–114.

Botwinick, J. (1984). *Aging and behavior.* New York: Springer.

Broca, P. (1861). Remarques sur le siège de la faculté du langue articulé suivies d'une observation d'aphémie (perte de la parole). *Bulletine Société Anatomique, 36,* 330–357.

Brown, R. (1973). *A first language: The early stages.* Cambridge, MA: Harvard University Press.

Chomsky, C. (1979). *The acquisition of syntax in children from 5 to 10.* Cambridge, MA: MIT Press.

Clayton, P., & Barrett, J. (Eds.). (1982). *Treatment of depression: Old controversies and new approaches.* New York: Raven Press.

Critchley, M. (1933). Discussion of the mental and physical symptoms of the presenile dementias. *Procedural Report of Social Medicine, 26,* 1077–1084.

Critchley, M. (1964). The neurology of psychotic speech. *British Journal of Psychiatry, 110,* 353–364.

Csikszentmihalyi, M., & Emery, O. (1979). Life themes: A theoretical and empirical exploration of their origins and effects. *Journal of Humanistic Psychology, 19,* 45–63.

Cummings, J., Benson, D., Hill, M., & Read, S. (1985). Aphasia in dementia of the Alzheimer type. *Neurology, 35,* 394–397.

Dale, P. (1976). *Language development: Structure and function.* New York: Holt, Rinehart, and Winston.

DeAjuriaguerra, H., Gainotti, J., & Tissot, R. (1969). Le comportement des déments du grand âge face à l'échec on au risque d'échec. *Journal de Psychologie Normale et Pathologique, 3,* 329–346.

DeRenzi, E., & Vignolo, L. (1962). The token test: A sensitive test to detect receptive disturbances in aphasics. *Brain, 85,* 665–678.

deSaussure, F. (1966). *Course in general linguistics.* New York: McGraw-Hill.

Eisdorfer, C., & Cohen, D. (1980). Diagnostic criteria for primary neuronal degeneration of the Alzheimer type. *Journal of Family Practice, 11,* 141–145.

Emery, O. (1982). *Linguistic patterning in the second half of the life cycle.* Unpublished doctoral dissertation, The University of Chicago, Committee on Human Development.

Emery, O. (1984). The regressive aphasia of senile dementia Alzheimer's type. In *New advances in Alzheimer's and treatable dementias.* (Audio-Transcript P 28-100-848). Washington, DC: American Psychiatric Association.

Emery, O. (1985). Language and aging. *Experimental Aging Research Monographs, 11* (1).

Emery, O. (1986). Linguistic decrement in normal aging. *Language & Communication, 6,* 47–64.

Emery, O. (in press). *Pseudodementia* (Western Reserve Geriatric Education Center Interdisciplinary Monograph Series).

Emery, O., & Csikszentmihalyi, M. (1981). The socialization effects of cultural role models in ontogenetic development and upward mobility. *Child Psychiatry and Human Development, 12,* 3–18.

Emery, O., & Emery, P. (1983). Language in senile dementia of the Alzheimer type. *Psychiatric Journal of the University of Ottawa, 8,* 169–178.

Ernst, B., Dalby, M., & Dalby, A. (1970). Aphasic disturbances in presenile dementia. *Acta Neurologica Scandinavia, 43* (Suppl.), 99–100.

Gewirth, L., Shindler, A., & Hier, D. (1984). Altered patterns of word associations in dementia and aphasia. *Brain and Language, 21,* 307–317.

Goodglass, H., & Kaplan, E. (1972). *The assessment of aphasia and related disorders.* Philadelphia: Lea & Febiger.

Grunhaus, L., Dilsaver, S., Greden, J., & Carroll, B. (1983). Depressive pseudodementia: A suggested diagnostic profile. *Biological Psychiatry, 18,* 215–225.

Head, H. (1926). *Aphasia and kindred disorders of speech.* Cambridge: Cambridge University Press.

Huff, F., & Corkin, S. (1984). Recent advances in the neuropsychology of Alzheimer's disease. *Progress in Neuropsychopharmacology and Biological Psychiatry, 8,* 643–648.

Irigaray, L. (1973). *Le Langage des déments.* The Hague: Mouton.

Jakobson, R. (1964). Towards a linguistic typology of aphasic impairments. In A. V. S. DeReuck & M. O'Connor (Eds.), *Disorders of language* (pp. 21–42). Boston: Little, Brown.

Joynt, R. (1984). The language of dementia. *Advances in Neurology, 42,* 65–69.

Kahn, R. (1971). Psychological aspects of aging. In I. Rossman (Ed.), *Clinical geriatrics* (pp. 107–114). Philadelphia: Lippincott.

Kahn, R., Goldfarb, A., Pollack, M., & Peck, A. (1960). Brief objective measures for the determination of mental status in the aged. *American Journal of Psychiatry, 117,* 326–328.

Kahn, R., & Miller, N. (1978). Assessment of altered brain function in the aged. In M. Storandt, I. Siegler, & M. Elias (Eds.), *Clinical psychology of aging* (pp. 43–70). New York: Plenum.

Kahn, R., Zarit, S., Miller, N., & Niederehe, G. (1975). Memory complaint and impairment in the aged: The effect of depression and altered brain function. *Archives of General Psychiatry, 32,* 1569–1573.

Kay, D., & Bergmann, K. (1980). Epidemiology of mental disorders among the aged in the community. In J. Birren & R. Sloane (Eds.), *Handbook of mental health and ageing* (pp. 34–56). Englewood Cliffs, NJ: Prentice-Hall.

Kertesz, A. (1979). *Aphasia and associated disorders: Taxonomy, localization, and recovery.* New York: Grune and Stratton.

Kirshner, H., & Freemon, F. (1982). *The neurology of aphasia.* Lisse, Holland: Swets and Zeitlinger.

Kirshner, H., Webb, W., Kelly, M., & Wells, C. (1984). Language disturbance: An initial symptom of cortical degeneration and dementia. *Archives of Neurology, 41,* 491–496.

Kral, V. (1962). Senescent forgetfulness: Benign and malignant. *Journal of the Canadian Medical Association, 86,* 257–260.

Luria, A. (1973). *The working brain.* New York: Basic Books.

Luria, A. (1980). *Higher cortical functions in man.* New York: Basic Books.

Martin, A., & Fedio, P. (1983). Word production and comprehension in Alzheimer's disease: The breakdown of semantic knowledge. *Brain and Language, 19,* 124–141.

McAllister, T. (1983). Overview: Pseudodementia. *American Journal of Psychiatry, 140,* 528–533.

Miller, E., & Hague, F. (1975). Some statistical characteristics of speech in presenile dementia. *Psychological Medicine, 5,* 255–259.

Newmeyer, F. (1980). *Linguistic theory in America.* New York: Academic Press.

Nielson, J. (1963). Geronto-psychiatric period–prevalence investigation in a geographically delimited population. *Acta Psychiatrica Scandinavia, 38,* 307.

Pearce, J., & Miller, E. (1973). *Clinical aspects of dementia.* Baltimore: Williams & Wilkins.

Pincus, J., & Tucker, G. (1985). *Behavioral neurology.* New York: Oxford University Press.

Post, F. (1975). Dementia, depression, and pseudodementia. In D. Benson (Ed.), *Psychiatric aspects of neurologic disease.* New York: Grune & Stratton.

Primrose, E. (1962). *Psychological illness: A community study.* Springfield, IL: Thomas.

Rochford, G. (1971). A study of naming errors in dysphasic and in demented patients. *Neuropsychologia, 9,* 437–443.

Schwartz, M., Marin, O., & Saffran, E. (1979). Dissociations of language function in dementia: A case study. *Brain and Language, 7,* 277–306.

Shamoian, C. (1984). *Biology and treatment of dementia in the elderly.* Washington, DC: American Psychiatric Press.

Spreen, I., & Benton, A. (1969). *The Token Test.* Victoria, B.C.: University of Victoria.

Stengel, E. (1964). Psychopathology of dementia. *Procedural Record of Social Medicine, 33,* 911–914.

Troll, L. (1985). *Early and middle adulthood.* Monterey, CA: Brooks-Cole.

U.S. Department of Health and Human Services. (1984). *Report of the Secretary's task force on Alzheimer's disease.* Washington, DC: U.S. Government Printing Office.

Wang, H. (1977). Dementia in old age. In W. Smith & M. Kinsbourne (Eds.), *Aging and dementia* (pp. 1–24). New York: Spectrum.

Wechsler, D. (1973). *A standardized memory scale for clinical use.* New York: The Journal Press.

Weschsler, D., & Stone, C. (1979). *Wechsler Memory Scale.* New York: The Psychological Corporation.

Wilson, R., Bacon, L., Fox, J., & Kaszniak, A. (1983). Word frequency effect and recognition memory in dementia of the Alzheimer type. *Journal of Clinical Neuropsychology, 5,* 95–104.

Woods, R., & Britton, P. (1985). *Clinical psychology with the elderly.* Rockville, MD: Aspen Systems.

Yngve, V. (1986). *Linguistics as a science.* Bloomington, IN: Indiana University Press.

Yudofsky, S. (1984). *New advances in Alzheimer's and treatable dementias.* (Audio-Transcript P 28-100-848). Washington, DC: American Psychiatric Association.

14　Patterns of language and memory in old age

Leah L. Light and Deborah M. Burke

The research discussed in the present volume indicates that language and memory do not decline uniformly in old age but that there are some aspects of each which are impaired and some which are spared. In this chapter, we focus on different approaches to understanding the patterns of impaired and spared functioning in language and memory in old age. The search for patterns that describe categories of behavior that share properties is prominent in several approaches to the study of memory and language. In experimental psychology, there is a tradition of concern for dissociations among different aspects of cognition (see Klatzky, this volume). Within the study of memory, distinctions have been made among a variety of memory systems (e.g., Atkinson & Shiffrin, 1968; Baddeley, 1986; Tulving, 1972, 1983). More generally, cognitive processes have been categorized as effortful or automatic (Hasher & Zacks, 1979). Within the neuropsychological literature, there is an attempt to identify patterns of behaviors that are impaired in particular neuropathological conditions (Squire, 1987). In the study of individual differences, the factor-analytic approach is widely used to identify patterns of association among specific abilities (Thurstone, 1938).

In this chapter, we consider what the experimental, neuropsychological, and individual-difference approaches contribute to our understanding of language and memory in old age. Within the experimental approach, we focus on certain memory distinctions, and, in our final section, on distinctions between automatic and effortful processes. In our discussion, we point out the implications of research on aging for theory development in cognitive psychology. Our treatment is not meant to be exhaustive, but rather to take up themes that emerge from a reading of other chapters in this book.

Memory systems and distinctions

In the study of memory there is general agreement that memory is not a unitary system, but there is no consensus on the nature of its subsystems (e.g., Anderson, 1985; Mandler, 1985; Tulving, 1984, 1985). Here we evaluate certain proposals

The authors contributed equally to this chapter; order of authorship was decided by a predetermined rotational system. Preparation of the chapter was supported by National Institute on Aging Grant 2 R01 AG02452. The authors thank Richard Lewis and Tim Salthouse for helpful comments on an earlier version.

244

about the structure of memory by reviewing how well they describe patterns of age-related change in adulthood. This is a common approach in reviews of experimental findings on aging (e.g., Burke & Light, 1981; Craik, 1977; Hartley, Harker, & Walsh, 1980; Parkinson, 1982), but these reviews have been concerned primarily or exclusively with performance on memory tests. We cast a broader net here and consider studies of language ability as well. After all, our knowledge of language is represented in memory. Further, it is hard to separate these two domains in everyday cognition. This fact is recognized at a theoretical level where it is often difficult to differentiate between linguistic and memory components of models of comprehension, production, and retention (Anderson, 1983; Dell, 1986; Kintsch & van Dijk, 1978; MacKay, 1987).

It is clear from the chapters in this volume that aging research has become increasingly concerned with the relation between memory and language. We have selected for evaluation three memory distinctions that seem most prominent in aging research and most promising for describing the interaction of memory and language. These are semantic versus episodic memory, new versus old information, and explicit versus implicit memory. These distinctions do not come with well-specified models concerning the nature of memory representations and processes involved in acquiring new memories and retrieving old memories. Nor do they include developmental mechanisms to account for sparing of one type of memory and impairment of another. They are helpful, however, in organizing findings so that we can discern patterns of spared and impaired function in old age.

Semantic and episodic memory

In an important paper elaborating the distinction between semantic and episodic memory, Tulving (1972) proposed that there are two memory systems containing different kinds of information. Episodic information consists of personally experienced, temporally dated episodes, while semantic information consists of world knowledge, including language. The systems were originally described as functionally independent, but more recently Tulving (1984) proposed that episodic memory is embedded in and functionally dependent on semantic memory.

With respect to aging, there is a body of literature that suggests that the episodic/semantic distinction may prove useful in characterizing the pattern of spared and impaired functioning in language and memory. Older adults consistently show impairment relative to younger adults on traditional laboratory episodic memory tasks, while their performance on semantic tasks such as vocabulary tests does not consistently show a decline. For example, a common result, and one that we find regularly in our own research, is that older adults have vocabulary scores that are the same as or higher than younger adults, but they have lower scores on an experimental task involving episodic memory. Indeed, on the Wechsler Adult Intelligence Scale, the verbal subtests show little decline with age (Botwinick, 1984). Such findings have led to a view that language, unlike other aspects of cognition, is stable in adulthood (Riegel, 1973). This is consistent with preservation of the semantic system in Tulving's model.

Salthouse (this volume), however, points out that older adults do show age-related declines on some vocabulary tests. Further, he demonstrates that the direction and magnitude of age-related differences depend on the nature of the vocabulary test. The source of deficits does not appear to be in changes in the structure or content of semantic knowledge. Salthouse suggests that some semantic processes may be affected by aging while others may be unaffected. A case in point is that older adults typically produce fewer items in verbal fluency tests (McCrae, Arenberg, & Costa, 1987; Obler & Albert, 1985; Schaie & Parham, 1977) and have increased word finding difficulties in spontaneous speech (Burke & Harrold, this volume; Burke, Worthley, & Martin, in press). Borod, Goodglass, and Kaplan (1980) reported a decline in confrontation naming in old age. Although Borod et al.'s findings may reflect the lower education level of their older adults, Van Gorp, Satz, Kiersch, and Henry (1986) found a small negative correlation between performance on the Boston Naming Test and age for adults aged 59–80+ who had equivalent education, suggesting that confrontation naming is sensitive to age. Thus, the simplest case of preservation of a semantic system and age-related declines in an episodic system is not supported. Rather an understanding of aging effects seems to require a more fine-grained analysis in which specific processes in each system are identified and measured.

Activation is one of the most important processes in the semantic system and is postulated to account for retrieval of semantic knowledge (e.g., Anderson, 1983). There is considerable evidence from studies of semantic priming that activation is constant across age in adulthood in both its magnitude and its rate of spreading (e.g., Balota & Duchek, 1988; Burke & Harrold, this volume; Howard, this volume). Interestingly, parallel findings are reported in studies of episodic priming. Howard (this volume) demonstrated that episodically related words prime each other in an episodic recognition task and that the magnitude of the effect is age invariant (see also Rabinowitz, 1986). Consistent with this, Light and Albertson (this volume) report that semantic priming between related words (i.e., coreferential nouns) also primes episodic information associated with one of the words so that it is responded to more rapidly on an episodic recognition task. Again, magnitude of episodic priming is comparable across age but, nonetheless, older adults have poorer retention of the sentences involved in the study. The fact that both episodic and semantic priming are age invariant supports the view that they involve a common process. However, these results do not rule out an episodic/semantic model because they are compatible with Tulving's notion of an episodic system that shares processes with a semantic system.

An analysis of aging research reveals another more fundamental problem with the semantic/episodic distinction. This distinction is easy to illustrate by contrasting memory for personally experienced events (e.g., memory for a particular list of words) with memory for word meaning (e.g., vocabulary tests). However, studies described in this volume are concerned with the role of memory for particular experiences in language comprehension or production. In these studies the boundaries between semantic and episodic information are difficult to draw. For example, the interpretation of word meaning in a sentence is influenced by the prior semantic context (Burke & Harrold, this volume). The prior context is the particular semantic information that was personally experienced and it influences on-line semantic encoding. Is the prior context episodic or semantic information? Similarly, prior linguistic context influences interpretation of anaphora (Light & Albertson; Zelinski, this volume) and the making of pragmatic inferences (Zacks & Hasher, this volume). Comprehension in these cases requires access to information whose relevance in making the necessary inference is based on recency and/or semantic and pragmatic knowledge. Again, the information seems to be both episodic and semantic, and it is unclear how these can be teased apart.

Similarly, the role of prior context in speech production has long been recognized. Certain errors in speech production provide a window on language processes affected by context as with, for example, *spoonerisms,* where there is a transposition of phonemes in nearby words. Spoonerisms can be induced in the laboratory by having subjects read silently word pairs followed by a target pair which is spoken aloud. The word pairs are similar to the spoonerized version of the target. For example, when word pairs like *back mud, bad mouth,* and *bat much* precede the articulation of *mad bug,* the spoonerism *bad mug* is frequently produced. Spoonerisms have also been induced by manipulating either linguistic or environmental semantic context. For instance, in a condition where there is a threat of electric shock, *shad bock* may be spoonerized into *bad shock* (Motley, Baars, & Camden, 1983). Models of speech production as well as some models of comprehension concerned with effects of prior context do not differentiate between episodic and semantic information. Rather, both semantic knowledge and personally experienced information are represented in the same system, and their retrieval involves the same activation mechanism (e.g., Anderson, 1983; Dell, 1986; MacKay, 1987).

Memory for old and new information

Another way of describing patterns of age-related change in adulthood involves the distinction between tasks that require use of old versus new information. For example, this distinction overlaps with the classification of intellectual abilities into crystallized intelligence, which is stable in old age, and fluid intelligence, which shows age-related declines (Horn, 1976). Our analysis of the interaction of memory and language suggests that the new/old distinction may be more useful than the episodic/semantic distinction in describing aging effects.

First, there is very consistent evidence demonstrating that older adults are less able than young adults to remember recent experiences when tested by recall or recognition of verbal information (e.g., Burke & Light, 1981). This memory problem can impair comprehension if older adults cannot remember relevant prior context (e.g., Light & Albertson, this volume; Zacks & Hasher, this volume). As we pointed out, it is hard to classify prior context as episodic or semantic information, but it clearly involves retention of new information.

Second, some of the aging effects attributed to differential decline on semantic and episodic tasks may be attributable to differential memory for new and old information. That is, tests of language ability involve information that typically has been learned at some time in the remote past, while laboratory episodic tasks require new learning. If older adults' memory problems are primarily in learning new information, this would produce age deficits in episodic but not semantic tasks. An example of this is Charness's (1981) study of chess players. Both age and chess skill predicted ability to remember recently seen chess positions, but only skill was a predictor of ability to choose a good move.

Untangling the confound of new/old information and episodic/semantic information calls for a comparison of young and older adults' memory for new and old semantic and episodic information. A number of investigators have attempted to compare young and older adults' memory for recent and remote world knowledge such as historical events (e.g., Botwinick & Storandt, 1980; Perlmutter, Metzger, Miller, & Nezworski, 1980), and for recent and remote episodic experiences such as high school classmates (Bahrick, Bahrick, & Wittlinger, 1975), and students taught in college courses (Bahrick, 1984). These studies describe the methodological problems that plague this research and that are perhaps responsible for the inconsistent findings on age differences (see also Burke & Light, 1981; Salthouse, 1982). In a study that avoids one of these problems by controlling retention interval, Bahrick (1984) has presented evidence that age differences are small in remembering names and faces of former students but substantial in learning face–name pairings when these have been forgotten or never learned.

In sum, there is insufficient evidence to decide whether age-related memory declines are best described as an episodic memory problem that involves both new and old information or as a problem in acquiring new memories that involves both episodic and semantic information.

However, memory for old information is not always spared and memory for new information is not always impaired in old age. In particular, older adults sometimes have difficulty accessing old information, as in the case of word finding problems. They also do not appear to have difficulty in accessing relatively new information when asked to produce autobiographical memories in response to cue words (Holding, Noonan, Pfau, & Holding, 1986; Rubin, Wetzler, & Nebes, 1986).

Explicit and implicit memory

Also, with respect to new learning, older adults have little or no decrement when tested by some implicit measures that tap the effects of prior experience without conscious recollection. In contrast, they generally do show decrements when tested by explicit measures of recall and recognition that require conscious recollection (e.g., Burke & Light, 1981). For instance, Moscovitch (1982) found that repetition priming in a lexical decision task was the same in young and older adults although recognition memory was better for the young. In his lexical decision task, the same words were presented on two occasions, and response latency was less for the second occurrence of a word. This task does not explicitly ask the subject to remember the prior experience, but the reduction in latency demonstrates that there is memory for the prior experience. Similarly, Light and Singh (1987) found that identification of perceptually degraded words was improved to the same extent in young and old by a prior exposure, but the old had poorer recall and recognition for the same words. However, not all implicit memory measures show such clear evidence for preserved new learning in old age. We return to this issue in the section on neuropsychological approaches.

The implicit/explicit distinction has been applied only to the domain of memory. In this book we have been considering memory in relation to language and this has led us to the realization that the implicit/explicit classification may be useful for language tasks as well. That is, there are tasks that do not require conscious awareness of semantic or syntactic interpretations of language for correct performance. In the semantic domain, lexical decisions are faster when word targets are preceded by semantically related words. The equivalence of this semantic priming effect in young and old adults is evidence for preservation of the semantic relations among words (Burke & Harrold; Howard, this volume). Similarly there are preserved effects of category dominance on latency to decide if an instance is a category member (Mueller, Kausler, Faherty, & Oliveri, 1980; Nebes, Boller, & Holland, 1986). This pattern of response times suggests preserved semantic structure within categories. However, the word-finding problems discussed above involve deliberate production of particular words and thus constitute evidence for impairment on explicit language tasks.

Older adults also show preserved syntactic and semantic analyses of sentences when tested implicitly. For example, older adults show even more priming than young adults in perceiving target words preceded by meaningful sentences as compared to control conditions (Cohen & Faulkner, 1983; Nebes et al., 1986). Similarly, young and older adults show the same effects of the semantic and syntactic content of word strings on recall (Stine, Wingfield, & Poon, 1987; Wingfield, Poon, Lombardi, & Lowe, 1985). However older adults show impaired performance when asked to interpret explicitly the syntactic structure of sentences in the Chomsky Test of Syntax (Emery, this volume). Young and older adults also show similar effects of the implicit causality of verbs on the interpretation of pronouns in a sentence completion task. This task does not require overt identification of the antecedents of pronouns, an ability that, under certain conditions, shows an age-related decline (Light & Albertson, this volume). We believe that these parallels in the relation of aging to implicit and explicit functions in memory and language suggest that this classification may provide a valuable analytic tool. At this time, however, our analysis of explicit and implicit tests of language must be regarded as only suggestive because of the lack of comparability of materials used in the two types of tasks.

Summary

In this section, we have evaluated three ways of describing patterns of language and memory in old age. Advocates of the episodic/semantic distinction argue that these are two inherently different types of information. We have argued that this approach has a problem at the theoretical level in that it is often hard in practice to decide whether some particular information is episodic or semantic, especially when considering natural language understanding and production. The distinction between old and new information, in contrast, is not inherent in a particular type of information. Rather, the old/new distinction suggests a problem in acquiring information in old age, regardless of the nature of the information.

As we have seen, the findings on older adults' impairments in language and memory do not map neatly onto either set of distinctions. We believe that the explicit/implicit distinction holds promise for describing patterns of spared and impaired function in old age. At this time, there are relatively few studies taking this approach to understanding memory in later life and none that we know apply it to language in old age. We have suggested that this distinction in fact describes the pattern seen in a number of studies of language and aging. There is, moreover, considerable evidence that the explicit/implicit distinction is useful for characterizing the pattern of memory loss in amnesia. We return to this issue in the next section.

The neuropsychological approach

The issue of whether the pattern of changes in memory and language that occur with normal aging are similar to patterns seen in conditions associated with neuropathology was examined in two of the chapters in this volume, namely those by Huff and Emery. This neuropsychological approach (Albert & Kaplan, 1980; Goldstein & Shelly, 1975; Moscovitch, 1982) is appealing because the changes that occur in the aging brain are not uniform. Rather, some areas are more affected than others, and we would expect cognitive functions depending on these areas of the brain to be most affected by normal aging. Some of the brain areas subject to change in aging are thought to underlie language and memory (e.g., Scheibel & Scheibel, 1975; Squire, 1987), and hence the question arises as to whether age-related declines in language and memory resemble those observed in aphasia and amnesia (Albert, 1981; Moscovitch, 1982; Squire, 1987).

A related set of questions can be asked about the nature of the disorder of language and memory found in senile dementia of the Alzheimer type (SDAT). That is, do the cognitive changes associated with Alzheimer's disease reflect an exaggeration of normal aging or do they show a qualitatively different pattern? The possibility that SDAT and normal aging might show some similarity in the pattern of cognitive deficits is suggested by findings that brains of older adults show some neuropathological signs associated with SDAT. For example, neurofibrillary tangles and plaque formation have been reported in the hippocampus of normal aged brains, and loss of neurons occurs in the hippocampus and some areas of cortex involved in language, that is, the superior temporal gyrus (Scheibel & Scheibel, 1975; Squire, 1987). Indeed, it has been suggested that the organic changes in the brains of normal old and SDAT patients are different quantitatively, but not qualitatively (Petit, 1982). In contrast to the situation in SDAT, the extent of both neuropathology and cognitive change is relatively small in normal aging.

Aphasia and normal aging

We first consider whether age-related changes in language resemble patterns of selective impairment found in aphasia. When young and old are compared on standardized neuropsychological batteries used to assess possible language deficits following brain damage, systematic age differences favoring the young are sometimes found, but this is not always the case (Bayles, Tomoeda, & Boone, 1985). Further, it is not clear whether the age-related differences that are found reflect true aging effects or whether they are secondary to cohort differences in education or hearing problems. Duffy, Keith, Shane, and Podraza (1976) found that performance on the Porch Index of Communicative Ability was positively related to education and negatively related to age and that the effect of education was greater than that of age. Similarly, Borod, Goodglass, and Kaplan (1980) found that scores on many of the subtests of the Boston Diagnostic Aphasia Examination were affected by both age and education while only two were affected by age alone. In both studies, the educational attainments of the oldest participants were lower than those of younger members of the sample and partial correlations were not reported, so there is a real possibility that age effects were due to educational differences across groups. Goldstein and Shelly (1984) found age differences on only one aspect of language-related measures derived from the Halstead–Reitan and the Luria–Nebraska batteries, auditory discrimination, and could not rule out the possibility that this difference was due to hearing impairment in the older subjects.

When age differences are found on neuropsychological tests of language, they do not consistently resemble any particular pattern of aphasia. The one area in which older adults may exhibit a pattern of loss that resembles a feature of aphasia is that of word finding and confrontation naming. Many aphasics have confrontation naming problems (e.g., Goodglass, 1980), and some residual anomia is said to be fairly common even in patients who have otherwise recovered quite well from their aphasia (Cummings, 1985). However, the naming disorder in aphasia has properties that have not been reported in normal aging. For example, a classic symptom of aphasia is paraphasia in which incorrect words or neologisms are used (e.g., Goodglass, 1980). Further research is needed to determine whether word finding problems represent a distinctive feature of language difficulties in old age or whether they are simply part and parcel of a general decline in language comprehension and production. Hence, the parallel between language deficits in aphasia and in normal aging in this area remains uncertain.

Amnesia and normal aging

In the case of memory and aging, there is evidence from a number of laboratories which suggests that there may be similarities in the nature of the memory deficit in amnesia and that in old age. More specifically, there are commonalities in the pattern of impaired and spared function seen in aging and in anterograde amnesia. The ability to acquire new information is severely impaired in anterograde amnesia while the ability to remember information learned in the remote past is affected less (Cohen & Squire, 1981; Zola-Morgan, Cohen, & Squire, 1983). Similarly, older adults show impairment in memory for new information, but there is no consistent evidence for age differences in remote memory (Salthouse, 1982). However, both older adults and amnesics have less trouble in learning paired associates when these consist of high-frequency associates than when they consist of unrelated pairs of words (Botwinick & Storandt, 1974; Canestrari, 1966; Kausler & Lair, 1966). This is consistent with the view that well-known information is preserved (e.g., word associations) while new learning is impaired in both amnesia and aging.

Anterograde amnesics have severely impaired memory for new information when memory is tested using conventional recall or recognition tests that require deliberate recollection of recently presented material. However, they are not unable to acquire new information. When tested by procedures that permit the effects of prior experience to be demonstrated without deliberate recollection, they often show normal or near normal retention together with complete inability to remember the learning situation and lack of awareness that they have acquired some new knowledge. These procedures, which include repetition priming (e.g., completing word fragments, perceptual identification of degraded words, and free association) have been called "implicit memory" tasks, to contrast them with the more traditional "explicit memory" measures of recall and recognition (Graf & Schacter, 1985).

A number of studies using these and other repetition priming paradigms have shown that, like amnesics, older adults have impaired explicit memory and preserved repetition priming (e.g., Howard, this volume; Light, 1988b; Light & Singh, 1987; Light, Singh, & Capps, 1986). Some caution is needed, however, in interpreting these results. In our studies of repetition priming, young and old do not differ reliably on measures of implicit memory, but in every case there is a trend toward an age difference favoring the young. Thus, there may be real, though small, age differences in repetition priming. Such differences may reflect true aging effects, or they may arise from the intrusion of conscious recollection into an implicit memory task because subjects have guessed the purpose of the experiment (Light & Singh, 1987). In either case, the validity of the explicit/implicit distinction for describing memory in old age would not be compromised because the age difference is always much greater in explicit than in implicit memory tasks.

Repetition priming is but one of several possible classes of implicit memory. Squire (1987) has suggested that there are several different types of implicit memory (his term for this is "procedural learning"), including cognitive skill learning, perceptual learning, motor skill learning, and classical conditioning as well as repetition priming, and that all of these forms of procedural learning are normal or relatively normal in anterograde amnesics. It thus becomes interesting to ask whether these other varieties of implicit memory are also spared in old age. Our review of the literature suggests that the evidence for sparing is not as clear-cut in these areas as it is in repetition priming.

With respect to cognitive skill learning, Cohen (1984) has reported normal acquisition of the solution to the Tower of Hanoi puzzle in amnesics despite poor memory for the learning experience itself. In normal older adults, however, Hartley and Kieley (1987) have found an age-related decline in performance on this task. Similarly, with respect to perceptual learning, Cohen and Squire (1980) studied mirror reading skills in amnesics and found that both acquisition and retention were normal when compared to nonamnesic controls though recognition memory was markedly inferior in the amnesics. Moscovitch, Winocur, and McLachlan (1986) found that older adults were slightly impaired relative to young adults in learning to read geometrically transformed scripts and had lower recognition memory scores. Taken together, these two pieces of evidence point to the lack of identical findings in amnesia and aging.

A number of studies have found evidence for learning and retention of perceptual motor skills in amnesics (e.g., Brooks & Baddeley, 1976; Cermak, Lewis, Butters, & Goodglass, 1973; Corkin, 1965, 1968; Starr & Phillips, 1970). However, neither the rate of acquisition nor the final asymptotic performance of amnesics is consistently as high as that of controls. A similar state of affairs exists in the aging literature. For instance, Salthouse and Somberg (1982) have shown that the effects of very protracted practice on the skills involved in playing a video game are quite similar in old and young but that the young were better at all stages of practice. Wright and Payne (1985) tested young and older adults on both mirror tracking and rotary pursuit tasks and found that both groups benefited from practice but that the young profited more. Welford (1985) has suggested that when the necessary motor movements are simple, older adults learn at least as fast as young adults, though they generally do not achieve equality with them, but that acquisition rates favor the young for more complex movements. Thus, the literature on neither amnesia nor aging is easy to characterize with respect to perceptual motor skills. The available evidence is, however, consistent with the view that both amnesics and older adults benefit from practice, but we would argue that it is not clear that skill acquisition is "normal" in either group.

Weiskrantz and Warrington (1979) examined classical conditioning of the eyeblink in two amnesics and found that both were able to acquire the conditioned eyeblink response though neither remembered much about the training procedure or apparatus. However, no control subjects were tested so there is no way of knowing whether performance was within the normal range. There is evidence that older adults do not develop the conditioned eyeblink response as readily as young adults (Braun & Geiselhart, 1959; Jerome, 1959; Kimble & Pennypacker, 1968; Woodruff-Pak, 1987). If classical conditioning is intact in anterograde amnesia but impaired in old age, this would suggest a dissociation between amnesia and aging. The existence of such a dissociation would not be too surprising, given that the cerebellum, which is thought to underlie eyelid conditioning (Woodruff-Pak, 1987), is one of the regions of the brain most affected by aging (Scheibel & Scheibel, 1975), whereas cerebellar damage is not invariably found in amnesia.

The results of studies of repetition priming suggest spared functioning in both amnesics and older adults, but the results of studies of other types of implicit memory do not, in our view, support the blanket conclusion that all aspects of implicit memory are perfectly preserved in old age or in amnesia. Part of the difficulty is that studies of amnesics often involve small numbers of patients with heterogeneous etiologies (e.g., Brooks & Baddeley, 1976; Moscovitch et al., 1986), making comparisons across studies problematic. What is needed at this juncture is a large-scale study of amnesics and normal older adults, using a variety of measures of both implicit and explicit memory. Only with such studies will we be able to make definitive statements about similarities between normal aging and amnesia.

We also want to offer a caveat. The apparent similarities between memory deficits in amnesia and in aging should not blind us to real differences that exist between them. First, the extent of memory impairment on explicit memory tasks is by no means as great in older adults as in amnesics; there is a real quantitative difference in the problem. Second, unlike amnesics, the healthy, normal older adults whom we have tested in memory experiments are fully aware of the fact that they have studied some material that they are being asked to remember and their memory does not seem to be memory without awareness. (It is, of course, possible that on an item-by-item basis older adults might be recovering more information without awareness than young adults, but overall they do seem to "know that they know.")

Third, although this may be a relatively rare state of affairs (Brooks & Baddeley, 1976), amnesics can have a quite circumscribed cognitive disorder. That is, their memory impairment may be accompanied by "preserved general intelligence as well as intact language, perceptual, and social skills" (Cohen, 1984, p. 98). For instance, amnesics do not have problems in confrontation naming or in word finding (Squire, 1987). In normal aging, however, there is an extensive literature demonstrating widespread changes in many aspects of cognition, including language, perception, attention, reasoning, and problem solving, in addition to memory. Thus, cognitive aging does not appear to be solely the aging of memory. What we do not know at this time is whether age-related changes in cognition, when they occur in a given individual, are across the board (i.e., whether the extent of any decline is the same for language, memory, problem-solving, etc.) or whether there are individuals who may show declines in some areas without accompanying declines in others. The neuropsychological approach encourages us to ask this question and to seek an answer to it by studying a broad spectrum of cognitive functions in the same individuals rather than by studying cognitive functions piecemeal in different groups of older adults.

SDAT and normal aging

In SDAT, the pattern of deficits in memory and language in the early stages of the disease show some similarity to the pattern seen in normal aging. We focus here on selective impairment in the early stages of SDAT because in later stages cognitive impairment is widespread and profound (e.g., Cummings & Benson, 1983) and testing of patients becomes difficult, if not impossible. As Huff (this volume) points out, a lexical impairment in the form of word-finding difficulties is a salient feature of SDAT and is often one of the earliest signs of the disease. In comparisons of early stage SDAT patients with age-matched controls, patients generate fewer instances of a specified category in verbal fluency tests (Bayles & Kaszniak, 1987; Benson, 1979; Nebes, Martin, & Horn, 1984) and have impaired confrontation naming on tests such as the Boston Naming Test (e.g., Harrold, 1986; Huff, this volume). Indeed, confrontation naming deficits have been reported in SDAT patients whose performance on other tests of language function remained normal (Kirshner, Webb, & Kelly, 1984). The spontaneous speech of SDAT patients also provides evidence of word finding difficulties compared to age-matched controls, as they have, for example, an excessive and inappropriate use of deictic terms, indefinite expressions, and pronouns (Cummings & Benson, 1983; Kempler, 1984).

As we noted earlier, word finding impairment has also been reported in normal aging. However, although this problem is a salient feature of old age, it remains to be shown that there is a specific lexical production impairment at a time when other aspects of language are relatively spared. Further, it is unclear that the same mechanism is involved in word-finding impairment in SDAT and normal aging. There is evidence that lexical comprehension, not just production, is impaired in SDAT (Bayles & Kaszniak, 1987; Emery, this volume; Huff, this volume; Kempler, 1984). This suggests that the lexical impairment may be related to a loss of semantic information corresponding to the lexical representation. Consistent with this, Huff (this volume) found that patients who had impaired confrontation naming also selected the name of a semantically similar object instead of the correct name for an object. In contrast, there is little evidence for a loss of semantic information in normal aging (Light, 1988a), and indeed, older adults' understanding of word meaning as measured by vocabulary tests shows little decline (Salthouse, this volume). Thus, it seems likely that normal older adults' word-finding difficulties are related to problems in retrieval of lexical code, not deficient semantic information (cf. Bowles & Poon, 1985). There is, however, evidence for a word-retrieval deficit in the absence of semantic deficits early in SDAT (Harrold, 1986; Huff, this volume). For example, Harrold demonstrated that early-SDAT subjects knew the functions of objects they could not name (but see Kempler, 1984). Further, phonemic but not semantic cues facilitated naming in SDAT and normal aging, suggesting that the deficit was in access to phonological information. Additional research is needed to determine if there is an early stage in SDAT with impaired access to phonological but not semantic information, followed by a loss of semantic information as well.

Impaired comprehension of syntax is not usually considered an early symptom of SDAT (Cummings & Benson, 1983) but nonetheless has been reported in a few mild-stage as well as more advanced-stage patients (Emery, this volume; Kempler, 1984). Emery presents evidence of declines in syntactic comprehension also in normal aging. Kemper (this volume) reports that older adults produce syntactically less complex sentences, while in SDAT there is some evidence that syntactic production is not impaired until late in the course of the disease (Kempler, 1984). Further, any impairment in syntactic production appears to be slight relative to impairment of naming (Appell, Kertesz, & Fisman, 1982).

It is interesting to note that in SDAT, as in normal aging, syntactic and semantic functioning appear to be preserved when performance is evaluated with implicit tests. As in normal aging, SDAT patients have preserved semantic priming in measures of reading latency both for single word and sentence primes (Nebes, Boller, & Holland, 1986; Nebes et al., 1984; see Tyler, in press, for a related finding in Wernicke's aphasia). Similarly, in normal aging and SDAT we see better recall when a string of words more closely approximates the semantic and syntactic structure of an English sentence (Nebes et al., 1984). In tasks that explicitly require syntactic and semantic interpretation, such as the Chomsky Test of Syntax or the Token Test, SDAT patients are severely impaired (Emery, this volume).

In addition to changes in language, another salient and early symptom of SDAT is impairment in memory for new information. Although SDAT patients do not always differ from normal age-matched controls on digit span (e.g., Vitaliano, Breen, Albert, Russo, & Prinz, 1984), they do appear to have smaller backward digit spans (Storandt, Botwinick, Danziger, Berg, & Hughes, 1985). Recall or recognition of word lists, sentences, and longer texts is impaired in SDAT (e.g., Storandt et al., 1985; Vitaliano et al., 1984). The impairment of memory for new information can be seen clearly in performance on the "Famous Faces" test (Moscovitch, 1982). Mild-stage SDAT patients did not differ from controls for the decades 1920–1960, but performance of normal adults improved for more recent years (1970s) while SDAT performance did not.

Older adults also have well-established declines in memory for new information. The pattern is similar to SDAT in that age differences are slight (though often reliable) on the forward digit span and larger on recall of words or texts (e.g., Burke & Light, 1981). The similarity between SDAT and normal aging here is hardly surprising, given that in both cases the hippocampus is affected. In addition, there is some evidence for preserved implicit memory in SDAT (Eslinger & Damasio, 1986; Knopman & Nissen, 1987; Moscovitch, 1982; but see Shimamura, Salmon, Squire, & Butters, 1987, for a different result). However, the similarity between the patterns of early SDAT and normal aging ends here. Older adults' memory problems appear to be limited to the acquisition of some types of new information, with the one exception of word-retrieval problems. SDAT patients, in contrast, show declines in memory for well-known information learned in the distant past before the onset of the disease, for example, the alphabet (Emery, this volume; Storandt et al., 1985).

Summary

In this section, we have compared patterns of changes in language and memory that occur in normal aging and in certain pathological conditions, namely the aphasias, anterograde amnesia, and SDAT. We see specific cognitive deficits in one or more of these conditions that are also found in normal aging, but the overall pattern of sparing and impairment in aging is not identical to any of them. Even in cases where there appear to be similar deficits in behavior, as in word-finding problems or the sparing of implicit memory, it is not clear that the underlying mechanisms involved are the same.

Our focus here has been on broad patterns of spared and impaired function in old age. Thus we have not been able to discuss all forms of focal neuropathological damage. There is considerable current interest in the similarity between aging and frontal lobe damage (e.g., Albert & Kaplan, 1980; Haaland, Vranes, Goodwin, & Garry, 1987; Moscovitch, 1982). However, we doubt that the pattern of cognitive impairment found in frontal lobe damage or in any other focal neuropathological condition will exactly match that associated with normal aging because brain changes are less localized in aging.

Individual differences

In cognitive psychology, the study of individual differences is motivated by a desire to understand why people show a wide range of abilities in different areas, particularly in complex skills such as reading comprehension. It is assumed that complex skills can be decomposed into more basic component abilities and that variations in these simpler underlying abilities can predict complex skill performance. The greater the spread of scores on component abilities and on the criterion task, the greater is the likelihood of detecting relationships among them. One widely held belief about aging is that older populations show greater variability in performance than younger populations (Krauss, 1980). Hence, older adults constitute an excellent population for the study of individual differences in complex skills. The inclusion of groups of different ages in research on basic mechanisms of cognition also permits an evaluation of the generality of hypothesized relationships among variables across the life-span (Hultsch, Hertzog, & Dixon, 1984). For instance, different patterns of correlations among tasks may arise because there are different proportions of young and old who use particular information-processing strategies (Hertzog, 1985). From the perspective of research on aging, discovery that different skill components are important in determining performance at different ages or that the relative contribution of different components varies across age could provide a window on the nature of cognitive aging. If, in addition to measures of component skills, researchers include measures of life-style variables such as occupation, health status, drinking habits, and leisure activities (e.g., reading, sports, hobbies, exercise levels), we may be able to get a handle on the importance of life-style choices to preservation of cognitive functions in later life (Arbuckle, Gold, & Andres, 1986; Craik, Byrd, & Swanson, 1987).

For these reasons there has been considerable recent interest in individual differences in cognitive aging. Within the experimental psychology tradition, this interest has been concentrated in two areas, namely the roles of processing resources and verbal ability in cognitive aging (see chapters by Cohen, Hartley, Howard, Kemper, Light & Albertson, and Salthouse). With respect to processing resources, the main research focus has been on determining whether memory and language impairments in old age are associated with reduced processing resources, for example, with lower attentional capacity or smaller working memory or reduced rate of processing (Salthouse, 1985). Thus, the research strategy is to obtain a measure or measures of processing resources as well as measures of performance on the skill of interest, such as comprehension or memory for prose (Hartley, this volume; Light & Anderson, 1985) or language comprehension (Kemper, this volume). The different age groups may be equated on measures of processing resources and then compared on the dependent variable under investigation; alternatively, statistical techniques may be used to assess the amount of variability in performance contributed by age and/or by processing resources. If processing resources in old age are reduced to the point where they are incapable of supporting mental operations crucial to efficient performance or lead to less efficient functioning, then one would expect to find that age differences disappear or are greatly reduced when the level of processing resources is held constant across age groups.

This approach has met with some success. For instance, Parkinson, Lindholm, and Urell (1980) reported that digit span predicted performance on a dichotic listening task and that young and older adults with similar spans did not differ in performance. Kemper (this volume) found that both digit span and ability to imitate complex sentences decreased with age and that these measures were correlated. Hartley (this volume) observed an increase in general slowing with age and found that slowing was of greater importance in predicting text recall in older groups of subjects. Although sentence span, a measure of working-memory capacity, did not vary across age groups, it was a reliable predictor of text recall for middle-aged and older adults though not for young adults. The only discrepant finding is that of Light and Anderson (1985), who found age-related drops in scores on several span measures and on paragraph memory scores but did not find the predicted relationships among span measures, paragraph memory, and age.

With respect to verbal ability, the research strategies have been similar to those used in the study of individual differences in processing resources. Thus, Hartley (this volume) included several measures of verbal ability in her study, including vocabulary (the most common index of verbal ability) as well as more basic measures of naming latency, word decoding speed, category access speed, etc. The major hypothesis about individual differences in verbal ability is that age differences in cognitive function will be smaller in groups of high verbal ability adults than in low verbal ability adults. Belief in this hypothesis is widespread, and although there are some studies that do not provide supporting evidence (e.g., Kemper, this volume), many studies do. Zelinski and Gilewski (in press) have conducted a meta-analysis of the literature on verbal ability and age differences in prose memory and have found that age differences were indeed smaller for high verbal ability groups than for low verbal ability groups.

Not only are the research strategies for both of these individual-difference variables similar, but also they share certain methodological and interpretive problems. For example, there are issues of how to measure the individual-difference variables. Both processing resources and verbal ability are rather global concepts. To choose a measure of processing resources, one must begin by deciding whether to think of processing resources in terms of speed, storage capacity, attention, or some combination of these such as working memory, and as Salthouse (this volume) points out, there are often no consensually validated measures for these concepts. Then one must decide whether to aim for a general measure of processing resources or for a skill-specific measure (see Salthouse, 1985, for a discussion). The problem that arises is that measures of processing resources that tap speed may not be highly correlated with measures of processing resources that tap storage capacity (see Hartley, this volume). Even measures that purportedly tap a single aspect of processing resources, such as speed or working-memory capacity, may not be highly correlated. Salthouse (1985) found correlations among measures of mental speed to average only about .3, and Light and Anderson (1985) found only modest correlations, roughly .3 to .5, among several span measures.

These results are not consistent with the view that that there is a single pool of processing resources for which a single general measure can be obtained (Navon, 1984; Neumann, 1987). Alternatively, there may be many pools of processing resources that are domain specific, modality specific, or perhaps even task specific. For instance, Salthouse (1985) suggested that it might be necessary to develop separate measures of rate for predicting performance on active and passive processing tasks. Similarly, in discussing the relation between speeds of young and older adults, Cerella (1985) pointed out that different functions might be needed for effortful and automatic tasks. Further, Hartley (this volume) found evidence for both a general speed factor and a task-specific speed factor. We return to this issue in the next section.

With respect to working memory, Baddeley, Logie, Nimmo-Smith, and Brereton (1985) compared the ability of two measures to predict reading comprehension. One measure was adapted from Daneman and Carpenter (1980) and required people to remember words in a series of sentences. The other was a counting span measure (Case, Kurland, & Goldberg, 1982) which required people to remember how many dots of a given color were on a series of notecards. Although both proved significant predictors of reading comprehension, the sentence span measure was the better of the two. As Baddeley et al. note, this leaves open the possibility that there may be "a specific language-based working memory system" (p. 130) which is not well tapped by the counting span task. If there is no single pool of processing resources drawn on by all mental operations, then it would not be surprising to find only weak correlations among various measures of processing resources, and attempts to find a single general index of processing resources are unlikely to meet with success.

Similar difficulties arise in choosing measures of verbal ability. As Hartley (this volume) points out, it is not clear just how we should define the concept of verbal ability. There is a long history of searching for pure measures of verbal ability (Anastasi, 1958). For instance, Thurstone (1938) differentiated between verbal relations, involving ideas and word meanings, as measured in part by vocabulary tests, and word fluency, as measured, for instance, by the number of words created from the letters in the word "generations." The current information-processing approach to verbal ability emphasizes both knowledge and simple mental operations underlying performance in particular tasks. For example, Hunt's (1978) formulation includes both vocabulary and speed measures of component processes. Consistent with Hunt's approach, it has been suggested that verbal ability measures that show age-related declines are those that seem to make greater demands on processing resources (Salthouse, this volume). In the research reported in this volume, Hartley used a variety of measures of verbal ability derived from Perfetti's (1985) model of reading skill, including vocabulary which taps knowledge and several measures of processing resources. Her results showed that for all age groups memory for text was related to a factor that included vocabulary and working-memory capacity while only older adults' recall was well predicted by a slowing factor.

Summary

We believe that results such as Hartley's call into question the usual practice of equating verbal ability with vocabulary scores or processing resources with single measures of working-memory capacity or speed. In addition, they highlight the importance of models that specify the mental operations underlying language and memory and that make clear the roles played by aspects of both verbal ability and processing resources. Only with such models will we be able to identify the particular cognitive processes responsible for age-related changes in performance.

Along these lines, we have one further point which is also well illustrated by Hartley's work. We assume that different cognitive structures and processes underlie different skills and, therefore, that those individual-difference variables that predict performance well for one skill will not necessarily be good predictors for another. Almost all of the many individual-difference measures taken by Hartley showed age differences. Yet not all of them contributed to factors that predicted text memory. It is important that we look for patterns such as these, in which the dependent measures of interest are related to some but not all possible predictors. Such patterns are informative because they allow us to pinpoint mechanisms underlying cognitive aging.

The role of processing resources in cognitive aging

One theme that runs throughout this volume is that age-related changes in language and memory are due to reduced processing resources in old age. This is not surprising, given that the processing resource hypothesis is currently the dominant account of cognitive decline in later life. Indeed, the importance of processing constraints has been noted by linguists as well as psychologists. For instance, Chomsky (1965) distinguished between *competence* and *performance*; the former term refers to a speaker/hearer's underlying knowledge of a language, while the latter refers to actual use of language which is constrained by such factors as memory limitations, distractions, and attentional lapses. In this section, we take up several questions that arise with respect to this approach. We consider the nature of the hypothesized resource limitation in old age. We then evaluate the processing resource approach in the light of aging research and suggest directions for theoretical development.

Conceptualizations of processing resources

Processing resources have been viewed in terms of limited capacity or in terms of speed of mental operations. One approach has been to identify processing resources with short-term or working-memory capacity. For instance, Baddeley (1986) has described working memory as "a system for the temporary holding and manipulation of information during the performance of a range of cognitive tasks such as comprehension, learning, and reasoning" (p. 34). In Baddeley's (1986) model, working memory consists of a central executive which "has attentional capacities and is capable of selecting and operating control processes" (p. 71) together with a set of slave systems which have specialized storage functions. Baddeley has focused on investigating the properties of the slave systems (the articulatory loop, the phonological store, the visuospatial scratch pad) though these aspects of his model have been largely unexplored by researchers in cognitive aging. It is the notion that lower capacity in the central executive constrains cognition in the elderly by placing limits on storage and/or manipulation of information that is reflected in the approach taken by many workers in cognitive aging. Similarly, Hasher and Zacks (1979) postulate that aging affects effortful processes, which require an expenditure of processing resources, but not automatic processes, which make little or no demand on attentional capacity.

The crucial assumptions here for aging research are that working memory has limited capacity, that there are individual differences in working-memory capacity, that on average greater age in adulthood is associated with diminished working-memory capacity, and that different cognitive operations make varying demands on working-memory capacity (e.g., Light & Anderson, 1985; Zacks & Hasher, this volume). An additional (hidden) assumption is that there is a single, undifferentiated pool of resources that can be drawn upon by all effortful processes. The general prediction is that age should interact with task demands, with tasks requiring more processing resources (working-memory capacity, attention, etc.) showing greater age-related demands. In this volume, this position is represented by the chapters of Cohen; Emery; Gillund and Perlmutter; Hartley; Kemper; Light and Albertson; and Zacks and Hasher.

An alternative way of conceptualizing processing resources is in terms of speed of mental operations. Because older adults are slower at most (though not all) cognitive tasks (Salthouse, 1985), it has been suggested that cognitive slowing underlies age-related cognitive impairment. It is unclear whether speed of mental operations should be viewed as a processing resource per se or whether the speed with which mental processes can be carried out is simply an index of the efficiency of these processes which is itself dependent on the amount of processing resources allocated to the task at hand. Several contributors to the present volume have discussed both capacity and speed in their treatment of processing resources (Burke & Harrold; Cohen; Howard; Light & Albertson; Salthouse). For instance, Salthouse has pointed out that within network models, working-memory capacity (storage) can be thought of in terms of the number of nodes simultaneously active in the network, available attentional capacity can be treated as the total amount of activation in the network at some moment, and speed can be conceptualized as rate of spreading activation.

As illustrated by the chapters in this volume, the processing resource framework has been embraced as an organizational device for making sense of a variety of findings of age-related changes in memory and language (see also Craik & Rabinowitz, 1984, Hasher & Zacks, 1979, and Light, 1988a, for reviews). It has also proven useful as a heuristic for choosing paradigms for new research. The development of theoretical ideas and the accumulation of empirical findings suggested by the processing resource approach has now reached a point where we need to sit back and contemplate future directions.

Problems with the processing resource approach

When we consider ways in which processing resources ideas have been used by researchers in cognitive aging, we are concerned by a tendency to use them as a post hoc means for categorizing phenomena into those that are effortful and those that are automatic rather than as a way of elucidating basic mechanisms that underlie language and memory. That is, behaviors that change with age are in some cases simply being labeled as "effortful" or "attentional" or "capacity demanding," whereas those that are not sensitive to age are labeled as "automatic." It could be argued that an empirical generalization based on findings in a number of short-term memory and attention tasks has been elevated to a theoretical postulate.

This classification strategy is inadequate because there are now several studies demonstrating that older adults do not have problems in all effortful tasks. For example, attentional aspects of semantic priming appear to be age constant (see chapters by Burke & Harrold and by Howard). Studies using dual-task procedures do not consistently find that older adults have larger deficits under dual-task conditions relative to single-task conditions (Duchek, 1984; Somberg & Salthouse, 1982; Wickens, Braune, & Stokes, 1987; but see Salthouse, Rogan, and Prill, 1984). Thus, the absence of age differences cannot be used as evidence that a particular task does not require effort. Further, assumptions have been made about the processing resource requirements of cognitive tasks without any independent measure of these requirements. Indeed, finding an age difference has been used as proof that some task is effortful, but this line of reasoning is clearly circular. Making age invariance a criterion for designating a task as automatic (Hasher & Zacks, 1979) does not avoid this problem. As we pointed out earlier (Burke & Light, 1981), the first step is to determine whether some process satisfies other criteria for automaticity or effortfulness but fails the developmental one. We think that this step has now been taken and that there is sufficient evidence to exclude developmental effects as markers for automaticity or effortfulness.

We think that the next task for researchers in cognitive aging is the explicit specification of models of cognition that lay out the mental operations underlying behavior. At the present time, there is a conspicuous absence of models that specify the precise nature or locus of capacity demands. Without such models, claims that particular age-related deficits are caused by reduced processing resources are not very convincing. For instance, we have reviewed evidence suggesting that there may be increased word-finding problems in old age. One could argue from these findings that word finding is effortful. On the other hand, one could just as easily argue that word-finding problems are due to temporary failures of automatic processes involved in accessing orthographic or phonological information from meaning. However, neither classification sheds any light on the nature of the processes that underlie word-finding difficulty.

A second example of this problem is the distinction between implicit and explicit memory. As discussed above, it appears that age differences are much greater on explicit than on implicit memory tasks and that implicit memory is relatively spared in amnesia. Some researchers have claimed (e.g., Squire, 1987) that these kinds of memory differ in their capacity requirements and that implicit memory depends on more automatic processes. However, the evidentiary basis for such claims is slim, and there is some evidence that amnesics can show learning on tasks that clearly require attentional capacity (Nissen & Bullemer, 1987). Skill acquisition also requires attention (e.g., Bahrick & Shelly, 1958), and both amnesics and older people sometimes show normal or near normal skill acquisition. Hence, the distinction between implicit and explicit memory may not lie in degree of automaticity. This is clearly an area that needs additional work.

Thus, we are in complete agreement with Zacks and Hasher's argument for explicit situation-specific models of cognitive activities. The need for more explicit models is made even clearer when we consider recent research that undermines some of the assumptions of the processing resource approach to cognitive aging. While it is agreed that, in general, cognitive operations make varying demands on resources, it is not always agreed whether *particular* mental activities do or do not require the allocation of capacity or whether, if some task involves automatic components, which ones these are (e.g., Jonides, Naveh-Benjamin, & Palmer, 1981; Kahneman & Treisman, 1984). Further, it is not clear whether attentional capacity should be thought of as involving a single pool of processing resources. We have reviewed findings in aging research, as well as in individual-differences research, that suggest that there may be a number of specific, independent attentional resources that are differentially involved in performance, depending on the task (e.g., Davies, Jones, & Taylor, 1984; Lansman & Hunt, 1982). This matter is of special concern to us because of the possibility that the operations underlying language comprehension may draw upon resources distinct from those involved in other cognitive activities (Baddeley et al., 1985). It has even been suggested recently that there may be so many identifiable separate pools of resources that the very concept may lose its usefulness as an explanatory device (Hirst & Kalmar, 1987; Neumann, 1987).

Finally, if old age is associated with reduced processing resources, *all* tasks on which performance is limited by amount of available resources should show greater decrements for older than for younger adults. As we have discussed above, however, this is not invariably the case. The obvious rebuttal to this criticism is that age differences should be found only on those tasks that really place a considerable strain on the available processing resources and that absence of age effects is simply diagnostic of the low demands made by a particular task. However, in both the semantic priming and dual-task studies reviewed above, there was evidence of capacity strain because of the presence of inhibitory effects in the former and decrements in primary task performance in the latter. Hence, the force of such rebuttals is weakened.

Older adults' unimpaired performance on effortful tasks need not be taken as contradictory to the processing resource approach because they can be accommodated if one assumes multiple pools of processing resources, with some of these affected by age and others not. This multiple-pool approach is vulnerable to the same problem of circularity that we have discussed unless there is a theoretically motivated way to define the boundaries of the different pools (Neumann, 1987). Further, there is no theoretical reason for postulating a developmental change in either unitary- or multiple-pool approaches to processing resources. Without a developmental mechanism to explain age-related declines in processing resources, such approaches merely rename a set of empirical findings.

In existing research where specific models have been used, it has been possible to locate the stage of processing that limits older adult's performance. For instance, Spilich (1983) used the Kintsch and van Dijk (1978) model to explain age differences in memory for prose. His analysis led to the conclusion that the limiting factor for his sample of normal older adults was size of short-term buffer, which was smaller for old than for young, rather than any difference in strategy use. Unfortunately, the generality of these results is unknown because Spilich's young and old samples were heterogeneous with respect to demographic variables such as education and residential status. However, we think his approach has much to recommend it. In other cases, specific models have been helpful in eliminating processing stages as sources of age decrements in performance. A number of researchers have used models of spreading activation to conceptualize attentional capacity (e.g., Burke & Harrold; Howard, this volume). Their analysis has led to the conclusion that the limiting factor for performance in older adults is neither rate nor amount of spreading activation.

If alternative conceptualizations of processing resources can be made specific enough, we can tell whether they lead to differential predictions in any experimental paradigms. For example, Zacks and Hasher (this volume) have proposed that for older adults reduced attentional capacity in working memory affects storage more than manipulation of information. Baddeley (1986) has suggested that in old age, limitations in working memory are due to general problems in reduced capacity rather than to allocation of attention. Specification of the mechanisms involved in these alternative views will allow us to test them empirically. In the course of working out predictions for alternative models, it may also become apparent that what appear to be quite different conceptualizations of processing resources in terms of speed and working memory are empirically indistinguishable (Salthouse & Prill, 1987). In addition, some theorists (MacKay, in press; Navon, 1984) have argued that with sufficient specification of mechanisms underlying performance, the need for talking about pools of resources may be eliminated. That is, the concept of resources may prove to be a placeholder that serves only until we understand the underlying structures that place limitations on performance.

Finally, like other theoretical positions, the processing resource approach limits our vision, both with respect to the nature of interesting questions to ask and with respect to classes of explanation. A case in point is the importance of social factors in language use. Two illustrations will suffice. Boden and Bielby (1986) found that older adults manage the flow of topics within a conversation very well but that the content of their conversations focuses on events in their past, something not observed in the conversations of young adults. One could hypothesize that the reason for this choice of topics is that in talking about one's own life history, retrieval demands are minimized so that processing resources are less taxed. Caporael (1981; Caporael & Culbertson, 1986) reported that caregivers in nursing facilities use a variety of baby talk in speaking to elderly patients who are less functionally able and less healthy. It could be argued that use of such a speech register reflects tuning of speech to the stereotypical or perceived cognitive capacity of patients.

In each of these examples, however, the processing resource account seems implausible. These appear to be interesting phenomena that have little to do with processing resources and that are better explained in other ways. Older adults may dwell on past events because these are milestones in their lives which are more salient or more distinctive than recent events or because recent events are less well remembered. Caretakers may speak in baby talk to patients to convey affection or to establish clear lines of authority. Whether one agrees with these conjectures is not critical here. What is important is that the processing resource approach does not seem to capture the richness or complexity of conversational interaction. Without an integrated approach which takes into account both cognitive and social psychological factors, our knowledge of language in old age is bound to be impoverished. Such an approach clearly goes beyond the scope of processing resource models as currently conceived.

Summary

The processing resource approach has been a valuable heuristic for detecting patterns of stability and change in cognitive aging. As is frequently the case in research, however, the accumulation of evidence reveals the shortcomings of this approach. Our analysis suggests that a fruitful direction for future research is the articulation of models that specify the locus of operation of processing resources in specific tasks so that the mechanisms underlying age-related changes in performance can be identified.

Conclusions

Our goal in this chapter has been to evaluate different approaches to identifying patterns of spared and impaired language and memory functions in old age. Aging research provides a rich testing ground for the usefulness of these approaches within cognitive psychology. Further, we see the identification of patterns of age-related changes in memory and language as the first step in understanding their nature. Within the experimental tradition, we have considered several distinctions. As our review demonstrates, we cannot sort spared and impaired aspects of language and memory into convenient bins labeled episodic and semantic memory, old and new information, or automatic and effortful processes. The implicit versus explicit distinction cuts across these dichotomies and may fare better as a way of characterizing cognitive changes in old age. The neuropsychological approach to cognition led us to an examination of similarities between patterns of function in normal aging and in pathological conditions such as aphasia, amnesia, and Alzheimer's disease. Although there is some overlap in impaired function between normal aging and one or more of these conditions, normal aging nonetheless cannot be described by any of the syndromes we have considered. The individual-differences approach is based on the assumption that there will be identifiable components of language and memory that are differentially affected by aging. There is not yet sufficient consistent evidence to permit the isolation of these components, but this approach is still in its infancy.

Our attempts to fit what we know about cognitive aging into categories have led us to identify methodological and conceptual problems that hamper efforts to develop some of these approaches into more full-fledged theoretical accounts of cognitive aging. We believe that progress in cognitive aging research depends on the development of models that take into account the interdependence of language and memory and that include theoretically motivated developmental mechanisms to account for spared and impaired function in old age.

References

Albert, M. L. (1981). Changes in language with aging. *Seminars in Neurology, 1,* 43–46.

Albert, M. S., & Kaplan, E. (1980). Organic implications of neuropsychological deficits in the elderly. In L. W. Poon, J. L. Fozard, L. S. Cermak, D. Arenberg, & L. W. Thompson (Eds.), *New directions in memory and aging: Proceedings of the George A. Talland Memorial Conference* (pp. 403–432). Hillsdale, NJ: Erlbaum.

Anastasi, A. (1958). *Differential psychology: Individual and group differences in behavior* (3rd ed.). New York: Macmillan.

Anderson, J. R. (1983). A spreading activation theory of memory. *Journal of Verbal Learning and Verbal Behavior, 22,* 261–295.

Anderson, J. R. (1985). *Cognitive psychology and its implications* (2nd ed.). San Francisco: Freeman.

Appell, J., Kertesz, A., & Fisman, M. (1982). A study of language functioning in Alzheimer patients. *Brain and Language, 17,* 73–91.

Arbuckle, T. Y., Gold, D., & Andres, D. (1986). Cognitive functioning of older people in relation to social and personality variables. *Psychology and Aging, 1,* 55–62.

Atkinson, R. C., & Shiffrin, R. M. (1968). Human memory: A proposed system and its control processes. In K. W. Spence & J. T. Spence (Eds.), *The psychology of learning and memory* (pp. 89–195). New York: Academic Press.

Baddeley, A. (1986). *Working memory.* Oxford: Oxford University Press (Clarendon Press).

Baddeley, A., Logie, R., Nimmo-Smith, I., & Brereton, N. (1985). Components of fluent reading. *Journal of Memory and Language, 24,* 119–131.

Bahrick, H. P. (1984). Memory for people. In J. E. Harris & P. E. Morris (Eds.), *Everyday memory, actions and absent-mindedness.* Orlando, FL: Academic Press.

Bahrick, H. P., Bahrick, P. O., & Wittlinger, R. P. (1975). Fifty years of memory for names and faces: A cross-sectional approach. *Journal of Experimental Psychology: General, 104,* 54–75.

Bahrick, H. P., & Shelly, C. (1958). Time sharing as an index of automatization. *Journal of Experimental Psychology, 56,* 288–293.

Balota, D. A., & Duchek, J. M. (1988). Age related differences in lexical access, spreading activation and simple pronunciation. *Psychology and Aging, 3,* 84–93.

Bayles, K. A., & Kaszniak, A. W. (1987). *Communication and cognition in normal aging and dementia.* Boston: Little, Brown.

Bayles, K. A., Tomoeda, C. K., & Boone, D. R. (1985). A view of age-related changes in language. *Developmental Neuropsychology, 1,* 231–264.

Benson, D. F. (1979). Neurologic correlates of anomia. In H. Whitaker & H. Whitaker (Eds.), *Studies in neurolinguistics* (Vol. 4, pp. 293–328). New York: Academic Press.

Boden, D., & Bielby, D. D. (1986). The way it was: Topical organization in elderly conversation. *Language & Communication, 6,* 73–89.

Borod, J. C., Goodglass, H., & Kaplan, E. (1980). Normative data on the Boston Diagnostic Aphasia Examination, Parietal Lobe Battery, and the Boston Naming Test. *Journal of Clinical Neuropsychology, 2,* 209–215.

Botwinick, J. (1984). *Aging and behavior: A comprehensive integration of research findings* (3rd ed.). New York: Springer-Verlag.

Botwinick, J., & Storandt, M. (1974). *Memory, related function and age.* Springfield, IL: Thomas.

Botwinick, J., & Storandt, M. (1980). Recall and recognition of old information in relation to age and sex. *Journal of Gerontology, 35,* 70–76.

Bowles, N. L., & Poon, L. W. (1985). Aging and retrieval of words in semantic memory. *Journal of Gerontology, 40,* 71–77.

Braun, H. W., & Geiselhart, R. (1959). Age differences in the acquisition and extinction of the conditioned eyelid response. *Journal of Experimental Psychology, 57,* 386–388.

Brooks, O. N., & Baddeley, A. D. (1976). What can amnesic patients learn? *Neuropsychologia, 14,* 111–122.

Burke, D. M., & Light, L. L. (1981). Memory and aging: The role of retrieval processes. *Psychological Bulletin, 90,* 513–546.

Burke, D. M., Worthley, J., & Martin, J. (1988). I'll never forget what's-her-name: Aging and tip of the tongue experiences in everyday life. In M. M. Gruneberg, P. Morris, & R. N. Sykes (Eds.), *Practical aspects of memory: Current research and issues* (Vol. 2, pp. 113–118). Chichester: Wiley.

Canestrari, R. F. (1966). The effects of commonality on paired-associate learning in two age groups. *Journal of Genetic Psychology, 108,* 3–7.

Caporael, L. R. (1981). The paralanguage of caregiving: Baby talk to the institutionalized aged. *Journal of Personality and Social Psychology, 40,* 876–884.

Caporael, L. R., & Culbertson, G. H. (1986). Verbal response modes of baby talk and other speech at institutions for the aged. *Language & Communication, 6,* 99–112.

Case, R., Kurland, M., & Goldberg, J. (1982). Operational efficiency and the growth of short-term memory span. *Journal of Experimental Child Psychology, 33,* 386–404.

Cerella, J. (1985). Information processing rates in the elderly. *Psychological Bulletin, 98,* 67–83.

Cermak, L. S., Lewis, R., Butters, N., & Goodglass, H. (1973). Role of verbal mediation in performance of motor tasks by Korsakoff patients. *Perceptual and Motor Skills, 37,* 259–262.

Charness, N. (1981). Aging and skilled problem solving. *Journal of Experimental Psychology: General, 110,* 21–38.

Chomsky, N. (1965). *Aspects of the theory of syntax.* Cambridge, MA: The MIT Press.

Cohen, G., & Faulkner, D. (1983). Word recognition: Age differences in contextual facilitation effects. *British Journal of Psychology, 74,* 239–251.

Cohen, N. J. (1984). Preserved learning capacity in amnesia: Evidence for multiple memory systems. In L. R. Squire & N. Butters (Eds.), *Neuropsychology of memory* (pp. 83–103). New York: Guilford Press.

Cohen, N. J., & Squire, L. R. (1980). Preserved learning and retention of pattern analyzing skill in amnesia: Dissociation of knowing how and knowing that. *Science, 210,* 207–209.

Cohen, N. J., & Squire, L. R. (1981). Retrograde amnesia and remote memory impairment. *Neuropsychologia, 19,* 337–356.

Corkin, S. (1965). Tactually-guided maze learning in man: Effects of unilateral cortical excisions and bilateral hippocampal lesions. *Neuropsychologia, 3,* 339–351.

Corkin, S. (1968). Acquisition of motor skill after bilateral medial temporal-lobe excision. *Neuropsychologia, 6,* 255–265.

Craik, F. I. M. (1977). Age differences in human memory. In J. E. Birren & K. W. Schaie (Eds.), *Handbook of the psychology of ageing* (pp. 384–420). New York: Van Nostrand Reinhold.

Craik, F. I. M., Byrd, M., & Swanson, J. M. (1987). Pattern of memory loss in three elderly samples. *Psychology and Aging, 2,* 79–86.

Craik, F. I. M., & Rabinowitz, J. C. (1984). Age differences in the acquisition and use of verbal information: A tutorial review. In H. Bouma & D. G. Bouwhuis (Eds.), *Attention and performance X: Control of language processes* (pp. 471–499). Hillsdale, NJ: Erlbaum.

Cummings, J. L. (1985). *Clinical neuropsychiatry.* Orlando, FL: Grune & Stratton.

Cummings, J. L., & Benson, D. F. (1983). *Dementia: A clinical approach.* Boston: Butterworths.

Daneman, M., & Carpenter, P. A. (1980). Individual differences in working memory and reading. *Journal of Verbal Learning and Verbal Behavior, 19,* 450–466.

Davies, D. R., Jones, D. M., & Taylor, A. (1984). Selective and sustained-attention tasks: Individual and group differences. In R. Parasuraman & D. R. Davies (Eds.), *Varieties of attention* (pp. 395–447). Orlando, FL: Academic Press.

Dell, G. S. (1986). A spreading-activation theory of retrieval in sentence production. *Psychological Review, 93,* 283–321.

Duchek, J. M. (1984). Encoding and retrieval differences between young and old: The impact of attentional capacity usage. *Developmental Psychology, 20,* 1173–1180.

Duffy, J. R., Keith, R. L., Shane, H., & Podraza, B. L. (1976). Performance of normal (non-brain injured) adults on the Porch Index of Communicative Ability. In R. H. Brookshire (Ed.), *Clinical aphasiology: Proceedings of the conference 1976* (pp. 32–42). Minneapolis: BRK Press.

Eslinger, P. J., & Damasio, A. R. (1986). Preserved motor learning in Alzheimer's disease: Implications for anatomy and behavior. *Journal of Neuroscience, 6,* 3006–3009.

Goldstein, G., & Shelly, C. H. (1975). Similarities and differences between psychological deficit in aging and brain damage. *Journal of Gerontology, 30,* 448–455.

Goldstein, G., & Shelly, C. H. (1984). Relationships between language skills as assessed by the Halstead–Reitan Battery and the Luria–Nebraska Language-Related Factor Scales in a non-aphasic patient population. *Journal of Clinical Neuropsychology, 6,* 143–156.

Goodglass, H. (1980). Disorders of naming following brain injury. *American Scientist, 68,* 647–655.

Graf, P., & Schacter, D. L. (1985). Implicit and explicit memory for new associations in normal and amnesic subjects. *Journal of Experimental Psychology: Learning, Memory, and Cognition, 11,* 501–518.

Haaland, K. Y., Vranes, L. F., Goodwin, J. S., & Garry, P. J. (1987). Wisconsin Card Sort Test performance in a healthy elderly population. *Journal of Gerontology, 42,* 345–346.

Harrold, R. M. (1986). *Object naming in Alzheimer's disease: What is the cognitive deficit?* Unpublished doctoral dissertation, The Claremont Graduate School, Claremont, CA.

Hartley, A. A., & Kieley, J. (1987). *Tests of a processing resource explanation for age differences in problem solving.* Unpublished manuscript.

Hartley, J. T., Harker, J. O., & Walsh, D. A. (1980). Contemporary issues and new directions in adult development of learning and memory. In L. W. Poon (Ed.), *Aging in the 1980s* (pp. 239–252). Washington, DC: American Psychological Association.

Hasher, L., & Zacks, R. T. (1979). Automatic and effortful processes in memory. *Journal of Experimental Psychology: General, 108,* 356–388.

Hertzog, C. (1985). An individual differences perspective: Implications for cognitive research in psychology. *Research on Aging, 7,* 7–45.

Hirst, W., & Kalmar, D. (1987). Characterizing attentional resources. *Journal of Experimental Psychology: General, 116,* 68–81.

Holding, D. H., Noonan, T. K., Pfau, H. D., & Holding, C. S. (1986). Date attribution, age, and the distribution of lifetime memories. *Journal of Gerontology, 41,* 481–485.

Horn, J. L. (1976). Human abilities: A review of research and theory in the early 1970s. In M. R. Rosenzweig & L. W. Porter (Eds.), *Annual Review of Psychology* (Vol. 27, pp. 437–485). Palo Alto, CA: Annual Reviews.

Hultsch, D. F., Hertzog, C., & Dixon, R. A. (1984). Text recall in adulthood: The role of intellectual abilities. *Developmental Psychology, 20,* 1193–1209.

Hunt, E. (1978). Mechanics of verbal ability. *Psychological Review, 85,* 109–130.

Jerome, E. A. (1959). Age and learning – experimental studies. In J. E. Birren (Ed.), *Handbook of aging and the individual: Psychological and biological aspects* (pp. 655–699). Chicago: University of Chicago Press.

Jonides, J., Naveh-Benjamin, M., & Palmer, J. (1981). Assessing automaticity. *Acta Psychologia, 60,* 157–171.

Kahneman, D., & Treisman, A. (1984). Changing views of attention and automaticity. In R. Parasuraman & D. R. Davies (Eds.), *Varieties of attention* (pp. 29–61). Orlando, FL: Academic Press.

Kausler, D. H., & Lair, C. V. (1966). Associative strength and paired-associate learning in elderly subjects. *Journal of Gerontology, 21,* 278–280.

Kempler, D. (1984). *Syntactic and symbolic abilities in Alzheimer's disease.* Unpublished doctoral dissertation, University of California, Los Angeles.

Kimble, G. A., & Pennypacker, H. S. (1968). Eyelid conditioning in young and aged subjects. *Journal of Genetic Psychology, 103,* 283–289.

Kintsch, W., & van Dijk, T. A. (1978). Toward a model of text comprehension and production. *Psychological Review, 85,* 363–394.

Kirshner, H. S., Webb, W. G., & Kelly, M. P. (1984). The naming disorder of dementia. *Neuropsychologia, 22,* 23–30.

Knopman, D. S., & Nissen, M. J. (1987). Implicit learning in patients with probable Alzheimer's disease. *Neurology, 37,* 784–788.

Krauss, I. K. (1980). Between- and within-group comparisons in aging research. In L. W. Poon (ed.), *Aging in the 1980s* (pp. 542–551). Washington, DC: American Psychological Association.

Lansman, E. & Hunt, M., (1982). Individual differences in secondary task performance. *Memory & Cognition, 10,* 10–24.

Light, L. L. (1988a). Language and aging: Competence versus performance. In J. E. Birren & V. L. Bengtson (Eds.), *Emergent theories of aging* (pp. 177–213). New York: Springer.

Light, L. L. (1988b). Preserved implicit memory in old age. In M. M. Gruneberg, P. Morris, & R. N. Sykes (Eds.), *Practical aspects of memory: Current research and issues* (Vol. 2, pp. 90–95). Chichester: Wiley.

Light, L. L., & Anderson, P. A. (1985). Working-memory capacity, age, and memory for discourse. *Journal of Gerontology, 40,* 737–747.

Light, L. L., & Singh, A. (1987). Implicit and explicit memory in younger and older adults. *Journal of Experimental Psychology: Learning, Memory, and Cognition, 13,* 531–541.

Light, L. L., Singh, A., & Capps, J. L. (1986). Dissociation of memory and awareness in young and older adults. *Journal of Clinical and Experimental Neuropsychology, 8,* 62–74.

MacKay, D. (1987). *The organization of perception and action: A theory for language and other cognitive skills.* New York: Springer-Verlag.

MacKay, D. (in press). Perception, action and awareness: A three body problem. In W. O. Prinz & O. Neumann (Eds.), *Relations between perception and action: Current approaches.* Berlin: Springer-Verlag.

Mandler, G. (1985). *Cognitive psychology: An essay in cognitive science.* Hillsdale, NJ: Erlbaum.

McCrae, R. R., Arenberg, D., & Costa, P. T. (1987). Declines in divergent thinking with age: Cross-sectional, longitudinal, and cross-sequential analyses. *Psychology and Aging, 2,* 130–137.

Moscovitch, M. (1982). A neuropsychological approach to perception and memory in normal and pathological aging. In F. I. M. Craik & S. Trehub (Eds.), *Aging and cognitive processes* (pp. 55–78). New York: Plenum.

Moscovitch, M., Winocur, G., & McLachlan, D. (1986). Memory as assessed by recognition and reading time in normal and memory-impaired people with Alzheimer's disease and other neurological disorders. *Journal of Experimental Psychology: General, 115,* 331–346.

Motley, M. T., Baars, B. J., & Camden, C. T. (1983). Experimental verbal slip studies: A review and an editing model of language encoding. *Communication Monographs, 50,* 79–101.

Mueller, J. H., Kausler, D. H., Faherty, A., & Oliveri, M. (1980). Reaction time as a function of age, anxiety, and typicality. *Bulletin of the Psychonomic Society, 16,* 473–476.

Navon, D. (1984). Resources – A theoretical soup stone? *Psychological Review, 91,* 216–234.

Nebes, R. D., Boller, F., & Holland, A. (1986). Use of semantic context by patients with Alzheimer's disease. *Psychology and Aging, 1,* 261–269.

Nebes, R. D., Martin, D. C., & Horn, L. C. (1984). Sparing of semantic memory in Alzheimer's disease. *Journal of Abnormal Psychology, 93,* 321–330.

Neumann, O. (1987). Beyond capacity: A functional view of attention. In H. Heuer & A. F. Sanders (Eds.), *Perspectives on perception and action* (pp. 361–394). Hillsdale, NJ: Erlbaum.

Nissen, M. J., & Bullemer, P. (1987). Attentional requirements of learning: Evidence from performance measures. *Cognitive Psychology, 19,* 1–32.

Obler, L. K., & Albert, M. L. (1985). Language skills across adulthood. In J. E. Birren & K. W. Schaie (Eds.), *Handbook of the psychology of aging* (pp. 463–473). New York: Van Nostrand Reinhold.

Parkinson, S. R. (1982). Performance deficits in short-term memory tasks: A comparison of amnesic Korsakoff patients and the aged. In L. S. Cermak (Ed.), *Human memory and amnesia* (pp. 77–96). Hillsdale, NJ: Erlbaum.

Parkinson, S. R., Lindholm, J. M., & Urell, T. (1980). Aging, dichotic memory and digit span. *Journal of Gerontology, 35,* 87–95.

Perfetti, C. A. (1985). *Reading ability.* New York: Oxford University Press.

Perlmutter, M., Metzger, R., Miller, K., & Nezworski, T. (1980). Memory of historical events. *Experimental Aging Research, 6,* 47–59.

Petit, T. L. (1982). Neuroanatomical and clinical neuropsychological changes in aging and senile dementia. In F. I. M. Craik & S. Trehub (Eds.), *Aging and cognitive processes* (pp. 1–21). New York: Plenum.

Rabinowitz, J. C. (1986). Priming in episodic memory. *Journal of Gerontology, 41,* 204–213.

Riegel, K. F. (1973). Language and cognition: Some life-span developmental issues. *Gerontologist, 13,* 478–482.

Rubin, D. C., Wetzler, S. E., & Nebes, R. D. (1986). Autobiographical memory across the life span. In D. C. Rubin (Ed.), *Autobiographical memory* (pp. 202–221). Cambridge: Cambridge University Press.

Salthouse, T. A. (1982). *Adult cognition: An experimental psychology of human aging.* New York: Springer-Verlag.

Salthouse, T. A. (1985). *A theory of cognitive aging.* Amsterdam: North-Holland.

Salthouse, T. A., & Prill, K. A. (1987). Inferences about age impairments in inferential reasoning. *Psychology and Aging, 2,* 43–51.

Salthouse, T. A., Rogan, J. D., & Prill, K. A. (1984). Division of attention: Age differences on a visually presented memory task. *Memory & Cognition, 12,* 613–620.

Salthouse, T. A., & Somberg, B. L. (1982). Skilled performance: Effects of adult age and experience on elementary processes. *Journal of Experimental Psychology: General, 111,* 176–207.

Schaie, K. W., & Parham, I. A. (1977). Cohort-sequential analyses of adult intellectual development. *Developmental Psychology, 13,* 649–653.

Scheibel, M. E., & Scheibel, A. B. (1975). Structural changes in the aging brain. In H. Brody, D. Harman, & J. M. Ordy (Eds.), *Aging* (Vol. 1, pp. 11–37). New York: Raven Press.

Shimamura, A. P., Salmon, D. P., Squire, L. R., & Butters, N. (1987) Memory dysfunction and word priming in dementia and amnesia. *Behavioral Neuroscience, 101,* 347–351.

Somberg, B. L., & Salthouse, T. A. (1982). Divided attention abilities in young and old adults. *Journal of Experimental Psychology: Human Perception and Performance, 8,* 651–663.

Squire, L. R. (1987). *Memory and brain.* New York: Oxford University Press.

Spilich, G. J. (1983). Life-span components of text processing: Structural and procedural differences. *Journal of Verbal Learning and Verbal Behavior, 22,* 231–244.

Starr, A., & Phillips, L. (1970). Verbal and motor memory in the amnestic syndrome. *Neuropsychologia, 8,* 75–88.

Stine, E. L., Wingfield, A., & Poon, L. W. (1987). How much and how fast: Rapid processing of spoken language in later adulthood. *Psychology and Aging, 1,* 303–311.

Storandt, M., Botwinick, J., Danziger, W. L., Berg, L., & Hughes, C. P. (1985). Psychometric differentiation of mild senile dementia of the Alzheimer type. *Archives of Neurology, 41,* 497–499.

Thurstone, L. L. (1938). *Primary mental abilities* (Psychometric Monograph No. 1). Chicago: University of Chicago Press.

Tulving, E. (1972). Episodic and semantic memory. In E. Tulving & W. Donaldson (Eds.), *Organization of memory* (pp. 381–403). New York: Academic Press.

Tulving, E. (1983). *Elements of episodic memory.* Oxford: Oxford University Press (Clarendon Press).

Tulving, E. (1984). Precis of elements of episodic memory. *Behavioral and Brain Sciences, 7,* 223–268.

Tulving, E. (1985). How many memory systems are there? *American Psychologist, 40,* 385–398.

Tyler, L. K. (in press). Locating the comprehension deficit in Wernicke's aphasia. *Cognitive Neuropsychology.*

Van Gorp, W. G., Satz, P., Kiersch, M. E., & Henry, R. (1986). Normative data on the Boston Naming Test for a group of normal older adults. *Journal of Clinical and Experimental Neuropsychology, 8,* 702–705.

Vitaliano, P. P., Breen, A. R., Albert, M. S., Russo, J., & Prinz, P. N. (1984). Memory, attention, and functional status in community-residing Alzheimer type dementia and optimally healthy aged individuals. *Journal of Gerontology, 39,* 58–64.

Weiskrantz, L., & Warrington, E. K. (1979). conditioning in amnesic patients. *Neuropsychologia, 17,* 187–194.

Welford, A. T. (1985). Practice effects in relation to age: A review and a theory. *Developmental Neuropsychology, 1,* 173–190.

Wickens, C. D., Braune, R., & Stokes, A. (1987). Age differences in the speed and capacity of information processing: 1. A dual-task approach. *Psychology and Aging, 2,* 70–78.

Wingfield, A., Poon, L. W., Lombardi, L., & Lowe, D. (1985). Speed of processing in normal aging: Effects of speech rate, linguistic structure, and processing time. *Journal of Gerontology, 40,* 579–585.

Woodruff-Pak, D. S. (1987, May). *Parallel studies of classical conditioning and aging in rabbits and humans.* Paper presented at the First Annual Meeting of the Cognitive Aging Conference, Atlanta, GA.

Wright, B. M., & Payne, R. B. (1985). Effects of aging on sex differences in psychomotor reminiscence and tracking proficiency. *Journal of Gerontology, 40,* 179–184.

Zelinski, E. M., & Gilewski, M. J. (in press). Memory for prose and aging: A meta-analysis. In M. L. Howe & C. J. Brainerd (Eds.), *Cognitive development in adulthood.* New York: Springer-Verlag.

Zola-Morgan, S., Cohen, N. J., & Squire, L. R. (1983). Recall of remote episodic memory in amnesia. *Neuropsychologia, 21,* 487–500.

Author index

Subject index

activation of memory (*see also* priming)
  automatic/effortful, 85–86
  spreading of, 5–6, 79–83, 103–110, 246, 264
  time course of, 83–86, 90, 94, 104-105
Alzheimer's disease
  anomia in, 210–219, 222–223, 255
  aphasia in, 219, 237–240
  clinical course of, 210
  demographics of, 221
  and depression, 224–225, 240
  fluency in, 212, 215–217, 218
  memory in, 226–228, 230, 231–232
  neuropathology of, 209, 250
  and normal aging, 228–229, 236–237, 254–256
  perceptual deficit in, 211–213, 215, 217
  phonology in, 210–211, 227, 228, 231–233, 255
  pronouns in, 227, 233
  semantics in, 210–211, 212–213, 216–218, 219, 223, 226, 227, 231, 233–235, 255
  severity and performance in, 217, 229–230, 235–237
  syntax in, 210–211, 223–227, 228–237, 255
amnesia, 91
  and normal aging, 251–254
anaphoric devices (*see also* inference)
  in Alzheimer's disease, 227, 233
  noun phrases, 123–129, 141–143
  pronouns, 9, 138–141, 143–146, 148–149, 179–180, 249
  and working memory, 9, 123–129, 143–146, 148–149
anomaly, detection of, 146–148, 184
aphasia (*see also* Alzheimer's disease), 102
  and normal aging, 250–251
articulation, 2
attentional processes, *see* processes: attentional
automatic processes, *see* processes: automatic

brain
  changes in Alzheimer's disease, 209, 250
  changes in normal aging, 250

classical conditioning, 253
coreference, 8, 119, 123–129, 138–146

dementia, *see* Alzheimer's disease
depth of processing, *see* levels of processing; text memory
discourse memory, *see* text memory

evoked potentials, 84

foregrounding, 127–129, 146–148

implication, logical vs. pragmatic, 134–139
individual differences (*see also* text memory; verbal ability: individual differences), 256–260
inference
  difficulty, 158–159, 161–168
  invited, 8–9, 134
  and working-memory capacity, 117–118, 134, 143–149, 157–159, 161–168, 180, 182–185
integration of information (*see also* coreference; inference; text memory), 8–9, 117–119, 123, 165, 166–167, 184–185
intonation and stress, 178

knowledge
  declarative/procedural, 4, 29–30, 252
  domain specific, 198–200
  generic (*see also* scripts), 119–123
  of material, *see* topic: familiarity
  sensorimotor, 4
  of task, 193

language comprehension, 8–11, 133–135, 249
language production (*see also* syntactic processing), 10
  imitation, 62–64
  spontaneous speech, 60–62
  and working memory, 64–67
  written, 67–73
levels of processing, 100–103, 182–185, 200–201
lexical access, 8, 40–41, 212–214, 216–219
lexical decision, 81–86, 103, 106, 157
lexicon, 4–5, 113

memory (*see also* text memory; working memory)
  autobiographical, 248
  episodic, 4, 245–248

280

Printed in the United Kingdom
by Lightning Source UK Ltd.
135972UK00002B/41/P